Current Topics in Pathology

Continuation of Ergebnisse der Pathologie

63

Editors

E. Grundmann · W. H. Kirsten

Pathology of the Gastro-Intestinal Tract

Contributors

A. C. Branfoot, I. M. P. Dawson, K. Elster
H. T. Enterline, M. I. Filipe, D. M. Goldenberg, Aa. Johansen
R. H. Riddell, J. M. Skinner, H. Thompson
R. Whitehead

Editor

B. C. Morson

With 155 Figures

Springer-Verlag Berlin · Heidelberg · New York 1976

E. Grundmann, Professor Dr., Pathologisches Institut der Universität, Westring 17,
D-4400 Münster/Westf., Germany

W.H. Kirsten, Professor Dr., Department of Pathology, The University of Chicago,
950 East 59th Street, Chicago, IL 60637, USA

B.C. Morson, Professor Dr., Pathology Department, St. Mark's Hospital, City Road,
London, ECIV 2PS, Great Britain

ISBN-13:978-3-642-66483-0 e-ISBN-13:978-3-642-66481-6
DOI: 10.1007/978-3-642-66481-6

Softcover reprint of the hardcover 1st edition 1976

Library of Congress Catalog Card Number 56-49162.

Contents

List of Contributors

A.C. Branfoot	Westminster Medical School, Udall Street Laboratories, Udall Street, London SW1P 2PP, Great Britain
I.M.P. Dawson	Department of Pathology, University of Nottingham, University Park, Nottingham NG7 2RD, Great Britain
K. Elster	Pathologisches Institut, Städtische Krankenanstalten, Kulmbacher Straße 23, D-8580 Bayreuth, Germany
H.T. Enterline	Hospital of the University of Pennsylvania, 3400 Spruce Street, Philadelphia, PA, USA
M.I. Filipe	Westminster Medical School, Udall Street Laboratories, Udall Street, London SW1P 2PP, Great Britain
D.M. Goldenberg	Division of Experimental Pathology, Department of Pathology, University of Kentucky, Lexington, KY 40506, USA
Aa. Johansen	Bispebjerg Hospital, Bispebjerg Bakke 23, 2400 Kobenhavn, NV., Denmark
R.H. Riddell	Department of Anatomic Pathology, University of Chicago, 950 East 59th Street, Chicago, IL 60637, USA
J.M. Skinner	School of Medicine, The Flinders University of South Australia, Bedford Park, South Australia 5042
H. Thompson,	The General Hospital, Department of Histology, Steelhouse Lane, Birmingham B4 6NH, Great Britain
R. Whitehead	School of Medicine, The Flinders University of South Australia, Bedford Park, South Australia 5042

Early Gastric Cancer

AA. JOHANSEN

The object of this paper is to describe the pathology of the particular stage of gastric cancer known as early carcinoma. The basis for the survey is the relevant literature. Since early gastric cancer is extremely common and has been extensively investigated in Japan, relatively many Japanese works available in English will be mentioned. The author's experience of 56 cases personally collected and investigated during the last 10 years will be included.

I. Definition and Nomenclature

Since precise definition and adequate names are presumed to prevent the confusion often met with in older literature, this subject will be treated in detail in this passage. During the last decade the common designation "early cancer" has concerning the stomach developed into a well defined term meaning a carcinoma which has not extended beyond the submucosal layer of the stomach wall. Most investigators use the name even if lymph node metastases are present. Therefore, a complete definition of early gastric cancer (egc) is: *a carcinoma limited to the mucosa or mucosa/submucosa regardless of the presence of lymph node metastases.* Just as the case is for carcinomas elsewhere invasive growth through the basal membrane of the crypts and the glands into the lamina propria is required. Egc should be separated from precancerous lesions including carcinoma in situ. The muscularis mucosae plays no role in the definition, but divides egc into two groups, *intramucosal* and *submucosal carcinomas*, both able to metastasize (Fig. 1).

To the pathologist who makes the diagnosis by histological examination the designation is not the best. "Early" is generally not much used in the vocabulary of pathology. Names based on facts related to the examination of the specimens would be preferable. Superficial carcinoma used e.g. by *Friesen* et al. (1962) or surface carcinoma (*Mason*, 1967) cover the pathology of such tumours better and are good collective names for the two clear and self-evident terms: intramucosal carcinoma and submucosal carcinoma. On the other hand egc has acquired a world-wide use and the Anglo-Saxon form is more or less used in many languages including German and even French. The term seems to be understood and accepted by all branches of gastroenterology, and realizing this, it is obvious that any change will only create confusion.

Whether egc always is an early stage of later advanced stomach cancer and therefore deserves its name has been commented on by *Okabe* (1971). The results of his investigations will be given later.

Who first used egc in its well defined meaning is unknown to the author, but there is no doubt that Japanese gastroenterology has played a considerable role for the use and the distribution of the term. According to *Murakami* (1971) the designation is a linguistic analogy to "early tuberculosis" which originally in Japan was used in the meaning tuberculosis which could be cured. Consequently egc should be looked upon as stomach carcinoma which can be cured.

Two other expressions are worth a comment: *superficial spreading type of carcinoma* introduced by *Stout* in 1942 for describing the superficial analogy to linitis plastica. The name is good, and if it is used within the limits of the definition of egc – which was not the case for a third of the cases published by *Stout* (1942) – it gives a good description of certain forms of Japanese type IIc and IIc + III carcinomas. Naturally it cannot always replace egc. The same sort of early cancer has been designated *superficial erosive carcinoma* (*Ewing*, 1936; *Konjetzny*, 1953).

In the German literature egc equals "Frühkarzinom" among others used by *Wiendl* and *Piger* (1971), *Hermanek* and *Rösch* (1973), *Jansen* (1974), *Elster* et al. (1975). The analogy to superficial carcinoma is "oberflächlicher Schleimhautkarzinome" used by *Versé* (1903, 1908), when egc first was described. The term was later used by *Konjetzny* (1940), when he had accepted (1937) that the "eigentümliche Schleimhautbefunde" previously described several times by himself (*Konjetzny*, 1913; *Anschütz* and *Konjetzny*, 1921; *Konjetzny*, 1938) were cancer. The expression has also been used by *Rössle* (1944) and *Abel* (1952).

In France "le cancer de l'estomac au début" or "précoce" (*Gutmann* et al., 1939; *Albot*, 1943; *Loutsch*, 1947; *Gutmann*, 1956, 1967) correspond closely to egc. Superficial car-

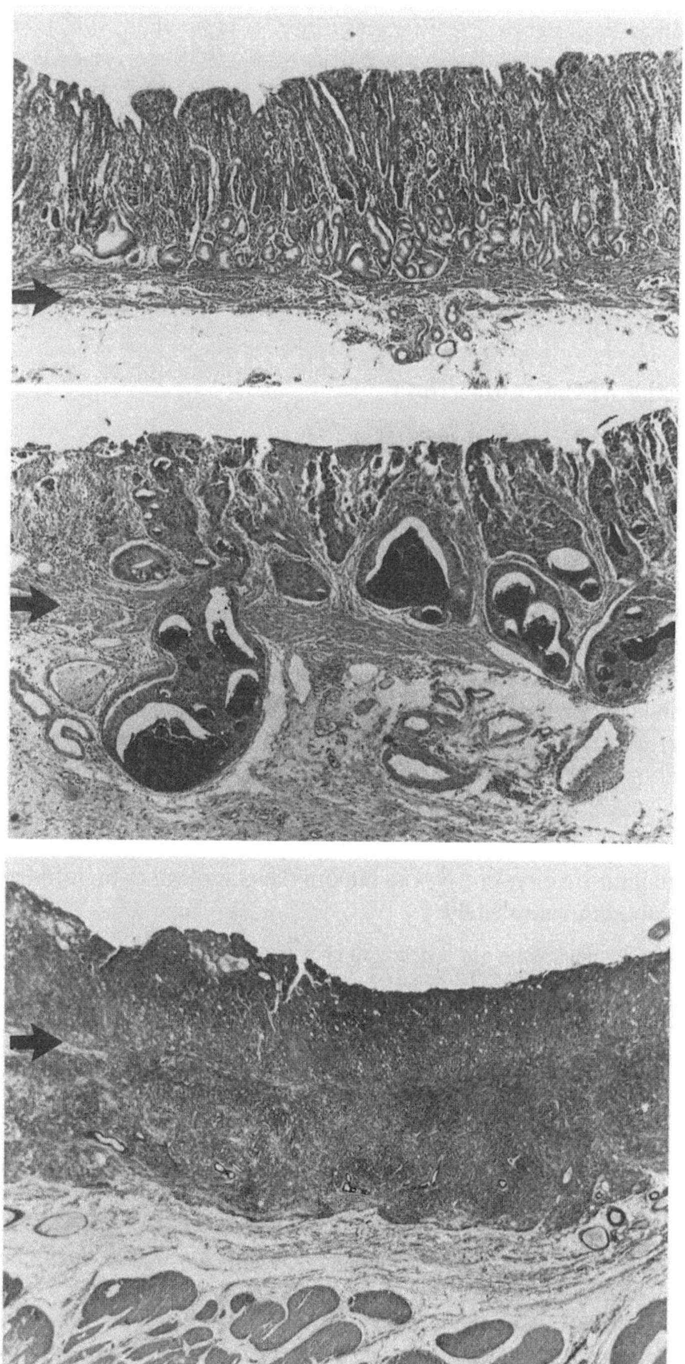

Fig. 1 a-c. Three forms of early gastric cancer: a) Intramucosal carcinoma. The carcinoma is mainly limited to the foveolar zone. H&E, x 25. b) Submucosal carcinoma with slight invasion. PAS, x 40. c) Submucosal carcinoma with extensive invasion. H&E, x 15. The arrows indicate the lamina muscularis mucosae cinomas are designated "cancer en surface" (*Cattan* et al., 1947). "Le cancer gastrique érosif a march lente" (*Gutmann* and *Bertrand*, 1938) corresponds to superficial erosive carcinoma.

Finally it should be mentioned that unfortunately some good examples of egc, mainly intramucosal carcinomas, have been published under the name of carcinoma in situ (*Mallory*, 1940; *Parturier-Lannegrace* et al., 1947; *Geffroy* and *Jouanneu*, 1951; *Osmond*, 1953; *Kuhlencordt*, 1951). As pointed out by *Bocian* and *Geschke* (1958) all these tumours invaded the lamina propria and could not be designated carcinoma in situ in the classical sense of *Schauenstein* (1908) and *Rubin* (1918).

II. The Author's Material

The material has been collected at Bispebjerg Hospital, Copenhagen. This hospital is not especially a cancer hospital, but a general municipal hospital with 1400 beds and two surgical departments subspecialized in gastroenterology. The hospital serves all districts of the city of Copenhagen and receives patients from all social classes. From 1964 all gastric resection specimens received in the department of pathology were investigated with special reference to egc. Up to 1972 inclusive, about 90 per cent of all the specimens were examined macroscopically and histologically by the author. During this period 54 specimens with egc were received. All – except two arriving during the authors absence – were primarily handled by himself. The material is consecutive and has by the pathologist been treated as prospective. In the same period two specimens with egc were received from other hospitals making a total of 56 cases (64 lesions).

No effort was spared to get the specimens as fresh as possible. About 75 per cent were sent to the department for frozen section diagnosis, most of them forwarded by means of a pneumatic tube system. Not so seldom the pathologist was at the operation ward and got the stomach immediately.

The specimens were photographed in a fresh state, pinned up on a corkboard and fixed usually in 10 per cent buffered formalin. It should be noticed that even 10 to 15 min of fixation will accentuate the contours of the lesions. After fixation the specimens were rephotographed (black/white and colour) and a sketch was drawn. Several blocks were made allowing examination of every irregularity of the mucosa and the degree of the gastritis in the pyloric, border, and body gland zone on both curvatures, the anterior and the posterior wall. In short, a procedure close to that prescribed by *Mochizuki* (1971) was carried out.

All the sections from specimens with egc were stained with haematoxylin-eosin, van Gieson, PAS, and Alcian blue. A double mucin staining namely the *Marks* and *Drysdale*'s (1957) modification of the *Zimmermann* (1925) reaction with added colloidal iron was considered most useful by the author who has great experience with it. The big battery of mucin stainings reflects the author's interest in this problem and is not considered necessary for daily use, but at least a PAS reaction should be carried out. Reticulin staining was sometimes used for investigating the basal membrane.

At this passage a comment should be given on the question: how many sections (blocks) should be taken? It is easier said than done to cut up the stomach completely and usually it is not necessary. Some compromises must be made. Supposing that a lesion is localized to the lesser curvature in the border zone – this is very often the case – those who are profoundly interested in egc must make a complete section of the whole lesser curvature side and the neighbouring part of the anterior and posterior wall, naturally including the lesion and a proper part of the adjacent mucosa. This usually leads to 50 to 75 blocks. Their position should be indicated on the sketch or the photo. Additional sections must be taken from the remaining part of the stomach for evaluating the gastritis. They can be made as "Swiss Rolls" (*Magnus*, 1937).

Lesions which are only slightly suspicious on macroscopic examination should be cut out from the specimen in such a way that – if malignancy is demonstrated – the position of the sections can be reconstructed. This method supplemented by some Swiss rolls can also be used by those who are only interested in the plain diagnosis of a macroscopically obvious egc, and the number of sections can be limited to less than twenty.

III. Frequency

The frequency and total number of gastric cancers diagnosed in its early stage can to some degree be estimated from the pertinent literature.

Versé (1908) found 12 cases of egc among 10,000 consecutive autopsies from Leipzig. *Bertrand* (1937) reported on 6 cases found among 120 gastric cancers during a period of 5 1/2 year in the Salpêtrière, Paris. *Gutmann* (1972) coworking with *Bertrand* mentioned 32 mucosal cancers found before and during World War II. In 1942 *Stout* presented 15 cases of superficial spreading carcinoma revealed among 69 stomach cancers in the Presbyterian Hospital 1937-1941. Later *Golden* and *Stout* (1948) calculated the frequency of this type of carcinoma to 14 per cent.

Hess (1956) estimated the frequency of egc to 3.3 per cent on the basis of 520 resection specimens with cancer investigated in a 6 1/2-year period in Basel. *Schade* (1962) reported that the frequency was 6 per cent among 282 stomach cancers diagnosed by cytology in Newcastle 1954-1958.

Mason (1965) related the frequency of egc to gastric ulcers. In 158 resection specimens with gastric or duodenal ulcer examined at Kings College Hospital 8 cases (5.1%) were disclosed. All were localized in specimens with gastric ulcers.

The frequency of egc in Scandinavia has been mentioned by *Myhre* (1953) who among 631 gastric cancer specimens investigated in Norway 1949-1952 found 8 cases of superficial spreading carcinomas. Among 378 gastric carcinomas not related to ulcers *Öhman* et al. (1972) found 23 (6%) which were submucosal carcinomas. Furthermore, among 21 ulcer cancers 7 (37%) were early.

The widespread use of fiber gastroscopy has caused a considerable rise in the number of egc diagnosed in the last few years. *Elster* et al. (1975) collecting gastric cancer from the Erlangen district demonstrated 119 cases from 1969 until the end of January 1975 with a clear increase in the frequency from year to year. In an interesting report *Miller* and *Kaufmann* (1975) collected information from 261 European endoscopic centers. Among 18,887 gastric cancers 1170 (6.2%) were early.

From the huge Japanese literature a few representative works are to be mentioned. On the basis of 200 gastric resection specimens collected at the Tohoku University, *Muto* (1965) and *Muto* et al. (1968) estimated the frequency of egc to 1.3 per cent at the beginning of the forties increasing to 36.4 per cent in 1965. In the same way *Kidokoro* (1971) at the Tokyo University Hospital found an increase of egc from 6.7 per cent in 1961 to 34 per cent in 1969, figures quite similar to those of *Kawai* (1971).

In an excellent report from Yokoyama Hospital and Aichi Cancer Center, Nagoya, *Nagayo* (1968) found 322 cases (13.3%) of egc among 2416 gastric cancers diagnosed from 1953 to 1966. *Nakamura* et al. (1967) reported on 144 (13.9%) superficial carcinomas among 1038 cases of gastric cancer.

The frequency of egc in Japan can also be estimated on the basis of mass surveys. From 1960 to 1967 422,025 patients were examined in the Sendai Prefecture (*Yamagata* et al., 1970). 794 cancers were found, 180 were egc. This was 27 per cent of the operated cases. In Miyagi Prefecture (*Nikaido* et al., 1970) 504,505 persons were examined 1960-1969. 776 cancers were found. The ratio of operated cases of gastric cancer to egc was 26.4 per cent. According to *Takahashi* (1971) and on basis of national statistics 1,573,667 persons in Japan were examined in 1969. 0.2 per cent had gastric cancer and about 30 per cent were egc.

In a more indirect way several works underline the extremely high frequency of egc in Japan. *Nagayo* and *Yokoyama* (1974) reported that among 4189 resected cancers 143 were scirrhus cancers in the fundic part of the stomach. Forty-two of the cases were egc. From 1964 to 1967 *Nakamura* et al. (1968) collected 33 egc of the microcarcinoma type, meaning that the diameter was less than 5 mm. This material had increased to 65 up to the end of 1973 (*Nakamura*, 1975). They were found more or less incidentally in 764 resection specimens examined in the Cancer Institute in Tokyo. Such illustrative numbers can only be found in Japan.

In conclusion it can be said that the frequency of gastric cancer in its early state in Europe is less than 10 per cent and in Japan about 30 per cent.

Author's material: It is difficult for a pathologist to estimate the frequency and number of egc in a hospital population. This can only be done on the basis of the material received for histological examination. The 54 patients from Bispebjerg Hospital were examined from 1964 to 1972. In the same period specimens from 476 patients with gastric cancer were examined. In 331 cases the material was resection or gastrectomy specimens. In 145 cases some sort of biopsy, preoperative, suction or fiber gastroscopic, from patients not resected. This means that egc formed 16 per cent of all resection specimens and 11 per cent of the total number of specimens from patients with histologically verfied carcinomas. The number of patients being admitted to the hospital in this period with gastric carcinoma without getting this histologically verfied is unknown to me. But according to general custom of the hospital this number must be negligible.

IV. Age and Sex Distribution

Gastric cancer is a rare disease before the age of 35. According to *Walthers* et al. (1943) investigating 10,890 cases from the Mayo Clinic, the fifties was the most common age group for the diagnosis of cancer. *Eker* and *Efskin* (1960) examining 1298 resection specimens from all parts of Norway showed that in this series the sixties was the most common age. This was also the case in a Finnish series (*Inberg* et al., 1972) and in a Danish report (*Nielsen* et al., 1974).

In 1964 *Oota* reported that the most common age of patients resected for gastric cancer was 50-60. *Nakamura* et al. (1967) in a series of 616 cases resected 10 years later found that the age had increased by 10 years. He did not find any age difference between advanced cancer and egc. The most common age in *Nagayo*'s (1965) material of 171 cases of egc was 50-60.

In their survey of European egc *Miller* and *Kaufmann* (1975) found that among 658 patients the most common age for men was the sixties (115 patients) or the fifties (114 patients). The sixties was the most common age for women followed by the seventies. As stressed by the authors it is noteworthy that the average age for egc decreased from Northern to Southern Europe. If the tenth degree of longitude is followed the average age for patients with egc was in Norway 68.9 years, in Denmark 63.8, in West-Germany 59.9, in Switzerland 57.8, and in Italy 53.4

Concerning sex distribution there is general agreement that gastric cancer and consequently egc is more common among men than among women. The relation is 2:1 to 3:2. There is no exception from this rule in any report referred to in this survey. Among the 1170 cases reported by *Miller* and *Kaufmann* (1975) 60 per cent were men and 40 per cent were women.

Author's material: The age distribution is given in Figure 2. The average age of men was 68.6 and of women 65.5. The eldest and the youngest patients (89 – 37 years) were both men. The average age of these patients compared with the age of patients with advanced cancer reported from Scandinavia was equal. The ratio of men to women was 1.8:1.

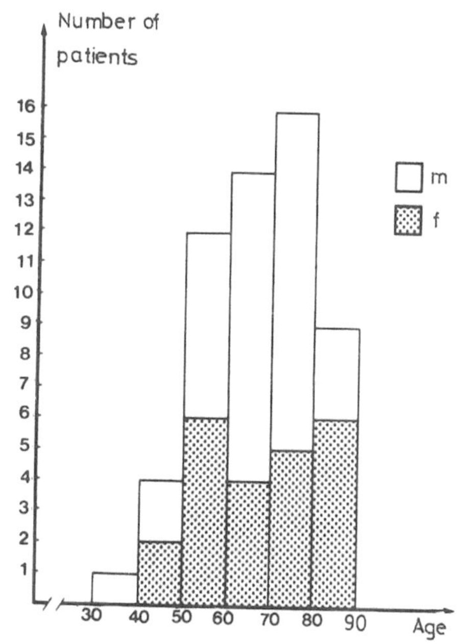

Fig. 2. Age and sex distribution of 56 patients with early gastric cancer

V. Macroscopic Features and Topography

1. Types and Classification Systems

The main principle for classifying gastric carcinomas macroscopically is closely related to the fact that the stomach is a hollow organ with a relatively thick wall. Only three basic types are possible: 1. The tumour tissue may grow into the lumen forming a polypoid, fungating or nodular carcinoma. 2. The tumour tissue may infiltrate the stomach wall as either linitis plastica or superficial spreading carcinoma. 3. The tumour tissue may grow outward penetrating the wall and invariably forming an ulcerating carcinoma.

Among the numerous classification systems which more or less modify this principle the classical one by *Bormann* (1926) is still in general use. Similar classifications are made by *Konjetzny* (1938), *Golden* and *Stout* (1948), *Eker* and *Efskin* (1966), *Guise* (1967), *Wanke* (1971), and *Morson* and *Dawson* (1972). The author agrees with the view of *Morson* and *Dawson* (1972) that too precise classification is of doubtful value. This is also underlined by *Stout* (1953) who classified 37 per cent of 470 carcinomas as of "no special" type.

The Japanese classification. Egc can hardly be dealt with without a profound study of the Japanese classification system.

When gastroenterologists in Japan realized that previous systems used for advanced carcinomas were insufficient or not applicable to egc they made a new system, based on exactly the same principles. This was inevitable, but a little disappointing.

The classification was established at the annual meeting of the Japan Gastroenterological Endoscopic Society in 1962. President was Professor Y. Tasaka. Details about the event are given by *Murakami* (1971). Egc was divided into three principles groups (Fig. 3):

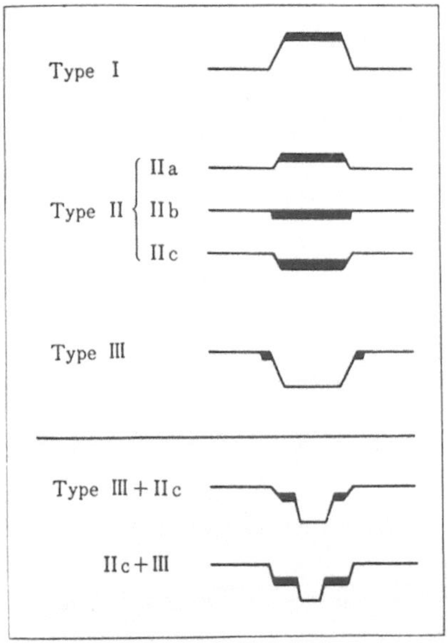

Fig. 3. The classification sketch given by the Japan Gastroenterological Endoscopic Society (from the journal: Stomach and Intestine)

Type I, *the protruded type:* the tumours project clearly into the lumen. This group contains all fungating, polypoid, papillomatous or nodular early carcinomas (Fig. 4).

Type II, *the superficial type:* where "unevenness of the surface is inconspicuous" (The official explanation given by the Endoscopic Society and always printed in the beginning

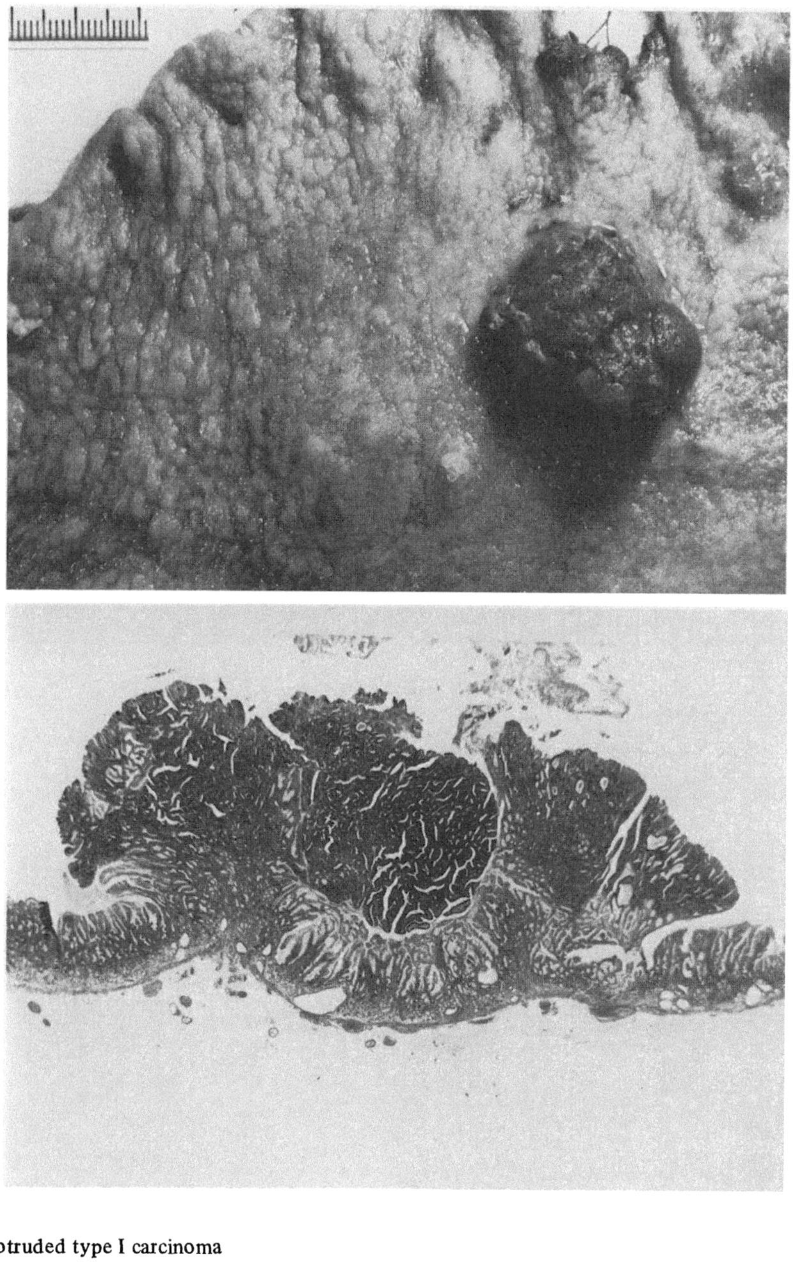

Fig. 4. The protruded type I carcinoma

of its journal "I to Cho" (Stomach and Intestine)). This type is further divided into three subtypes: type IIa, *the elevated type* (Fig. 5), where the tumour is elevated less than the thickness of the adjacent gastric mucosa (*Kobayashi* et al., 1972). Type IIb, *the flat type*, where no elevation or depression is seen. There might be some colour change in the surface epithelium, but for all practical purposes this subgroup contains incidentically found, macroscopically invisible carcinomas. Type IIc, *the depressed type* (Fig. 6), where the surface level is slightly depressed. The depression should not exceed the level of the sub-

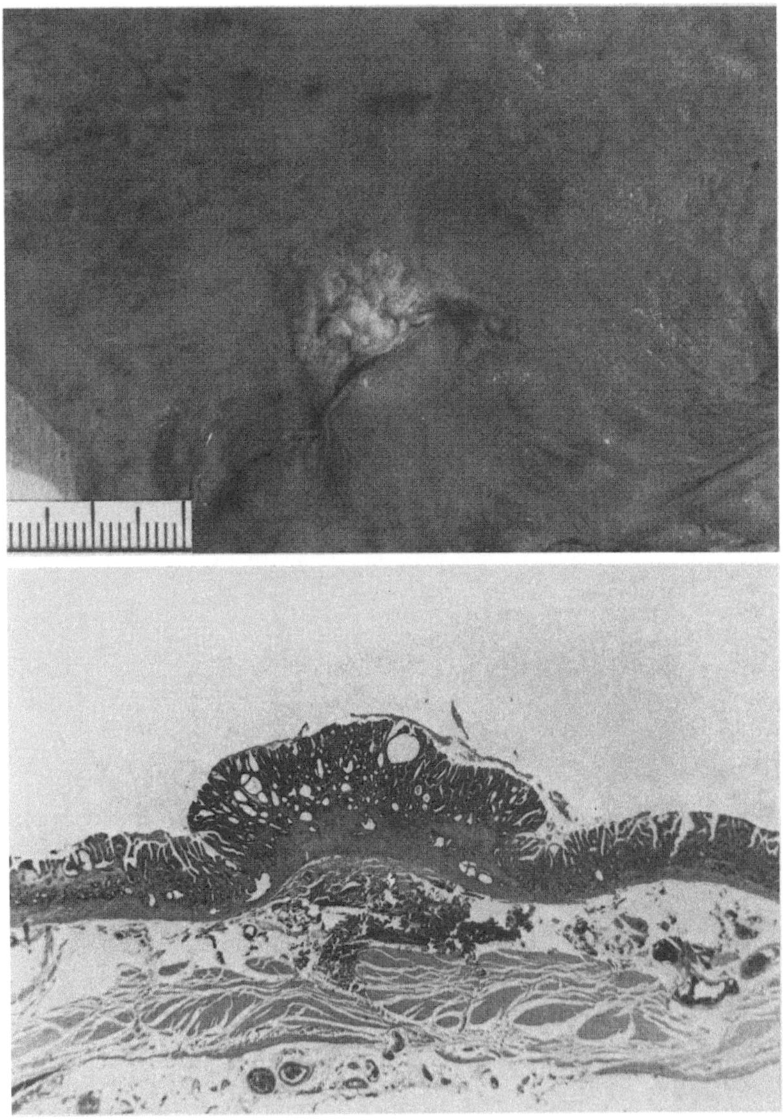

Fig. 5. The superficial, elevated type IIa carcinoma

mucosa. The depressed area often shows another colour than the adjacent mucosa. Sometimes it is covered by mucous or fibrin presenting itself as an erosion. The natural folds of the mucosa are disrupted (Fig. 13), and if the depressed area is large, as often seen, small islands of mucosa of normal height may be observed in it.

Type III, *the excavated type* (Fig. 7), shows a prominent excavation of variable depth in the gastric wall.

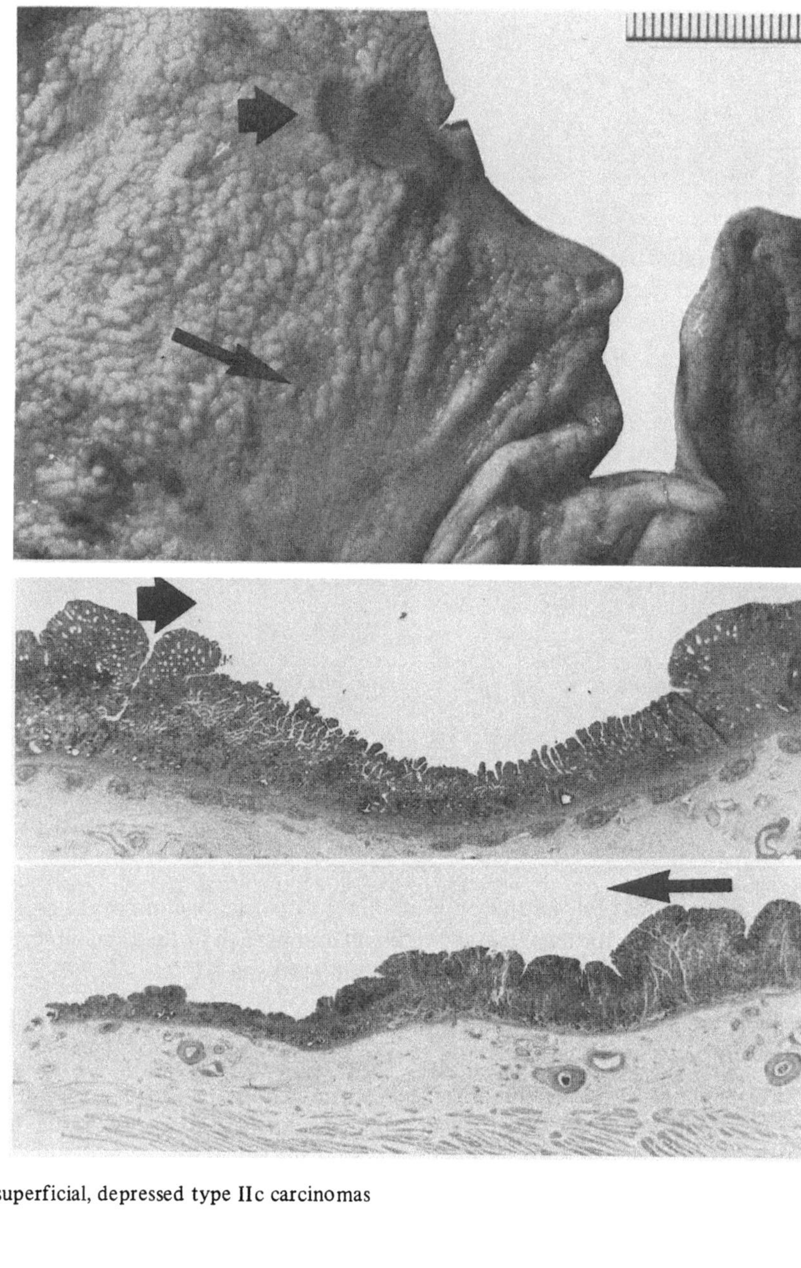

Fig. 6. Two superficial, depressed type IIc carcinomas

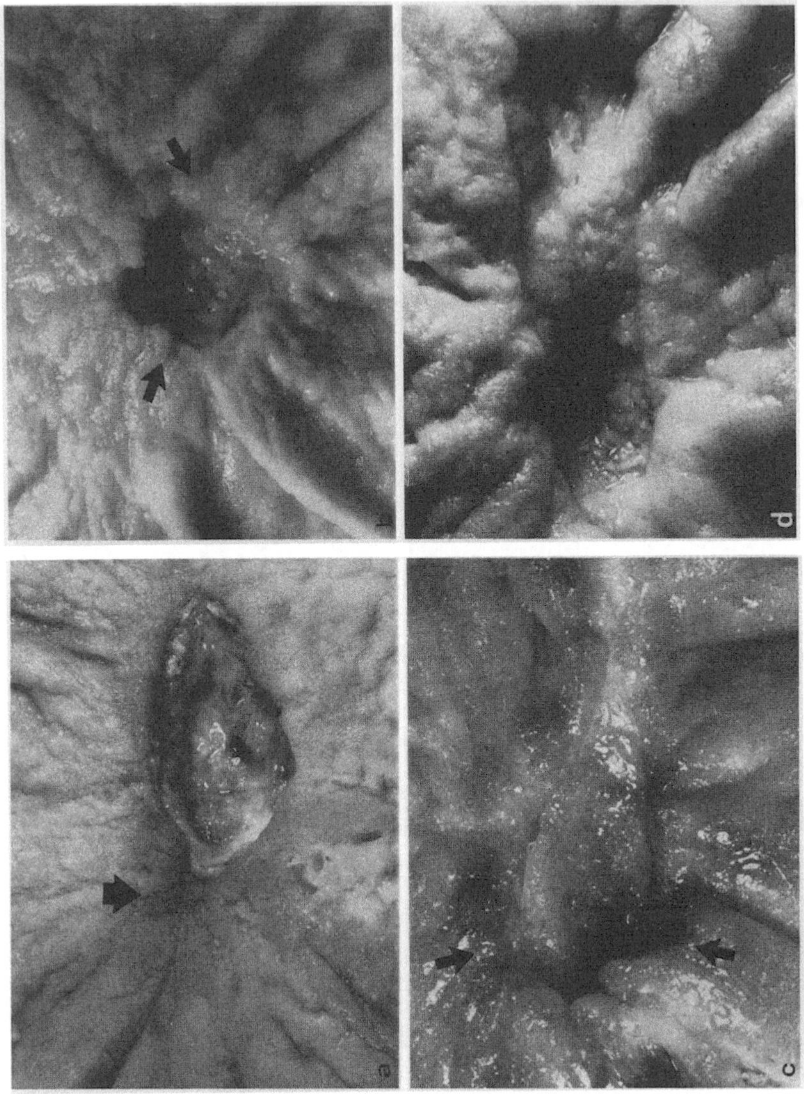

Fig. 7a-d. Four early ulcer-cancers: a) III + IIb. Apparently a benign ulcer. The arrow indicates the carcinoma which was macroscopically invisible except for a slightly darker colour. b) III + IIc. The carcinoma is situated below the arrows. The ulcer margin here "gnawn off". c) III + IIc. The carcinoma is right to the arrows and ends in a fissure-like lesion. d) III + IIc. Chronic ulcer to the left. Rectangular depressed carcinoma right to the ulcer

As far as the author can see this originally three step classification works as a five step classification. Both for daily use and in the literature each of the three subtypes of type II is handled on an equal footing with the main types I and III.

To facilitate the routine use of the classification the roman letters instead of the names are nearly always used.

The different types can be combined. Some combinations are more common than some of the pure forms. When two types are combined, e.g., III + IIc (Fig. 8), the predominant type is placed first. All possible combinations of the five types are met, but naturally with different frequencies. Combinations between type I and the others are rare, whereas those between type III and the others are common. Even combination forms containing three types are sometimes seen.

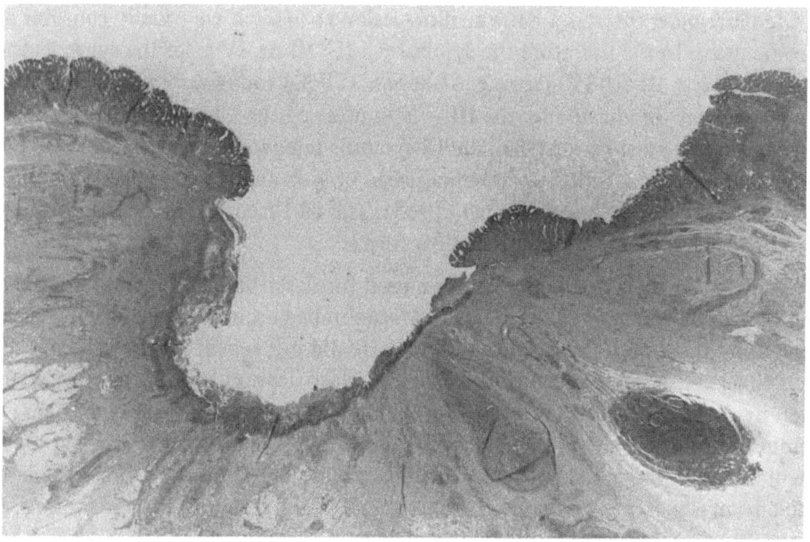

Fig. 8. Example of a section through a III + IIc carcinoma

As mentioned the classification was made by an *endoscopic* society. There are strong reasons to suppose that although the system can be used by any gastroenterologist it is primarily designed for the endoscopist. It is important to realize that Japanese endoscopists use it in such a way that they classify exactly what is seen without making any histogenetic consideration.

The classification system is widely adopted in Japan and is also in common use among European endoscopists. It has been criticized by some. The most weighty objections have been given by *Hermanek* and *Rösch* (1973) who, comparing the number of the different types published from different Japanese hospitals, revealed a considerable variation, probably on account of the subjective interpretion. Reducing the classification to "an interesting graphic improvement", *Gutmann* (1972) underestimated its importance considerably. There is no doubt that the clear definition given in the classification, especially for cases of type II, has occasioned that a great number of these lesions have been diagnosed.

Pathologists must have knowledge of this system to be able to keep up with the literature and to give the endoscopists relevant service.

Whether we should use it too in the routine must be decided individually for the departments, but a minimum of cases is required to make its advantages clear.

Since pathologists are concerned with the definitive diagnoses of the specimens I do not think we should use the classification in its original, non-histogenetic way, but on the contrary in our descriptions stress – if possible – that e.g. a type I lesion is a malignant transformed sessile adenoma or villous papilloma, and that all type III lesions are ulcer carcinomas and not only excavations. In this respect it is essential to understand that in Japan, gastric ulcer most often is a more shallow lesion than what we usually consider a classical chronic ulcer. In the literature the symbols Ul-II, -III or -IV after the symbols for the tumour, e.g. IIc + III (Ul-IV) [see e.g. *Shirakabe* (1968) and *Nakamura* (1970)] mean that the excavation – indicated by the III – is an ulcer of the Ul-IV type. This seems a little complicated to most Europeans. The Ul-symbols refer to an ulcer classification made by *Murakami* and *Oota*, unfortunately published only in Japanese. Explanation in English is given by *Sano* (1971) and *Nagayo* (1965). The Ul-IV corresponds to an ordinary deep, chronic ulcer, the other ones are shallow forms.

Naturally *other classifications* have been used for describing and facilitating the recognition of egc. *Konjetzny* (1938) divided "Magenkrebs in seinen ersten Anfängen" in five groups and illustrated the cases beautifully. He did not repeat his division in his English survey (1953). A comparison of the Japanese classification and that of *Konjetzny* has been given by *Hermanek* and *Rösch* (1973). The same authors have suggested (1973) a very simple and clear classification only differentiating between two forms: the polypoid and the ulcerous. Although simple classifications always are attractive I think there are considerable advantages in preserving the Japanese type II – the superficial carcinoma – as a main group. In my opinion this group is the essence of the whole problem. Using only two steps such carcinomas will disappear between great polyps and deep ulcers and the main benefit of the classification will be weakened or disappear. This benefit is primarily a didactic one. The different classifications do not tell much about the prognosis, since concerning egc this is always excellent, but they help us to recognize the lesions and teach others about them.

Author's material: Classifying my own material I have used the Japanese system in its most plain form and with only a little modification. For years I have especially been guided by the excellent and clear works of Professor *Nagayo* from Aichi Cancer Center in Nagoya (*Nagayo*, 1961, 1965, 1966). As previously mentioned I have considered the recognition of the type II carcinomas, the superficial type (which I should have preferred to call surface carcinoma) as the most important because they are so easily missed. According to my conception type III lesions are chronic gastric ulcers surrounded – totally or partly – by one of the type II superficial carcinomas. The most common form surrounding the ulcer is the depressed type IIc. If the ulcer looks completely benign and no differences in level are found at the margin, I think it is most logical to designate this surrounding carcinoma type IIb, and in the same way, if the ulcer margins are slightly elevated type IIa. This means that I do not use the designation type III alone realizing that it is not the excavation, but its margins which demonstrate the carcinoma. Therefore, my early *ulcer* cancers are divided into three forms (Fig. 9): III + IIc, III + IIb, corresponding to what is generally called III, and III + IIa which unfortunately is hypothetical for me as I have no examples myself, but it has been described [e.g. *Yamagata* and *Masuda* (1973) and *Elster* et al. (1975) using III + I]. I have not used other combination forms, but recently I have considered using the combination IIc + IIa (Fig. 13) which seems useful and characteristic. In the present material this combination is registered as pure type IIc.

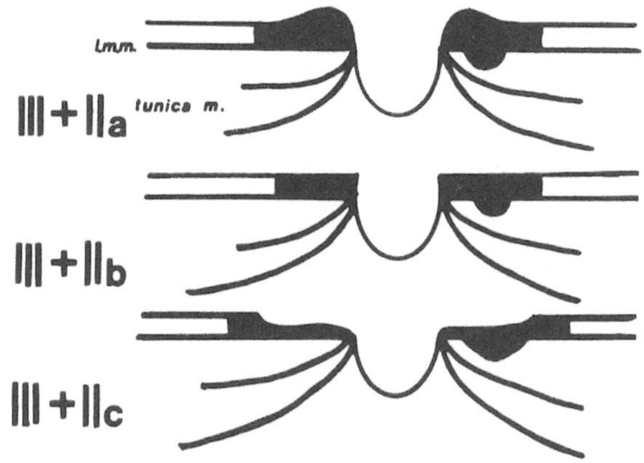

Fig. 9. Sketch indicating the author's classification of early *ulcer* carcinomas. A chronic ulcer is surrounded by the three types of superficial carcinomas IIa, IIb and IIc. To the left is demonstrated intramucosal carcinomas, to the right submucosal carcinomas

The distribution of 64 lesions in 56 stomachs together with the degree of penetration is given in Table 1. In Table 2 a representative Japanese material (*Nagayo*, 1968) and a German material (*Elster et al.*, 1975) are compared with the author's. The European material contained more elevated carcinomas than the Japanese. In my own material IIb lesions are relatively numerous. Four of the six cases are "the second" lesions in stomachs containing two separated tumours. The most marked difference between the European and the Japanese material is found for the ulcer-cancers which are far more often seen in the latter. According to the drawings of *Nagayo* (1968) some of the ulcers in his material might have been very shallow. *Nakamura* et al. (1967) found that if strict criteria were applied to a material of 144 superficial carcinomas 3.5 per cent were ulcer-cancers. Using *Oota*'s criterion including shallow ulcers on the same material this percentage would arise to 32 per cent.

It should be noticed that the sum of IIc and ulcer-cancers, in which way they may be indicated, are the same in *Elster*'s and my own material.

Table 1. Macroscopic type and degree of penetration

		total	intramucosal	submucosal 35	
				slight	extensive
		64	29	14	21
I protruded		10	3	2	5
II superficial	a elevated	3	1	–	2
	b flat	6	4	1	1
	c depressed	12	9	1	2
III chr. ulcer +	IIb flat carc.	10	5	2	3
	IIc depres. carc.	23	7	8	8

Table 2. The occurrence of different macroscopic types in one Japanese and two European series expressed in percentages

	Nagayo, 1968 n = 322	*Elster* et al., 1975 n = 90	*Johansen*, 1975 n = 64
I protruded	9.0%	14.4%	15.6%
II superficial a elevated	0.9%	7.8%	4.7%
II superficial b flat	1.9%	6.7%	9.4%
II superficial c depressed	15.8%	31.1% [a]	18.7%
III pure and all combination forms	72.4%	40.0%	51.6%

[a] included one case IIa + IIc

Concerning penetration I have divided the submucosal carcinomas into two groups (Fig. 1): those with only a few scattered cells or a gland imitation under the muscularis mucosae and those with a more extensive invasion. The group containing most intramucosal carcinomas was type II. This is in accordance with *Elster* et al. (1975). In *Nagayo*'s material (1968) type III carcinomas were also most often intramucosal.

2. Size

Many not familiar with the problem look upon egc as extremely small tumours. This is in no way the case. There is no size limitation in the definition of egc and many of the carcinomas are rather extensive although naturally the majority are small. *Konjetzny* (1938) stressed that many of the flat eroded carcinomas often have a diameter of 8 cm or more. Among the cases mentioned by *Golden* and *Stout* (1948) the smallest was about 1 cm^2 and the largest one occupied 180 cm^2. *Friesen* et al. (1962) reported that among their 65 lesions 8 per cent involved an area of 2 cm^2 or less. Seventy-two per cent measured from 2-30 cm^2, in 17 per cent the carcinomas replaced 30-100 cm^2, and in 2 cases the total specimen was involved in an irregular fashion. *Nagayo* (1968) subdivided his type IIc carcinomas into two groups: one group (31.4%) with carcinomas having well defined margins and diameters of less than 3 cm, and another group (68.6%) with ill defined boundaries and involving areas often measuring more than 5x5 cm.

Okabe (1971) in an interesting report related the horizontal diameter of egc to the depth of the carcinomatous infiltration. For elevated carcinomas the largest diameter was less than 60 mm and most of the tumours were intramucosal. For elevated carcinomas with a central depression (IIa + IIc) the largest diameter was less than 50 mm, but the majority of these tumours were submucosal. The largest cancers were found among the depressed ones, and there was no correlation between size and depth infiltration nor was this the case for ulcer-cancers which all had a diameter of less than 50 mm.

On the other hand, as already mentioned, *Nakamura* (1975) was able to collect 65 cases of microcarcinomas all having a diameter of less than 5 mm.

Author's material: I have divided the 64 lesions in my material into 6 groups according to their largest diameter (Table 3 and 4). More than half of the lesions had a largest diameter of 2 cm or less. Among tumours larger than 4 cm five were ulcer-cancers (Fig. 10) and two papillomatous tumours of type I.

There was nearly a direct correlation between the size of the tumour and the degree of penetration (Table 4).

Table 3. Macroscopic type and size (largest diameter)

		total	<1 cm	1.1-2cm	2.1-3cm	3.1-4cm	4.1-5cm	>5 cm
		64	17	17	11	11	5	3
I protruded		10	2	3	2	1	–	2
II superficial	a elevated	3	1	–	1	1	–	–
	b flat	6	4	1	–	1	–	–
	c depressed	12	3	4	3	1	1	–
III chr. ulcer +	IIb flat carc.	10	3	1	2	2	1	0
	IIc depres. carc.	23	4	8	3	5	3	1

Table 4. Degree of penetration and size (largest diameter)

		total	<1 cm	1.1-2cm	2.1-3cm	3.1-4cm	4.1-5cm	>5 cm
		64	17	17	11	11	5	3
Intramucosal		29	13	10	4	1	1	–
submucosal	slight	14	3	2	4	3	1	1
	extensive	21	1	4	3	7	3	2

3. Localization

It has to be stressed that the localization of gastric cancer can be given in relation to the traditional anatomical parts of the stomach which are the pyloric channel, the antrum, the body, the fundus, and the cardia. A more attractive way, especially from a histogenetic point of view, is to relate the localization to the type of the mucosa, either the pyloric gland mucosa or the body mucosa, separated by an intermediary or border zone mucosa often several cm in width. A combination of the two principles is often used. In this respect it has to be remembered that the pyloric mucosa always is most extensive at the lesser curva-

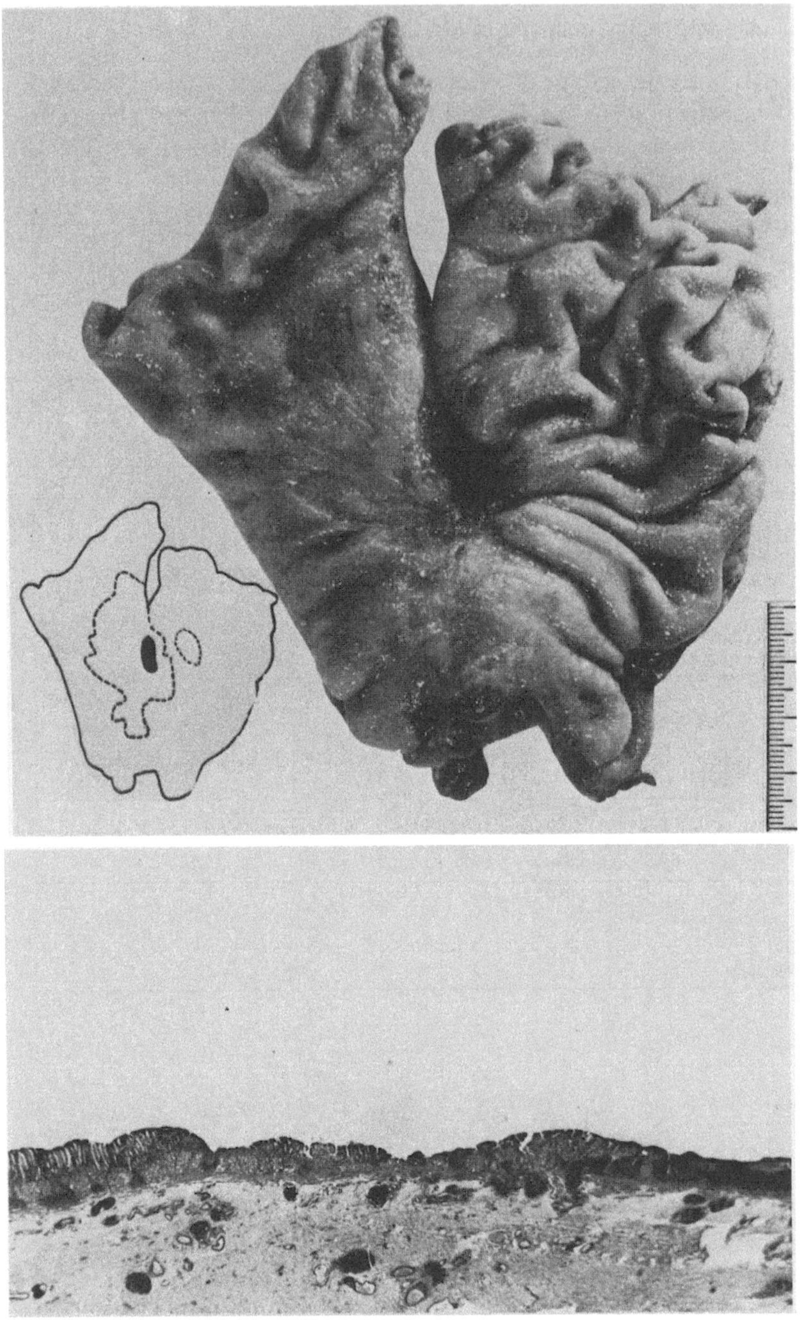

Fig. 10. Two type III + IIc lesions. The superficial carcinomas have ill defined borders and are both several cm^2 of extension

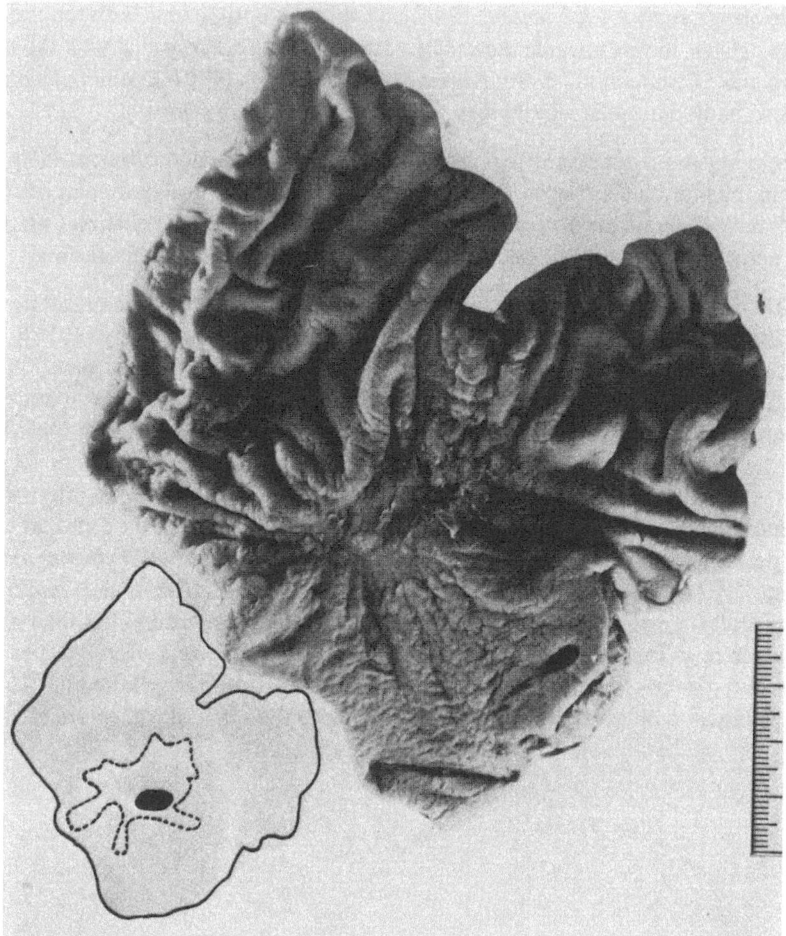

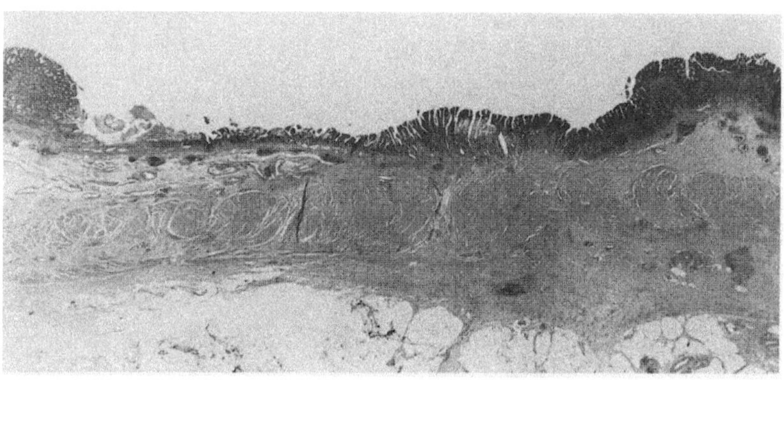

Fig. 10 (continued)

ture side (*Landboe-Christensen*, 1944) and that the border zone between the pyloric and body glands moves towards the cardia with increasing age, especially on the lesser curvature side (*Kimura* et al., 1970; *Kimura* and *Takemoto*, 1970). In older persons representative body mucosa is seldom seen at the lesser curvature side at all.

There is general agreement that gastric cancer is most often localized in the pyloric zone or in the intermediary zone. When localized in the anatomical body part of the stomach it is nearly always on the lesser curvature side at the top of the extended atrophic pyloric mucosa or in the atrophic body mucosa associated with pernicious anemia.

All the cases reported by *Hess* (1956) were localized to the pyloric or intermediary mucosa close to the lesser curvature. This was also the case in *Mason*'s study (1956). *Nagayo* et al. (1965) demonstrated that although the majority of 161 egc were localized in the pyloric and intermediary zone there was a slight difference between the three main types. More than half of type I carcinomas were localized in body mucosa. Among type II carcinomas only one was situated in that area. Concerning type III carcinomas about 10 per cent were localized to the body mucosa, but the majority were localized to the intermediary zone, especially on the lesser curvature side in good accordance with the fact that this is the region where gastric ulcers most often are seen (*Oi* et al., 1969; *Stadelmann* et al., 1970). *Sano* (1971) divided 300 cases of egc into 2 groups: cancers with ulcer and cancers without ulcers. Among those without ulcers 39.3 per cent were found less than 4 cm from the pyloric ring. The corresponding figures from those with ulcers were 19.8 per cent. In both cases 13 per cent were found more than 8 cm away from the pyloric ring. This is in good accordance with *Nagayo*'s work (1965) and with the work of *Nakamura* (1970) who found

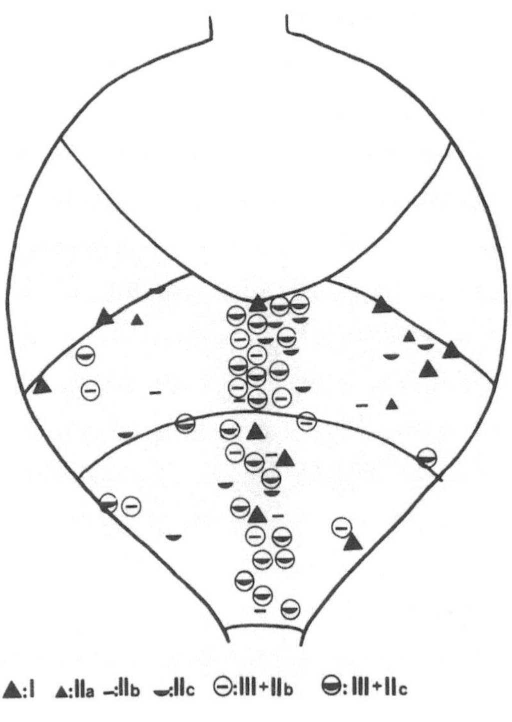

Fig. 11. Sketch indicating the localization of 64 early gastric carcinomas. The mid zone corresponds to the intermediary-type mucosa

a considerable number of undifferentiated carcinomas in the fundic mucosa. Actually it seems that the traditional view that gastric cancer is more common in the pyloric mucosa (ref. *Wanke*, 1971) has to be reviewed. In the retrospective study of 1170 cases of egc (*Miller* and *Kaufmann*, 1973) 49 per cent were localized in the body/fundic area. Among 4189 cases of resected stomach cancers from Aichi Cancer Center 14.9 per cent were classified as scirrhus carcinomas, 28 per cent of these were developing in the body/fundic area (*Nagayo* and *Yokoyama*, 1974). Recently *Nakamura* et al. (1975) among 173 cases of linitis plastica cancers collected from 1954-1974 found that 88 cases were localized in the body/fundic mucosa.

Author's material: The localization of the different types of 64 lesions is given in Figure 11. It is seen that practically all tumours were localized to the pyloric zone or to the intermediary zone. Indeed hardly any lesion was found in proven body mucosa. In two cases a relatively large number of parietal cells was revealed distal to the tumour, but they were found together with many pseudopyloric glands and comparing such areas with proven body mucosa it was the impression that the lesions were localized to the uppermost part of the intermediary zone.

The localization indicated on the sketch refers to the centre of the lesion. As mentioned, many tumours were very extensive and involved all three histological zones. Eleven lesions extended into the body mucosa where they were limited to the foveolar zone, but in all cases they originated from the intermediary mucosa. None of the lesions extended into the duodenal or cardiac mucosa.

4. Multiplicity

Gastric cancer is often a multifocal lesion. According to *Wanke* (1971) upto 1961 186 such cases have been published. The diagnostic criterions for multiplicity have been outlined by *Moertel* (1957). He demanded that (1) each lesion must be of pathologically proven malignancy, (2) the tumours must be separated from each other by intervals of microscopically normal gastric wall, and (3) the possibility that one of the lesions represents a local extension or a metastatic tumour must be ruled out beyond any reasonable doubt.

An important contribution to the problem has been given by *Collins* and *Gall* (1952) who investigated 117 specimens with gastric carcinoma: "In 26 stomachs (22%) multiple, independent, neoplastic lesions were found. Four (3.4%) of these were grossly appreciated, the remainder 22 (19%) were microscopic in size and preinvasive in character". There is no doubt that among these 22 cases some were precancerous lesions, but some might have been "carcinoma in situ" cases in the sense of *Mallory* (1940) meaning that they were intramucosal carcinoma in a modern concept.

The multiplicity of egc has been demonstrated by many authors. *Hess* (1956) revealed a multicentric origin in 11 cases out of 17. *Friesen* et al. (1962) demonstrated the presence of two or more regions of carcinoma separated by benign mucosa in 33 (51%) of 65 superficial carcinomas. Nine cases of 12 surface carcinomas reported by *Mason* (1965) showed multifocal origin. *Wiendl* and *Piger* (1971) found 7 multicentric cases among 220 gastric cancers, most of them in early stage. Among 66 cases of egc reported by *Elster* et al. (1975) 3 showed multiple carcinomas.

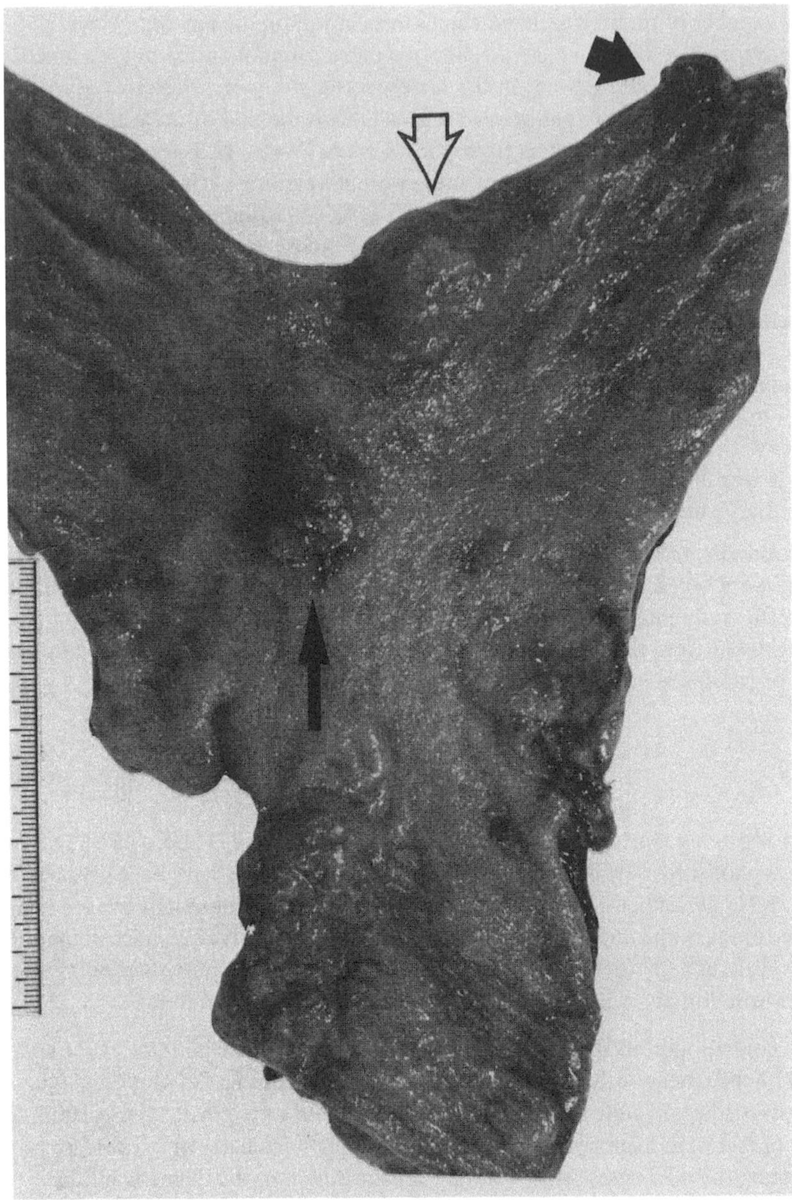

Fig. 12. Multifocal carcinomas. Three type I lesions are indicated by the arrows. Furthermore, an adenoma in the pyloric channel is seen

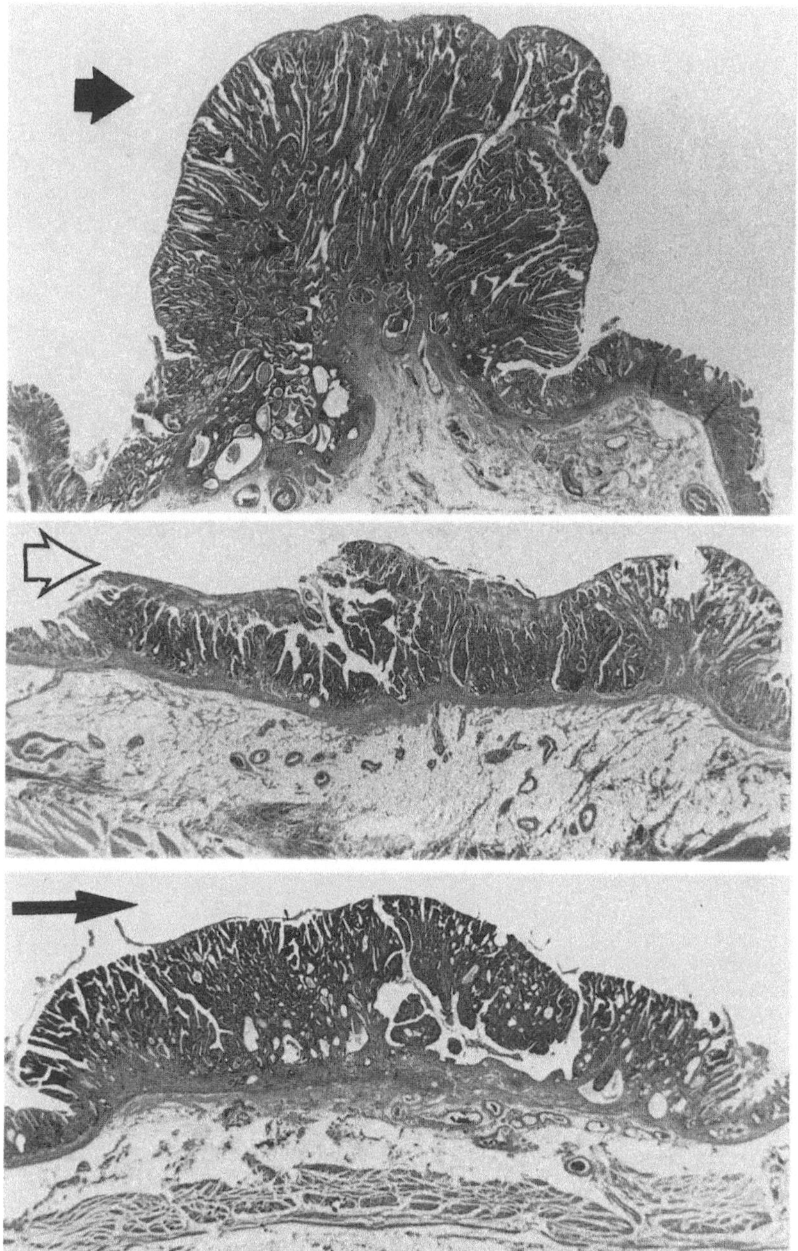

Fig. 12 (continued)

The same high frequency of multiplicity are met in the Japanese works. Among 171 cases of egc reported by *Nagayo* et al. (1965) 12 cases were multifocal. Especially the protruded tumours were multiple. This was also the case in *Sano*'s (1971) material where multiple

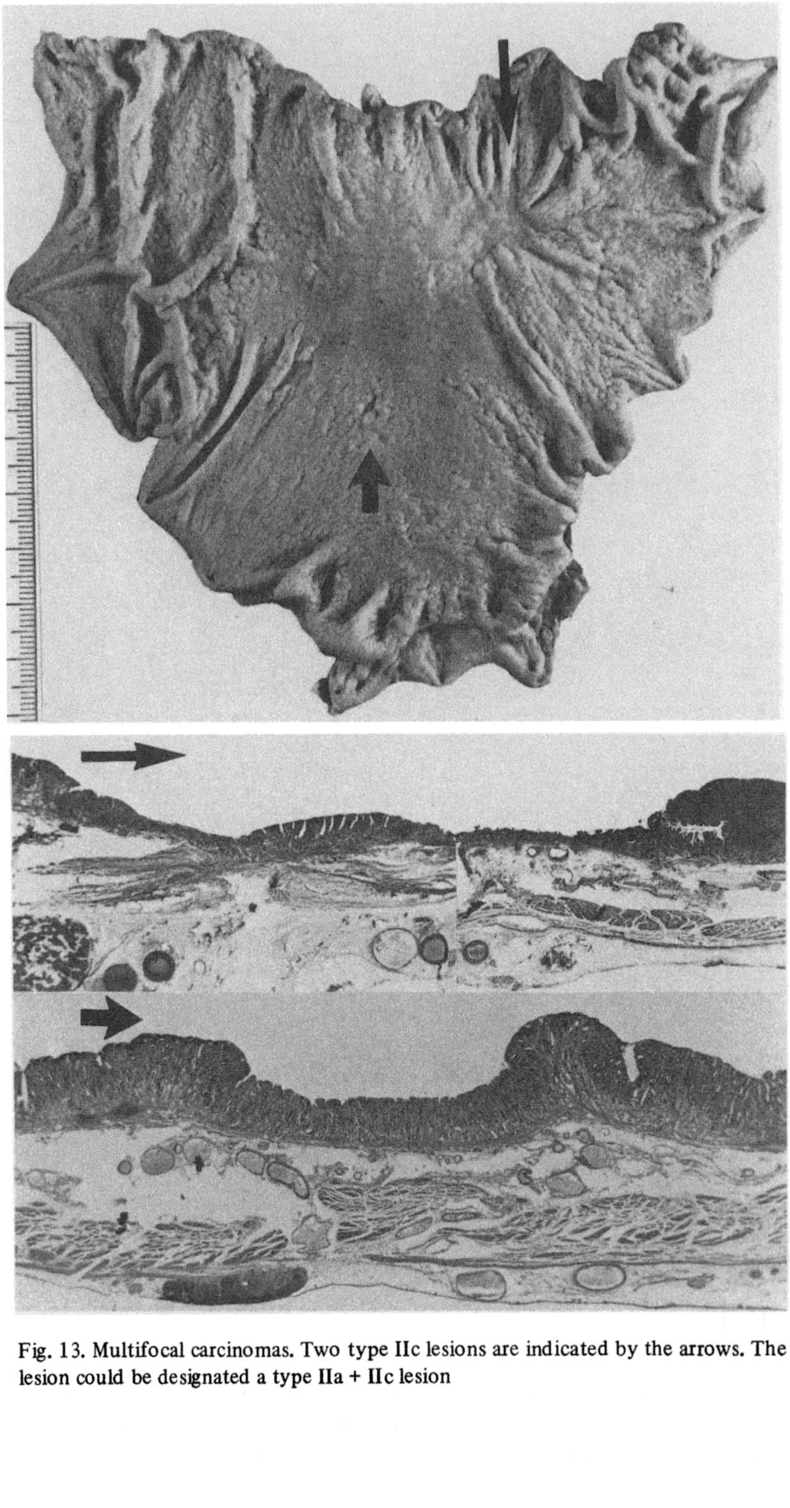

Fig. 13. Multifocal carcinomas. Two type IIc lesions are indicated by the arrows. The most distal lesion could be designated a type IIa + IIc lesion

cancers were found in 12.4 per cent in egc-specimens without ulcers and in 5.2 per cent in those with ulcers. *Nakamura* et al. (1967) found 7 cases with multiple cancers among 162 egc. Furthermore, multiplicity has been demonstrated in several of the 95 cases of egc reported by *Majima* et al. (1955, 1963, 1965).

Author's material: Among the 56 resection specimens 7 demonstrated multifocal lesions. In one case (Fig. 12) three protruded type I carcinomas were found together with a pyloric adenoma disclosing severe precancerous changes. In three stomachs lesions of type IIc were accompanied by another type IIc lesion (Fig. 13) in 2 cases, and in one case by a type IIb lesion. In three cases type IIb lesions were found separated from ulcer-cancers.

VI. Microscopic Appearance

1. Type and Grade

Although the histological picture of egc hardly can be described in detail without making histogenetical considerations, some general information about the microscopic appearance will be given here. All egc are adenocarcinomas. Epidermoid carcinomas and adenoacanthomas have – to the best of my knowledge – never been described at an early stage in the stomach.

Gastric carcinomas have been divided according to two different principles. The carcinomas have been classified in *types* as carcinoma adenomatosum, solidum, simplex, medullare, colloides, scirrhosum etc. based on their morphology and growth pattern, or according to their *grades* of differentiation into the wellknown four groups of Broders. Concerning egc the latter division is most important. All grades of differentiation are seen in egc.

Nagayo and *Komagoe* (1961) divided their 42 cases of pure intramucosal cancers into three groups according to differentiation: (1) Highly differentiated, where the cells had clearly preserved their polarity. The cells were most often cylindrical and their mucous secretion was low. The cells were arranged in tubular or glandular imitations, sometimes disclosing papillary structures. (2) Less differentiated, where the cells were more cuboidal but had still preserved some degree of polarity. Their mucous secretion was scanty. They were arranged in small cords or trabeculae which sometimes formed a network. (3) Undifferentiated, where the tumour cells had completely lost their polarity, their shape was round or polygonal and very often they secreted an abundant amount of mucus (signet ring cells). The cells were disseminated, without any system, into the surrounding stroma.

It may seem a little rigid to base degrees of differentiation on a relatively firm histological pattern. On the other hand, from a didactic point of view, it makes the classification easier, if the pathologist has the morphological prototypes, given in Table 5, in his mind. This sequence could be divided into two, three or even the four classical groups of Broders, although the last possibility is not recommended.

Table 5. Prototypes of carcinoma

Carcinoma papillare
carcinoma tubulare
carcinoma glandulare
carcinoma reticulare
carcinoma trabeculare
carcinoma globocellulare (signet ring cells)
carcinoma monocellulare (anaplasticum)

Sometimes the prototypes are found in nearly pure form, but naturally transition between neighbouring types is often seen. Coexistence of types located at each end of the sequence may also be seen. In such cases one type usually predominates making a grading of the differentiation possible. Should, however, each type be represented in equal amount the carcinoma must be considered to be of a mixed type, and it is very difficult or impossible to grade it exactly.

When deciding the degree of differentiation of a tumour considerable weight is placed on the appearance of the nuclei and the cytoplasmic/nuclear ratio together with the number of mitoses and their degree of atypism. The nuclei must be carefully studied in all cases, especially when advanced gastric cancers are to be graded, but they seem of lesser importance when classifying egc. Certain highly differentiated tubular early carcinomas have large and atypical nuclei and frequently many mitoses. On the other hand the nuclei of typical anaplastic cells are often small and – as known from the frozen section laboratory – can easily be confused with those of inflammatory cells. If the cells are of the signet ring type mitoses are practically never seen.

Stromal reaction is sparse and is hardly seen in intramucosal carcinomas. In poorly differentiated, particularly submucosal, carcinomas some fibrosis is seen. Evaluating the histology of 144 egc *Nakamura* et al. (1967) designated 14 (9.7%) as scirrhus cancers.

The different macroscopic types of egc are related to the degree of differentiation in a relatively constant way. Type I carcinomas are nearly always highly differentiated adenocarcinomas often with a papillary component. All the 21 type I carcinomas reported by *Nagayo* et al. (1965) were highly differentiated. Among 13 type I carcinomas, *Elster* et al. (1975) found only one undifferentiated. Exactly the same is the case concerning the type IIa carcinomas. The histology of type IIb carcinomas was in the before mentioned work by *Nagayo* also dominated by highly differentiated carcinomas in contrast to *Elster*'s material, where undifferentiated carcinomas were conspicuous.

Concerning type IIc lesions *Elster* et al. (1975) found among 28 cases, 8 highly, 1 poorly, and 5 undifferentiated of the signet ring type. Furthermore, 13 were of mixed types. *Nagayo* (1968) examined 51 cases of type IIc and found that 25 were well, 15 moderately, and 11 poorly differentiated. But in the group of small type IIc carcinomas with well demarcated borders, previously mentioned, all except one were highly differentiated.

Among 36 cases of type III carcinomas and their combination forms *Elster* et al. (1975) found 11 cases highly, 5 poorly, and 10 undifferentiated. Furthermore, 10 were of the mixed type. In 68 purely intramucosal type III carcinomas classified by *Nagayo* et al. (1965) 23 were highly, 8 moderately, and 8 poorly differentiated. Thirty were of the mixed type. *Nakamura* et al. (1967) found nearly a similar distribution. Summarizing this it can be said that the elevated carcinomas nearly always are highly differentiated, the flat ones may contain both groups, and the depressed carcinomas and especially the ulcer-cancers demonstrate a higher number of undifferentiated carcinomas.

Author's material: I have divided my cases into three groups according to the degree of differentiation. Although mixed types were present one type always predominated so that it was possible to place each case in one of the three groups. The first group contains highly differentiated carcinomas with a papillar or tubular pattern. The second group –

the moderately differentiated – contains carcinomas, where the tubular or glandular pattern can only be glimpsed. The cells are often collected in trabeculae. In the third group, which contains poorly or undifferentiated carcinomas, are found mainly signet ring cell carcinomas but also totally anaplastic carcinomas nearly without mucous secretion.

Table 6. Macroscopic types and degree of differentiation

		total	Degree of differentiation high	moderate	poor or no
		64	31	10	23
I protruded		10	9	1	–
II superficial	a elevated	3	3	–	–
	b flat	6	1	1	4
	c depressed	12	7	1	4
III chr. ulcer +	IIb flat carc.	10	5	1	4
	IIc depres. carc.	23	6	6	11

In Table 6 the groups of differentiation are related to the macroscopic types. It is seen that the results are nearly identical to the above mentioned, but the greatest part of my ulcer cancers belongs to the poorly or undifferentiated group. In Table 7 the three groups are related to the degree of penetration. The distribution did not reveal any conclusive pattern. Some examples of the microscopic pictures are given in Figure 14.

Table 7. Degreee of penetration and degree of differentiation

		total	Degree of differentiation high	moderate	poor or no
		64	31	10	23
Intramucosal		29	14	5	10
Submucosal	slight	14	8	3	3
	extensive	21	9	2	10

2. Histogenesis

Egc offers fairly good possibilities for studying the histogenesis of gastric carcinoma, since the original structure of the mucosa more frequently can be recognized than in advanced carçinomas. There is general agreement that there is a clear relationship between atrophic gastritis and the development of gastric carcinoma, and particularly intestinal metaplasia has been referred to as a precancerous lesion in the broad sense of the word. This subject has for years been thoroughly investigated and only some landmarks will be mentioned here.

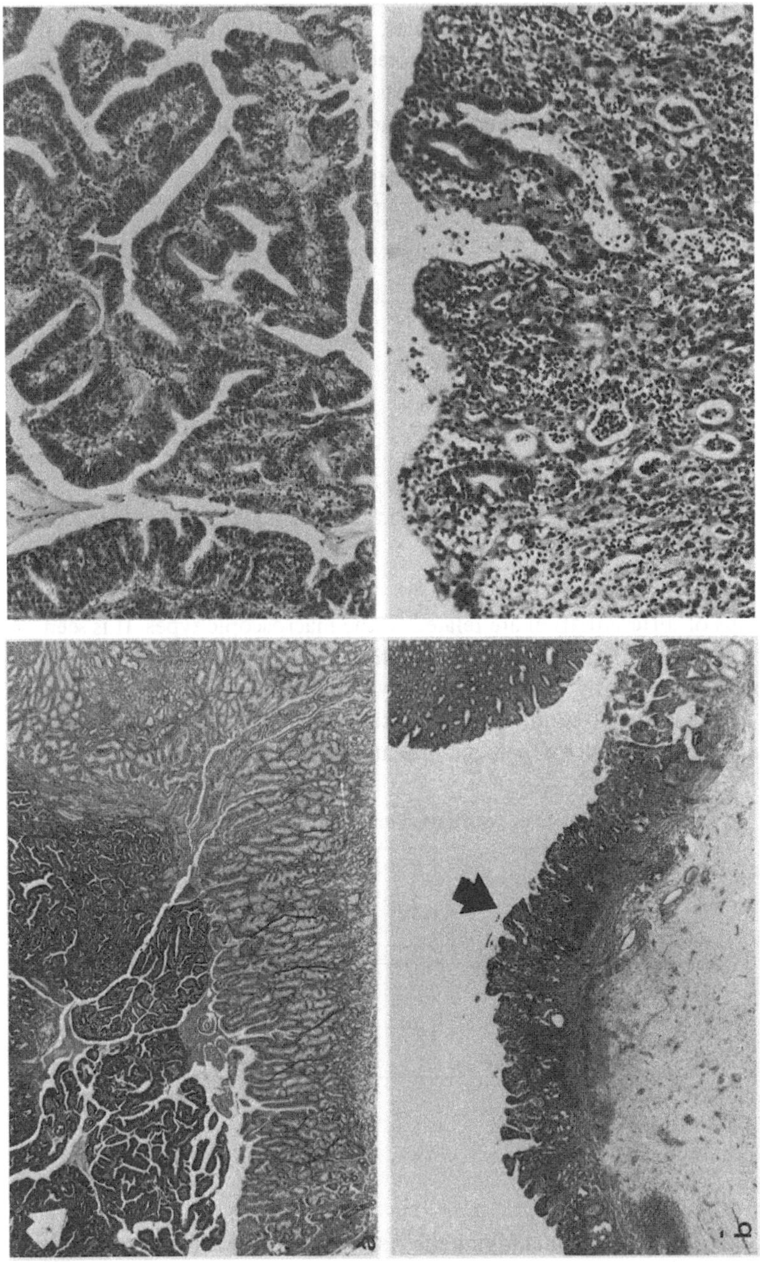

On the basis of 184 advanced gastric cancers and 6 papillomas *Järvi* and *Laurén* (1951) introduced the hypothesis that gastric cancers often originate from intestinal metaplastic epithelium and even do so "in the majority of cases". In his well known work *Laurén* (1965) divided 1344 cases of gastric cancer into two groups: intestinal-type carcinoma,

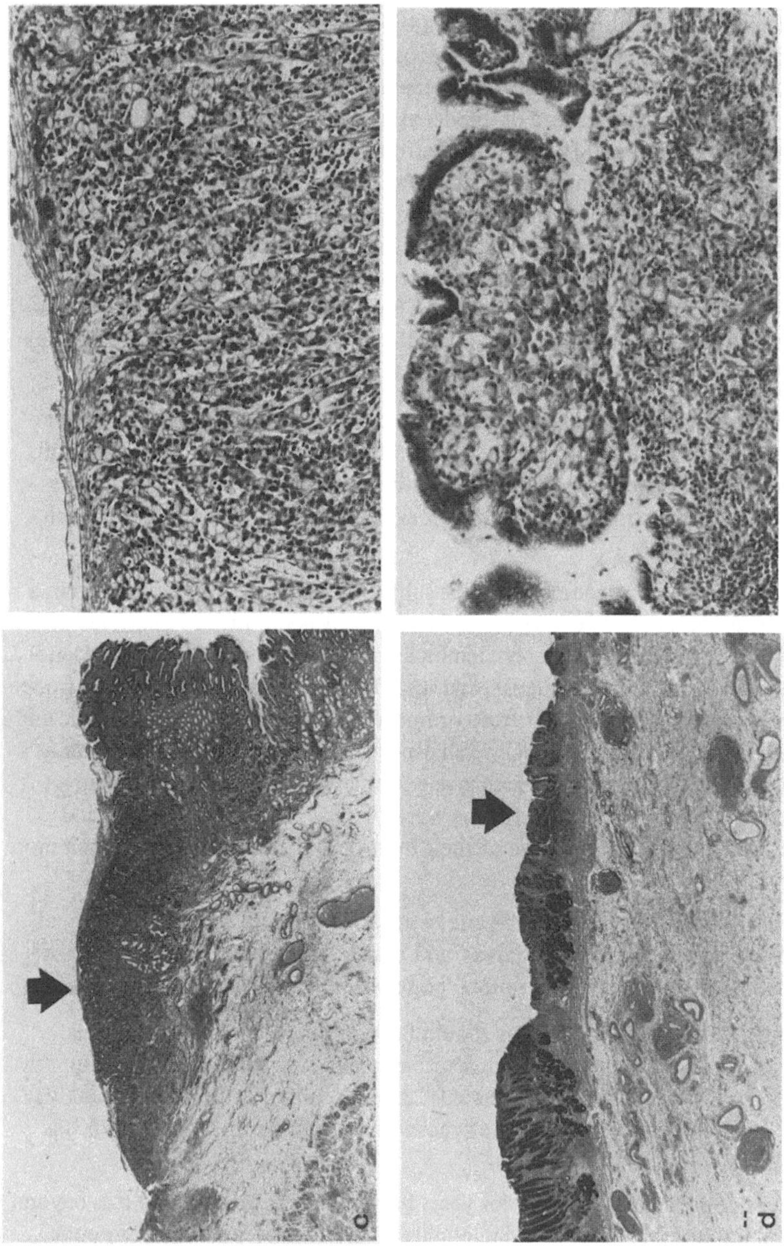

Fig. 14a-d. Different histological patterns of early gastric carcinomas: a) Highly differentiated adenopapillary carcinomas (from the type I carcinoma of Fig. 6). H&E, x 10 and x 100. b) Moderately differentiated adenocarcinoma of type IIb. H&E, x 10 and x 100. c) Low differentiated carcinoma with slightly trabecular pattern. From a III + IIc lesion. H&E, x 10 and x 60. d) Low differentiated carcinoma of the signet ring cell type from a IIc lesion. PAS, x 10 and H&E, x 100

accounting for 53 per cent, and diffuse carcinoma accounting for 33 per cent. Fourteen per cent showed a structure which did not allow any classification. As indicated by the name, intestinal-type carcinoma was considered to develop from intestinal metaplastic epithelium. Although not directly stated the diffuse carcinomas had consequently developed from the original unchanged mucosa. *Morson* (1955a) showed that intestinal metaplasia was most commonly found in the pyloric mucosa and on the lesser curvature side in all sorts of gastric diseases and that intestinal metaplasia was seen more often in stomachs with carcinoma than in those with gastric or duodenal ulcers. Investigating 107 resection specimens with carcinoma, *Morson* (1955b) found strong evidence that about 30 per cent of gastric cancers arise from intestinal metaplastic areas. In the same year he (1955c) showed that intestinal metaplasia is very common in gastric polyps. Later *Morson* and *Dawson* (1972) summarized the evidence for the precancerous role of intestinal metaplasia. They divided gastric carcinoma into three groups: carcinoma of intestinal epithelial pattern, diffuse carcinoma, and carcinoma of gastric epithelial pattern. The classification is not strictly a histogenetic one, but naturally the names indicate that the authors presume that a carcinoma can develop from both gastric epithelium and intestinal epithelium.

In Germany the pathology of intestinal metaplasia has been carefully studied by *Elster* et al. (1960) and *Heinkel* et al. (1960). In Japan *Nagayo* et al. (1965) found that highly differentiated adenocarcinomas were found together with severe degrees of intestinal metaplasia, and that this sort of gastritis was seldom among the low or undifferentiated carcinomas.

The investigator who has contributed most to this subject in Japan is *Nakamura* who in a series of works (*Nakamura* et al., 1966, 1968, 1971, 1975; *Nakamura*, 1970) arrived at the conclusion that highly differentiated adenocarcinomas (tubular and papillotubular adenocarcinomas) arise from intestinalized mucosa, and undifferentiated adenocarcinomas (mucocellular and anaplastic adenocarcinomas) from ordinary mucosa of the pyloric, fundic and cardiac type. The reports of *Nakamura* analyse all aspects of the problem and are mainly based on the study of microcarcinomas which give extremely good conditions for such studies. These reports are in accordance with the work of *Järvi* and *Laurén* (1951) and can be considered as a sort of confirmation of their hypothesis, carried out on a much more favourable material.

It must be underlined that *Nakamura* (1975) stresses that differentiated carcinomas in all cases originate from intestinal metaplastic areas, and that he rules out the possibility that such carcinomas also may originate from normal non-metaplastic foveolar epithelium.

Finally, *Konjetzny*'s (1938) life-long studies should be mentioned. It is especially this author who has put forward the concept that gastric cancer never develops in healthy gastric mucosa. He considered what he designated "atrophisch-hypertrophische" gastritis, often dominated by intestinal metaplasia, as a precancerous condition. *Schade* (1963) is of the same opinion.

Histogenetic studies of gastric cancer have for years been my main interest and it is beyond the limit of this survey to report my work in detail (this is under preparation for publication). It is my conviction that gastric carcinoma often is intimately related to metaplastic epithelium. In early carcinomas unmistakable transitions from such elements to carcinoma of the highly differentiated type may easily be observed (Fig. 15). Indeed it is true that a great number of tumours, early as well as advanced, demonstrate areas where more or less well developed brush borders and goblet cells let presume that the origin is intestinal metaplastic epithelium. It is observations of this kind made on ordinary stained specimens (*Morson*, 1955a) and specimens stained by different mucin (*Stiller* and *Stiller*, 1964; *Lev*, 1966;

Gad, 1969) or enzyme histochemical (*Wattenberg*, 1959; *Planteydt* et al., 1962) reactions which support the hypothesis. Studying the literature one gets the impression that the hypothesis is based on the following sequence: normal gastric foveolar epithelium → fully developed intestinal epithelium (or at least intestinal epithelium demonstrating brush borders and goblet cells) → precancerous epithelium with an appearance often like that known from adenomas in the colon → carcinoma. In my opinion, based on the constant use of double mucin stained specimens, this theory is far too simple.

In the first place many transitional forms between a normally developed gastric foveola with cylindrical, PAS-positive cells and a completely metaplastic intestinal crypt with non-

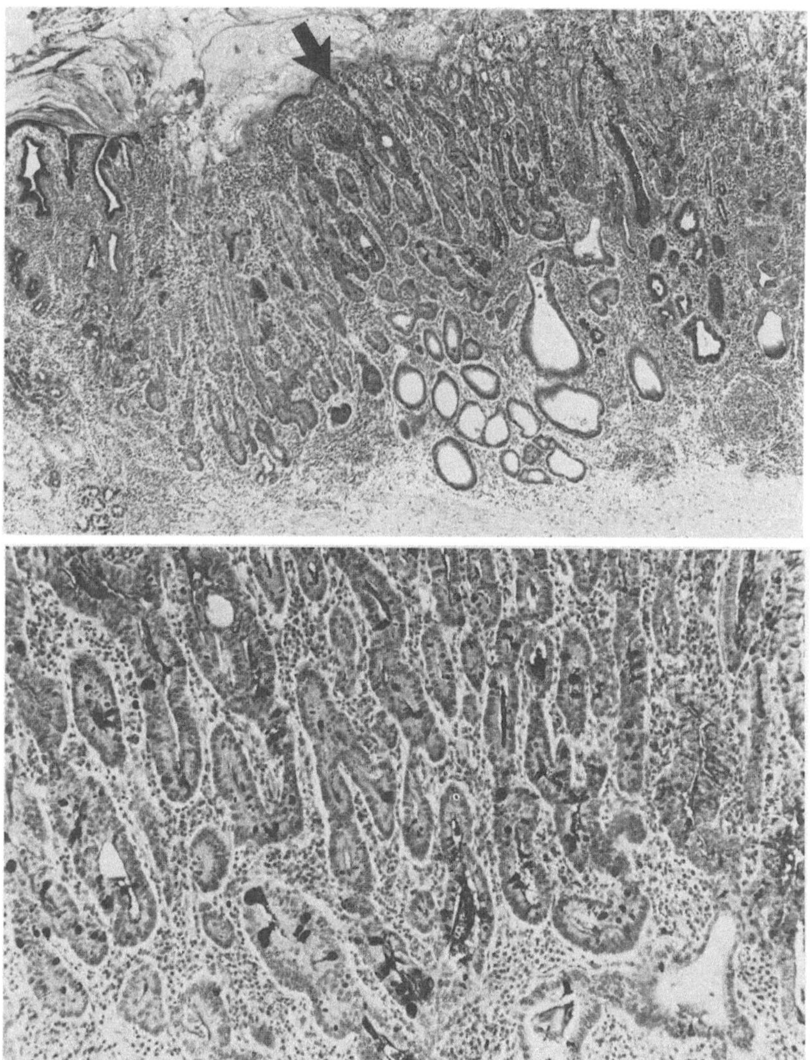

(a)

(b)

Fig. 15a and b. Transition from intestinal metaplastic epithelium to intramucosal carcinoma: a) PAS, x 40. b) PAS, x 100. The arrow indicates the position of b) mucin secreting, absorptive cells, provided with a brush border, and barrel-shaped goblet cells are seen. Classical goblet cells are often seen interposed between apparently normal PAS-positive cells (*Ming* et al., 1967). Other transitional forms may also be demonstrated. In the second place it is of great importance to realize that the cells situated at the bottom of the foveola, in the isthmus or neck region (depending on nomenclature) differ from other foveolar cells. These cells have been considered as being undifferentiated. Certain identification of them can only be made by electron microscopy (*Johnson* and *Young*, 1967; *Rubin* et al., 1968). Nevertheless, the presence of immature cells in this particular region, where also mitoses are common (*Teir* and *Räsänen*, 1961), and labelling indices and other cell division parameters (*Willems*, 1972) are high, has been acknowledged for years (*Babkin*, 1950; *Steven* and *Leblond*, 1953). The light microscopist can identify the cells by their low columnar shape, their large basally situated nucleus with prominent nucleoli and, most important, by the absence of an appreciable amount of mucin. The little which can be identified in the cells and in the neighbouring deep foveolar cells, for which they may be precursors, are in addition to being PAS-positive also stainable with methods for acid mucin, in my experience most constantly and strongly with colloidal iron.

(a)

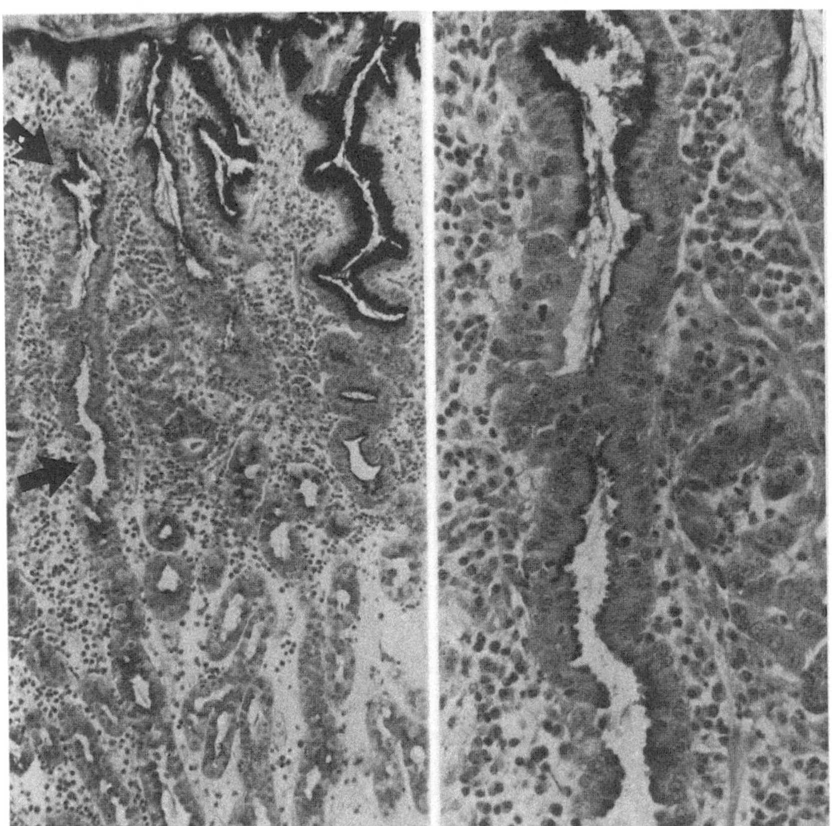

(b)

Fig. 16a and b. Intermediary-type mucosa with a few parietal cells: a) Demonstrates 4 foveolae of non-metaplastic type. The two to the right are nearly normal, the two to the left are abnormal with an undifferentiated pattern and severely reduced and even abolished mucus secretion. PAS, x 100. b) Foveolae indicated by arrows in a). PAS, x 250

One of the most conspicuous electron microscopic features of the cells is their prominent microvilli which in my opinion sometimes are so numerous that they light microscopically may form an indistinct brush border.

These are the cells on which the attention should be focused. Under *normal* circumstances they migrate towards the surface differentiating in such a way that the amount of PAS-positive mucus continuously increases until a maximum of differentiation is reached. This

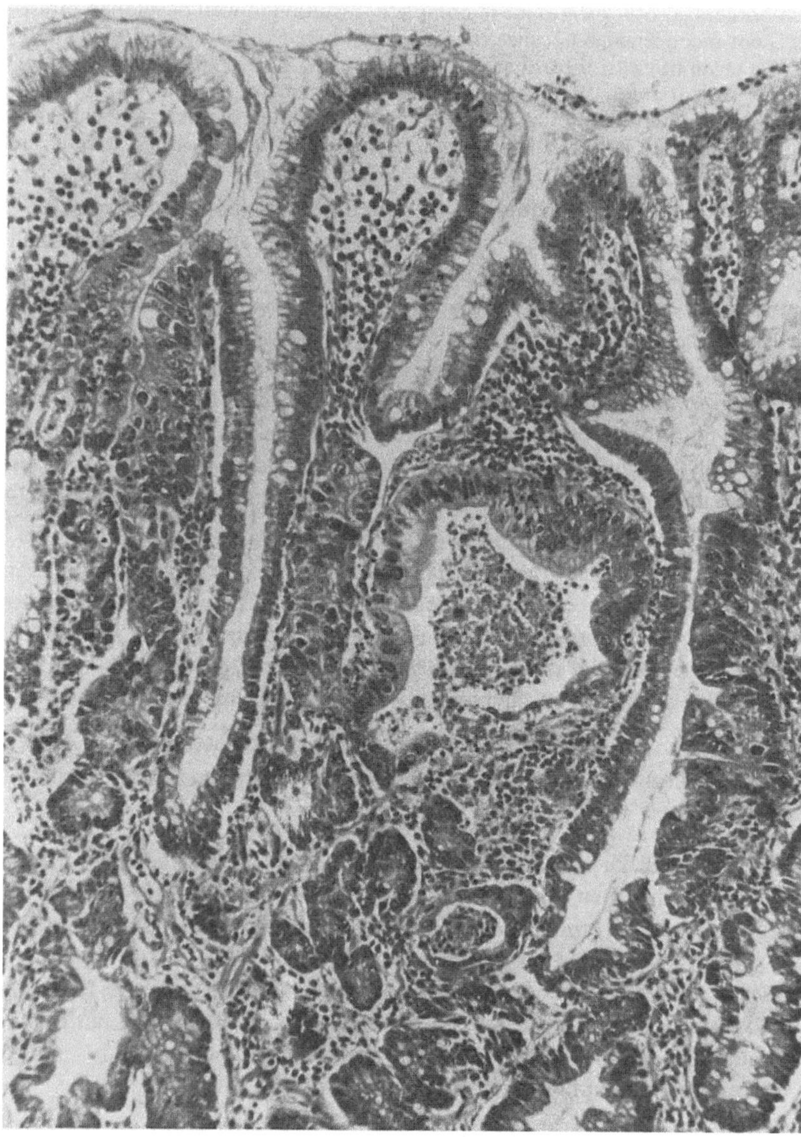

Fig. 17. A differentiated adenocarcinoma originating from foveolae demonstrating transition form between normal PAS-positive cylindrical epithelium and intestinal epithelium with goblet cells. H&E, x 100

usually happens at the point where the foveolar epithelium reaches the surface. During this differentiation they have at an early stage lost their stainability for acid mucus.

Under *abnormal* circumstances this migration may take place without a correspondingly normal differentiation, and the whole foveola will in some cases be covered with immature-looking cells hardly secreting mucus (Fig. 16). In other cases the whole or at least the greater part of the foveola is lined by cells having preserved the ability to secrete acid mucus. In still other cases the migration proceeds concomittantly with a differentiation towards intestinal epithelium. Sometimes this may be incomplete leading to cells with indistinct, badly defined brush borders, at other times more complete, resulting in well developed intestinal crypts. This is not inconceivable because the undifferentiated cells in the stomach may be one link of a chain of gastrointestinal cells (*Trier*, 1963; *Silva*, 1966; *Johnson* and *Young*, 1968) able to differentiate in different directions when abnormal influences affect them. Such influences are unfortunately unknown just as it is completely unknown whether the forces causing a neoplastic differentiation are not only quantitatively but also qualitatively different.

In my opinion there is little doubt that the undifferentiated cells and some of their first descendants may transform into malignant cells with an appearance determined by the above mentioned pattern. Carefull microscopy of egc and the adjacent mucosa will show the presence of some of the abnormal foveolar patterns (Fig. 16) and the transition to obviously malignant cells. Sometimes two different forms are found in neighbouring foveolae and I cannot therefore believe that differentiated carcinomas only originate in intestinal metaplastic epithelium. I hold the opinion that highly differentiated carcinomas may originate from both the metaplastic and the original epithelium and perhaps especially from their not fully developed forms (Fig. 17). In correspondence with this, undifferentiated carcinomas may originate from the gastric epithelium and – although rarely – also from intestinal epithelium.

I agree with the view that intestinal epithelium is most commonly found in stomachs with carcinoma, and is more common in those with highly differentiated than in those with poorly differentiated carcinomas but this does not necessarily mean that the tumours originate in the intestinal crypt. Intestinal metaplasia may just as well be an indicator of maladjusted regeneration on the basis of which neoplasia more easily takes place.

As mentioned a total statement of my histogenetic studies will not be given at this place, but in accordance with other reports the degree of gastritis and the extension of intestinal metaplasia will be mentioned.

Author's material: The occurrence of intestinal metaplastic epithelium in the corporic and pyloric mucosa has been divided into four groups in addition to the two conditions where intestinal metaplasia is totally absent or makes up the mucosa 100 per cent. These groups are related to the different macroscopic types (Table 8 and 9). As in all similar investigations high degree of intestinalization is found for type I and IIa carcinomas. For depressed cancer and ulcer-cancer hardly any metaplasia is found in the body mucosa, but in pyloric mucosa intestinalization is still extensive. As mentioned previously one should – in my opinion – be very careful in interpreting this histogenetically.

In the following Table 10 the degree of gastritis – of which intestinal epithelium is only one important side – is for the body mucosa related to the different types of carcinomas. The degree of gastritis has been estimated according to *Motteram* (1951) and *Christiansen* and *Johansen* (1966). It is seen that a considerable number of egc are accompanied by

Table 8. Distribution of intestinal metaplasia in the body mucosa in relation to the macroscopic types

		total	0	1-25%	26-50%	51-75%	76-99%	100%	corporic mucosa not present
		64	26	22	3	4	4	2	
I protruded		10	–	1	1	1	4	2	1
II superficial	a elevated	3	–	1	–	1	–	1	–
	b flat	6	2	3	–	1	–	–	–
	c depressed	12	4	6	1	1	–	–	–
III chr. ulcer +	IIb flat carc.	10	5	4	1	–	–	–	–
	IIc depres. carc.	23	15	7	–	–	–	–	–

Table 9. Distribution of intestinal metaplasia in the pyloric mucosa in relation to the macroscopic types

		total	0	1-25%	26-50%	51-75%	76-99%	100%	pyloric mucosa not present
		64	0	3	6	16	35	3	
I protruded		10	–	–	–	1	6	3	–
II superficial	a elevated	3	–	–	–	1	1	–	1
	b flat	6	–	–	–	2	4	–	–
	c depressed	12	–	1	1	5	5	–	–
III chr. ulcer +	IIb flat carc.	10	–	1	2	3	4	–	–
	IIc depres. carc.	23	–	1	3	4	15	–	–

Table 10. Macroscopic types related to the degree of gastritis in the body mucosa

		total	Normal	Superficial	Atrophic slightly	Atrophic severely	Atrophic maximal	corporic mucosa not present
		64	2	21	25	12	3	1
I protruded		10	–	–	1	6	2	1
II superficial	a elevated	3	–	–	1	1	1	–
	b flat	6	–	1	4	1	–	–
	c depressed	12	–	4	6	2	–	–
III chr. ulcer +	IIb flat carc.	10	1	3	5	1	–	–
	IIc depres. carc.	23	1	13	8	1	–	–

normal or only slightly changed mucosa. In 50 patients an augmented histamine test has been performed preoperatively. From Figure 18 is seen that more than half of the patients showed normal or hyperacidity. In Table 11 the pyloric gastritis has been divided into three groups. It is seen that nearly all macroscopic types of carcinomas are attended by severe pyloric gastritis.

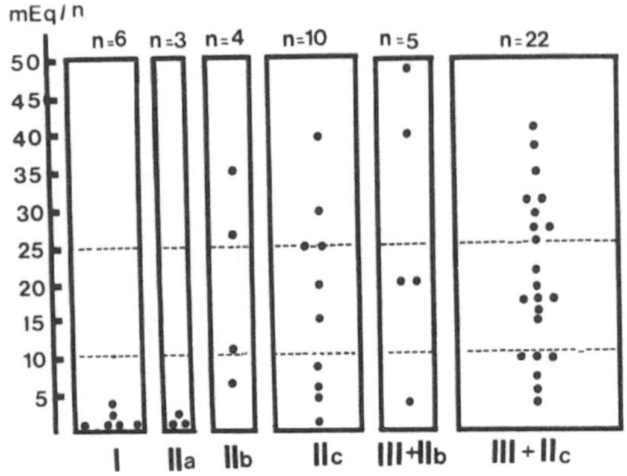

Fig. 18. Results of augmented histamine test in 50 patients (the test was not performed in 16 patienst)

Table 11. Macroscopic types and the degree of gastritis in the pyloric mucosa

		total	Normal	light	moderate	severe	pyloric mucosa not present
		64	0	6	8	49	1
I protruded		10	–	1	2	7	–
II superficial	a elevated	3	–	–	–	2	1
	b flat	6	–	1	1	4	–
	c depressed	12	–	2	1	9	–
III chr. ulcer +	IIb flat carc.	10	–	1	1	8	–
	IIc depres. carc.	23	–	–	3	19	–

VII. Lymph Node Involvement

A careful search for lymph nodes must be made in all specimens suspicious for egc and naturally all nodes from proven cases must be histologically examined. The presence of metastases does not exclude the diagnosis of egc, but – as mentioned later – the prognosis will be aggravated a little.

It is of historical interest that *Konjetzny* (1938) first accepted intramucosal carcinomas when he revealed a case with lymph node metastases. *Sano* (1971) found lymph node metastases in 4 per cent of intramucosal carcinomas connected with ulcer. For submucosal carcinomas an incidence of 16.3 per cent and 24.7 per cent was found for egc with and without connection with ulcer respectively.

Author's material: None of the intramucosal carcinomas demonstrated lymph node metastases. Three submucosal carcinomas had one lymph node each with metastasis. The lymph node capsules were not pervaded. One of the patients died without metastases. The two others have survived for 4 and 8 years.

VIII. Prognosis

Advanced carcinoma of the stomach has a poor prognosis despite all advances in surgical treatment. The following figures are considered representative (*Inberg* et al., 1971).

In the years 1946 to 1965, 1963 cases of gastric carcinoma were diagnosed at the University Hospital in Turku, Finland. Fifty-eight per cent were operated. Twenty-six per cent were resected. The 5-years survival rate for all resected cases was 19.6 per cent. If the resection was estimated as curative the 5-years survival rate was 23.8 per cent, and the 10-years survival rate 14.6 per cent. 5.1 per cent of all patients were alive after 5 years. The postoperative mortality (early mortality) was for normal partial resections 6.2 per cent, for gastrectomies and upper resections 18.3 per cent. This work reflects to some degree other Scandinavian reports (*Eker* and *Efskin*, 1960; *Öhman* et al., 1972; *Nielsen* et al., 1974). In Denmark 1229 cases of gastric cancer were registered in 1968 and 1075 died of the disease in the same year. The total 5-years survival has been estimated at 9.4 per cent (*Nielsen*, 1973). The before given figures are also in line with a report by *Hawley* et al. (1970) from England. A survey of the results in some American hospitals are given by *McNeer* and *Pack* (1967).

Generally speaking, the literature shows that among gastric cancer patients admitted to hospital on average 50 per cent are operated, and less than 30 per cent curatively resected. The operative mortality is usually higher than 10 per cent with some remarkable exceptions from Japan: *Nakayama* (1969) 1.5 per cent in 1762 patients and *Fujimaki* et al. (1972) 5.4 per cent in 431 patients). The 5-years survival rate is generally below 10 per cent with some notable exceptions, e.g. *Zacho* and *Fischermann* (1966) on special selected materials.

Gastric cancer in its early phase has a much more favourable prognosis. Although a limited number of follow-up series are available one gets the impression that the 5- and even the 10-years survival rate for intramucosal carcinomas is very close to 100 per cent and for submucosal carcinomas about 90 per cent. Based on a survey of the results from 22 institutions where 2364 cases of early gastric cancer were operated in the years 1962 to 1968 the 5-years survival rate was calculated to be, for intramucosal carcinomas without lymph node metastases 93.4 per cent and with lymph node metastases 91.5 per cent. The corresponding figures for submucosal carcinomas were 89 and 80.5 per cent. Lymph node metastases were found in 5.3 per cent of intramucosal carcinomas and in 19.6 per cent of submucosal carcinomas (*Hayashida* and *Kidokoro*, 1969, 1970).

The role of egc for the prognosis of gastric cancer as a whole has been shown by *Muto* (1965) and *Muto* et al. (1968). Their 5-years survival rate improved from 23 per cent to 44 per cent in a 25-years period where egc increased from 1.3 to 36.4 per cent in the material.

Author's material: On account of the very limited number of cases in my material the survival rate will be given in the following way. All the patients could be followed. Among the 56 one patient died from his carcinoma 6 years and 1 month post-operatively. Autopsy showed metastases to the lymph nodes and the liver. The primary carcinoma was a highly differentiated adenocarcinoma with moderate invasion into the submucosa. Two other patients died apparently of gastric cancer. One had 3 separate carcinomas (Fig. 12) one intramucosal and two submucosal, all highly differentiated. He died 9 months postoperatively at home. He also suffered from severe pulmonary tuberculosis and cor pulmonale. No autopsy was performed. The other patient had a highly differentiated submucosal ulcer carcinoma with only 5 small glands below the muscularis mucosae. He died 6 months postoperatively in a mental hospital. He constantly had blood in his stools and suffered a severe loss of weight. No autopsy was performed. Five patients (2.8%) died postoperatively within 20 days. Fifteen patients, in whom a total hospital autopsy was performed, died of other diseases unrelated to gastric cancer from 2 months to 9 years postoperatively. In no cases were recurrences or metastases found. Four patients, in whom no autopsy was performed, died of other diseases from 13 months to nearly 8 years postoperatively in their homes. They had been controlled twice a year and no signs of recurrence had been found. Gastric cancer was not mentioned on their death certificates. Twenty-nine patients were alive and in good state on 17th November 1975. The longest period of survival is 10 years and 9 months.

Using the decrement method (*Chiang*, 1968) and not excluding postoperatively dead patients, the cumulative 5-years and 10-years survival rate were 61.4 and 47.1 per cent respectively (Fig. 19).

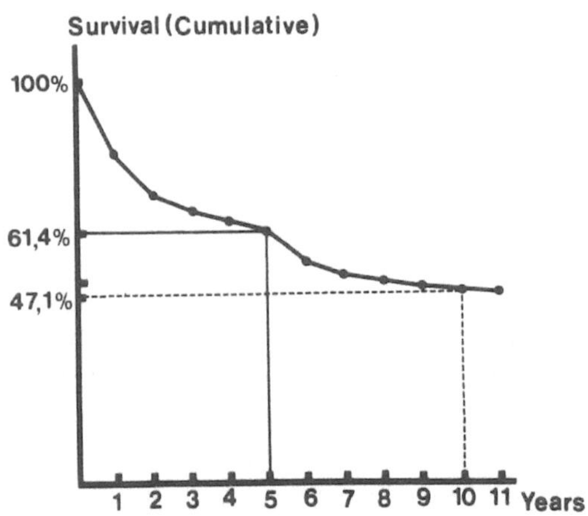

Fig. 19. Cumulative survival (decrement method) postoperatively dead included in the calculations

Referring to my own material it conclusively can be said that only one patient has died of his carcinoma with absolute certainty. Six others (4 + 2) may have died of gastric cancer since no autopsy was performed to exclude this, but in only two patients does it seem probable. The rest of the patients have died without any sign of recurrence or are alive.

IX. Clinical Remarks

Clinical investigations are beyond the limit of this survey and only a few remarks will be given especially to the diagnostic procedures to which pathologists can contribute. The methods, classical as well as new, for diagnosing gastric cancer are the same for all stages of the disease, but have for egc been brought to perfection.

Radiological examination has succeeded in demonstrating superficial and small early cancers in the western world for years (*Prévot*, 1937; *Golden* and *Stout*, 1948; *Grogg*, 1956; *Gutmann*, 1956), but the extremely advanced level, reached by Japanese radiologists (*Shirakabe* et al., 1968, 1971; *Maruyama*, 1971) is at least not common in Europe. Using double contrast (*Kumakura*, 1971) small and minute lesions of all kinds are demonstrated so clearly that the X-ray photo resembles photos of pathological specimens.

Endoscopic examination is without any doubt the most important improvement. The technical progress of the modern fiber gastroscopes has made careful examination of every part of the stomach wall possible. According to *Miller* and *Kaufmann* (1975) the basic material for diagnosing 1170 egc in Europe was 317,816 endoscopic examinations. *Rösch* (1970) has reported on the diagnostic role of endoscopy for egc, and this is also mentioned in the survey of *Pedersen* (1971) and by *Whitehead* (1973). Among the numerous Japanese works the report of *Takagi* (1971) and of *Kawai* (1972) should be consulted.

Gastrocamera examination is a special type of endoscopy where a small camera is passed into the stomach so that every part of the wall can be photographied. Its significance for egc has been given especially by *Sakita* (1968) and *Sakita* and *Oguro* (1971). Gastrocamera pictures of an unusually high quality are found in the book by *Demling, Ottenjann* and *Elster* (1972). Unfortunately none of the pictures illustrate early gastric cancer, although some of them are very close to it. Gastrocamera pictures play an important and exciting role in the communication between pathologists and endoscopists.

Gastric cytology has for the diagnosis of egc been applied in different ways: 1) Ordinary lavage cytology which is no longer used. 2) The abrasive balloon method still in use for diagnosing type IIb lesions. 3) Lavage cytology under direct fiber gastroscopic observation, where the washing solution is vigorously flushed out against the lesion under visual control, is a very effective method (*Kasugai*, 1968; *Kobayashi* et al., 1969; *Kasugai* and *Kobayashi*, 1974). 4) Smear cytology, where small pieces of tissue are taken by fiber gastroscopy and smeared out on slides, should according to *Shida* (1971) be an excellent method for diagnosing minute egc. 5) Finally brush cytology (*Kobayashi* et al., 1970; *Serck-Hanssen* et al., 1974) where a small brush is placed on a fiberscope and the lesion directly brushed, has given very good results.

Fiber gastroscopic biopsies are the diagnostic procedure most intimately involving pathologists. The close similarity between polyps, papillomas, erosions, and ulcers and the different forms of egc has made the bioptical confirmation of the diagnosis urgently important. I absolutely agree with the view of *Hermanek* (1973) that the diagnosis early cancer versus advanced cancer cannot be made by biopsies. Nevertheless, these may give the experienced pathologist reason to believe that an early cancer is a possibility. He can therefore ensure that he gets the specimen fresh for proper photography, pinning up and fixation.

On the other hand I do not agree with *Hermanek* (1973) that classification of carcinomas on the basis of biopsies should be avoided. On the contrary, if a gastric ulcer not suspicious to the clinician has been examined by biopsies and e.g. only one biopsy of seven has shown carcinoma, it is understandable that the clinician should want frozen sections for confirmation of the diagnosis. In such cases knowledge of the histological type will facilitate this procedure considerably. Correlation between the histological diagnosis of biopsies and of the egc themselves has been carried out by *Elster* et al. (1975) who found good correlation, especially between highly differentiated adenocarcinomas and signet ring cell carcinomas.

The diagnostic accuracy of fiber gastroscopic biopsies is high. According to *Takemoto* et al. (1971) the percentages of cases diagnosed as early gastric cancers through biopsy is reported to reach 95-97.5 per cent in Japan. *Kasugai* and *Kobayashi* (1974) found correct positive diagnoses in 98.3 per cent of 238 egc. According to the investigation of *Miller* and *Kaufmann* (1975) egc in 578 patients were diagnosed by endoscopic biopsies with an accuracy of 90 per cent. The best result was obtained from type IIc and III lesions. Moreover, this authors in contrast to others (*Johansen* and *Sikjär*, 1975) found a positive relationship between the diagnostic significance and the number of biopsies up to 12 per examination.

Author's material: Only 19 patients underwent fiber gastroscopic biopsy examination, since this procedure first was regularly used from 1970. On the first examination one or several biopsies from 16 patients showed carcinoma, from two patients the biopsies demonstrated precancerous changes, but no invasive carcinoma, and all the biopsies from one patient showed benign conditions. The three last mentioned examinations were repeated, and carcinoma was disclosed in two of them, but the third still showed precancerous changes. This carcinoma was type I.

X. Conlusion

In conclusion it can be said that egc occurs with a frequency great enough to make the knowledge of its pathology very essential to every pathologist. It demonstrates some rather well defined macroscopic types, is often multifocal and, although most common in pyloric or intermediary zone mucosa at the lesser curvature, it is sometimes seen in body and fundic mucosa. It measures from a few milimeters to several centimeters. Its histological picture range from highly differentiated to completely undifferentiated forms and it may develop from ordinary as well as from intestinalized mucosa. When surgically treated its prognosis is excellent even if lymph node metastases are present.

As mentioned several times egc is a stage of the development of ordinary gastric carcinoma. Between precancerous changes – which will not be discussed here – and early invasive carcinoma, transitions are often met, and it might be difficult to determine whether invasion into the lamina propria has taken place, especially for highly differentiated carcinomas. On the other hand, every pathologist, searching for egc, has experienced that a few additional sections from a block have forced him to reject the case as an early cancer and transfer it to the large group of advanced cancers. In this connection the important question should be asked: Do the different forms of egc mentioned in the survey represent early stages of all types of advanced cancer, or are they some special, slowly progressive forms, which seldom or never give rise to remote metastases? The question is applicable to other regions of the body. It has been commented on by *Okabe* (1971) who investigated the duration of symptoms and the growing and invading patterns of early as well as of advanced cancer. He reached the conclusion that two forms of gastric cancer exist. One which grows and invades rapidly and insidiously without symptoms before distant metastases are present. The type IIa + IIc might be the only known early stage of this form. And another more slowly growing form often detectable in its early stage. Especially type IIc + III belongs to this group and is by *Okabe* considered as a type of carcinoma which remains in an early stage for years. Unfortunately this type of carcinoma accounts for only 10 per cent of gastric cancers.

The study of *Okabe* (1971) ist thought-provoking, but is based on macroscopic types and tumour size studies. It does not take the histological pattern into consideration. To the author it is relevant that all degrees of differentiation and all histological types met in advanced gastric cancer, also are found in the early types. Even completely undifferentiated forms demonstrate many years of survival if treated in the early stage. If some gastric carcinomas grow extremely fast I think the explanation shall be found more in the host reaction than in the epithelial tumour tissue. Host reaction in gastric cancer has been investigated (*Larmi* and *Saxén*, 1963; *Hawley* et al., 1970) but egc would offer a good opportunity for further study of this phenomenon.

References

Abel, W.: Oberflächlicher Schleimhautkrebs des Magens. Fortschr. Röntgenstr. 77, 743-744 (1952).

Albot, G.: Les début du cancer l'estomac. Livre jubilaire de la Ligue francaise contre le Cancer, pp. 17-23. Paris: Masson et Cie 1943.

Anschütz, W., Konjetzny, G.E.: Die Geschwülste des Magens. Dtsch. Chir. 46f. I 1. Stuttgart: Enke 1921.

Babkin, B.P.: Secretory mechanism of the digestive glands. New York: Hoeher Medical Division. Harker and Row 1950.

Betrand, I.: Diagnostic histologique précoce du cancer de l'estomac. Deuxième Congrès de la Société Internationale de Gastro-Enterologie. Brussel 1937.

Bocian, J.J., Geschke, A.E.: Carcinoma in situ of the stomach. Arch. Path. 65, 6-12 (1958).

Bormann, R.: Geschwülste des Magens und Duodenum. In: Handbuch der speziellen pathologischen Anatomie und Histologie (ed. *F. Henke, O. Lubarsch*) Vol. IV/1. Berlin: Springer 1926.

Cattan, R., Baumann, J., Frumusan, F., Attal, C.: Un cas de cancer de l'estomac en surface. Arch. Mal. Appar. dig. 36, 295-299 (1947).

Chiang, C.L.: Introduction to stochastic processes in biostatistics. New York: Wiley 1968.

Christiansen, P.M., Johansen, AA.: Single gastric biopsy in subjects with low acid secretion after maximal histamine stimulation. Scand. J. Gastroent. 1, 86-93 (1966).

Collins, W.T., Gall, E.A.: Gąstric carcinoma: A multicentric lesion. Cancer 5, 62-72 (1952).

Demling, L., Ottenjann, R., Elster, K.: Endoscopie und Biopsie der Speiseröhre und des Magens. Stuttgart-New York: F.K. Schatthauer 1972.

Eker, R., Efskin, J.: The pathology and prognosis of gastric carcinoma (based on 1314 partially and totally resected cases). Acta chir. scand. Suppl. 264 (1960).

Elster, K., Kolaczek, F., Shimamoto, K., Freitag, H.: Early gastric cancer-experience in Germany. Endoscopy 7, 5-10 (1975).

Elster, K., Reiss, S., Heinkel, K.: Histotopographische Untersuchungen über die intestinale Metaplasie in Karzinom- und Ulkusmägen. Z. inn. Med. 15, 1053-1061 (1960).

Ewing, J.: The beginnings of gastric cancer. Amer. J. Surg. 31, 204-205 (1936).

Friesen, G., Dockerty, M., Remine, W.: Superficial carcinoma of the stomach. Surgery 51, 300-312 (1962).

Fujimaki, M., Soga, J., Wada, K., Tani, H., Aizawa, O., Kawaguchi, M., Ishibashi, K., Maeda, M., Kanai, T., Omori, Y., Muto, T.: Total gastrectomy for gastric cancer. Clinical considerations on 431 cases. Cancer 30, 660-664 (1972).

Gad, A.: A histochemical study of human alimentary tract. Mucosubstances in health and disease. I. Normal and tumour. Brit. J. Cancer 23, 52-63 (1969).

Geffroy, Y., Jouanneau, P.: Évolution décevante d'un cas de cancer gastrique "in situ". Arch. Mal. Appar. dig. 40, 76-82 (1951).

Golden, R., Stout, A.P.: Superficial spreading carcinoma of the stomach. Amer. J. Roentgenol. 59, 157-167 (1948).

Grogg, E.: Über Frühstadien des Magenkarzinoms. Radiol. clin. (Basel) 21, 10-19 (1952).

Guiss, L.W.: Pathology of gastric neoplasms. In: Neoplasms of the stomach (ed. *G.McNeer, G.T. Pack*), pp. 388-407. Philadelphia: J.B. Lippincott Company 1967.

Gutmann, R.A.: Le diagnostic du cancer d'estomac a la période utile. Paris: G. Doin & Cie 1956.

Gutmann, R.A.: Diagnostic du cancer gastrique précoce et avancé. Paris: G. Doin & Cie. 1967.

Gutmann, R.A.: Forty years of early gastric cancer. Stomach Intestine 6, 112-114 (1972).

Gutmann, R.A., Betrand, I.: Le cancer gastrique érosif a marche lente. Presse méd. 46, 814-817 (1938).

Gutmann, R.A., Bertrand, I., Peristiany, T.J.: Le cancer de l'Estomac au Debut. Paris: G. Doin & Cie 1939.

Hawley, P.R., Westerholm, P., Morson, B.C.: Pathology and prognosis of carcinoma of the stomach. Brit. J. Surg. 57, 879-883 (1970).

Hayashida, T., Kidokoro, T.: End results of early gastric cancer collected from 22 institutions. Stomach Intestine 4, 1077-1085 (1969).

Hayashida, T., Kidokoro, T.: End results of early gastric carcinoma. Advance abstracts p. 279. 4th World Congress of Gastroenterology. Copenhagen 1970.

Heinkel, K., Henning, N., Coninx, G.: Häufigkeit und Bedeutung von Becherzellen in der menschlichen Magenschleimhaut. Gastroenterologia 93, 269-278 (1960).

Hermanek, P.: Gastrobiopsy in cancer of the stomach. Endoscopy 5, 144-147 (1973).

Hermanek, P., Rösch, W.: Critical evaluation of the Japanese "early gastric cancer" classification. Endoscopy 5, 220-224 (1973).

Hess, R.: Early cancer of the stomach. Gastroenterologia 86, 365-369 (1956).

Inberg, M.V., Vouri, J., Viikari, S.J.: Carcinoma of the stomach, a follow-up study of 1963 patients. Acta chir. scand. 138, 195-201 (1972).

Jansen, H.H.: Magen. In: Organpathologie (*W. Doerr*, ed.), Vol. II, pp. 4-51–4-73. Stuttgart: Thieme 1974.

Johansen, AA., Sikjär, B.: Gastroscopic biopsy. Reliability of histological diagnosis with special reference to the single biopsy. Scand. J. Gastroent. 10, 453-458 (1975).

Johnson, F.R., Young, B.A.: Undifferentiated cells in gastric mucosa. J. Anat. (Lond.) 101, 617-618 (1967).

Johnson, F.R., Young, B.A.: Undifferentiated cells in gastric mucosa. J. Anat. (Lond.) 102, 541-551 (1968).

Järvi, O., Laurén, P.: On the role of heterotopias of the intestinal epithelium in the pathogenesis of gastric cancer. Acta path. microbiol. scand. 29, 26-43 (1951).

Kasugai, T.: Evaluation of gastric lavage cytology under direct vision by the fiber gastroscope employing Hank's solution as a washing solution. Acta cytol. (Philad.) 12, 345-351 (1968).

Kasugai, T., Kobayashi, S.: Evaluation of biopsy and cytology in the diagnosis of gastric cancer. Amer. J. Gastroent. 60, 199-203 (1974).

Kawai, K.: Validity rate of concerted diagnosis using various methods. In: Early Gastric Cancer (*T. Murakami*, ed.), pp. 273-280. Baltimore–London–Tokyo: University Park Press 1971.
Kawai, K.: The significance of endoscopy for gastric diseases. Endoscopy 4, 39-43 (1972).
Kidokoro, T.: Frequency of resection, metastasis and five-years survival rate of early gastric carcinoma in a surgical clinic. In: Early Gastric Cancer (*T. Murakami*, ed.), pp. 45-49. Baltimore–London–Tokyo: University Park Press 1971.
Kimura, K., Takemoto, T.: An endoscopic recognition of the pyloric-fundic gland border and its significance in chronic gastritis. Advance abstracts p. 370. 4th World Congress of Gastroenterology. Copenhagen 1970.
Kimura, K., Takemoto, T., Kondo, T.: Chronical transitional of the pyloric-fundic gland border in chronic gastritis. Advance abstracts p. 400. 4th World Congress of Gastroenterology. Copenhagen 1970.
Kobayashi, S., Kasugai, T., Yamaoka, Y., Yoshii, Y., Naito, Y.: Improved technique for gastric cytology utilizing simultaneous lavage and fiber gastroscopy. Gastrointest. Endoscopy 15, 198-203 (1969).
Kobayashi, S., Prolla, J.C., Kirsner, J.B.: Brushing cytology of the oesophagus and stomach under direct vision by fibroscopes. Acta cytol. (Philad.) 14, 219-223 (1970).
Kobayashi, S., Sugiura, H., Kasugai, T.: Reliability of endoscopic observation in diagnosis of early carcinoma of the stomach. Endoscopy 4, 61-65 (1972).
Konjetzny, G.E.: Über die Beziehungen der chronischen Gastritis mit ihren Folgeerscheinungen und des chronischen Magenulkus zur Entwicklung des Magenkrebses. Bruns' Beitr. klin. Chir. 85, 455-519 (1913).
Konjetzny, G.E.: Der Magenkrebs. Stuttgart: Enke 1938.
Konjetzny, G.E.: Der oberflächliche Schleimhautkrebs des Magens. Chirurg 12, 192-202 (1940).
Konjetzny, G.E.: The superficial cancer of the gastric mucosa. Amer. J. dig. Dis. 20, 91-96 (1953).
Kuhlencordt, F.: Das Carcinoma in situ des Magens und der kleine Magenkrebs. Dtsch. med. Wschr. 84, 2111-2115 (1959).
Kumakura, K.: Improvement and advances in double contrast studies. In: Early Gastric Cancer (*T. Murakami*, ed.), pp. 113-117. Baltimore–London–Tokyo: University Park Press 1971.
Landboe-Christensen, E.: Extend of the pylorus zone in the human stomach. Acta path. microbiol. scand. Suppl. 54, 671 (1944).
Larmi, T.K.I., Saxén, L.: "Host reactions" in gastric cancer. A preliminary study of 119 cases of gastrectomy. Acta chir. scand. 125, 144-146 (1963).
Laurén, P.: The two histological main types of gastric carcinoma: Diffuse and so-called intestinal-type carcinoma. Acta path. microbiol. scand. 64, 31-49 (1965).
Lev, R.: The mucin histochemistry of normal and neoplastic gastric mucosa. Lab. Invest. 14, 2080-2100 (1966).
Loutsch, H.: A propos d'un cas de cancer de l'estomac au début. Arch. Mal. Appar. dig. 36, 197-202 (1947).
Magnus, H.A.: Observations on the presence of intestinal epithelium in the gastric mucosa. J. Path. Bact. 44, 389-397 (1937).
Majima, S.: Histopathological studies of gastric ulcercarcinoma. Tohoku J. exp. Med. 62, 53-73 (1955).
Majima, S., Yoshida, K., Teshima, T., Karube, K.: Histopathological study on gastric polyps and their malignant degeneration. Tohoku J. exp. Med. 80, 355-369 (1963).

Majima, S., Yamaguchi, I., Karube, K., Teshima, T., Yoshida, K.: A histopathological study of the origin of early carcinoma of the stomach. Tohoku J. exp. Med. 86, 348-365 (1965).

Mallory, T.: Carcinoma in situ of the stomach and its bearing on the histogenesis of malignant ulcers. Arch. Path. 30, 348-362 (1940).

Marks, J.N., Drysdale, K.M.: A modification of Zimmermann's method for differential staining of gastric mucosa. Stain Technol. 32, 48-50 (1957).

Maruyama, M.: Diagnostic limits for early gastric cancer by radiography. In: Early Gastric Cancer (*T. Murakami*, ed.), pp. 119-130. Baltimore–London–Tokyo: University Park Press 1971.

Mason, M.K.: Surface carcinoma of the stomach. Gut 6, 185-193 (1965).

McNeer, G., Pack, G.T.: Neoplasms of the stomach. Philadelphia: J.B. Lippincott Company 1967.

Miller, G., Kaufmann, M.: Das Magenfrühkarzinom in Europa. Dtsch. med. Wschr. 100, 1946-1949 (1975).

Ming, S-C., Goldman, H., Freiman, D.G.: Intestinal metaplasia and histogenesis of carcinoma in human stomach. Cancer 20, 1418-1429 (1967).

Mochizuki, T.: Method for histopathological examination of early gastric cancer. In: Early Gastric Cancer (*T. Murakami*, ed.) pp. 57-62. Baltimore–London–Tokyo: University Park Press 1971.

Moertel, C.G., Bargen, A., Soule, E.H.: Multiple gastric cancers. Gastroenterology 32, 1095-1103 (1957).

Morson, B.C.: Intestinal metaplasia of the gastric mucosa. Brit. J. Cancer 9, 365-376 (1955a).

Morson, B.C.: Carcinoma arising from areas of intestinal metaplasia in the gastric mucosa. Brit. J. Cancer 9, 377-385 (1955b).

Morson, B.C.: Gastric polyps composed of intestinal epithelium. Brit. J. Cancer 9, 550-557 (1955c)

Morson, B.C., Dawson, I.M.P.: Gastrointestinal pathology. Oxford–London–Edinburgh–Melbourne: Blackwell Scientific Publications 1972.

Motteram, R.: A biopsy study of chronic gastritis and gastric atrophy. J. Path. Bact. 63, 389-397 (1951).

Murakami, T.: Pathomorphological diagnosis. In: Early Gastric Cancer (*T. Murakami*, ed.), pp. 53-55. Baltimore–London–Tokyo: University Park Press 1971.

Murakami, T., Nakamura, S., Urushibara, H., Miyashita, Y.: Chiryo 42, 261 (1960). Cited by *Nakamura* et al., Gann 58, 377-387 (1967).

Muto, M.: Surgical treatment of gastric cancer (an analysis of five years survival figure in 2014 cases). Fukushima J. med. Sci. 12, 17-21 (1965).

Muto, M., Maki, T., Majima, S., Yamaguchi, I.: Improvement in the end results of surgical treatment of gastric cancer. Surgery 63, 229-235 (1968).

Myhre, E.: Superficial spreading type of carcinoma of the stomach. Acta chir. scand. 106, 392-398 (1953).

Nagayo, T.: Mode of origin of gastric mucosal cancer with special reference to that of "superficial spreading type". In: Epidemiological, Experimental, and Clinical Studies on Gastric Cancer (*R. Kinosita* et al., eds.), pp. 113-122. Tokyo: Maruzen Co. 1968.

Nagayo, T., Komagoe, T.: Histological studies of gastric mucosal cancer with special reference to relationship of histological pictures between the mucosal cancer and the cancer-bearing gastric mucosa. Gann 52, 109-119 (1961).

Nagayo, T., Ito, M., Yokoyama, H., Komagoe, T.: Early phases of human gastric cancer: Morphological study. Gann 56, 101-120 (1965).

Nagayo, T., Yokoyama, H.: Scirrhus carcinoma occurring in the corpus (body) of the stomach. Acta path. jap. 24, 797-814 (1974).

Nakamura, K.: Histogenesis of cancer in the upper segment of the stomach. Stomach Intestine 5, 47-55 (1970).

Nakamura, K.: personal communication 1975.

Nakamura, K., Sugano, H., Takagi, K., Fuchigami, A.: Histopathological study on early carcinoma of the stomach: Criteria for diagnosis of atypical epithelium. Gann 57, 613-620 (1966).

Nakamura, K., Sugano, H., Takagi, K., Fuchigami, A.: Histopathological study on early gastric cancer of the stomach: Some considerations on the ulcer-cancer by analysis of 144 foci of the superficial spreading carcinomas. Gann 58, 377-387 (1967).

Nakamura, K., Sugano, H., Takagi, K.: Carcinoma of the stomach in incipient phase: Its histogenesis and histological appearance. Gann 59, 251-258 (1968).

Nakamura, K., Sugano, H., Takagi, K., Kumakura, K.: Conception of histogenesis of gastric carcinoma. Stomach Intestine 6, 9-21 (1971).

Nakamura, K., Sugano, H., Maruyama, M., Sugiyama, N., Takagi, K.: Histopathological study of primary locus of linitis plastica. Stomach Intestine 10, 79-86 (1975).

Nakayama, K.: Gastric cancer: The success of early detection by a coordinated program of periodic gastric mucosal X-ray studies and gastroscopic and gastric camera observations. Surgery 65, 227-231 (1969).

Nielsen, J.: personal communication 1974.

Nielsen, S. AA. D., Amdrup, E., Christiansen, P., Fenger, C., Jensen, H-E., Lindskov, J., Nielsen, J.: Carcinoma of the stomach, an analysis of 385 cases treated 1955-64. Acta chir. scand. 140, 313-320 (1974).

Nikado, N.: Early diagnosis of stomach cancer by the mass-survey. Advance abstracts p. 274. 4th World Congress of Gastroenterology. Copenhagen 1970.

Öhman, V., Wetterfors, J., Moberg, A.: Primary gastric cancer and its prognosis. Acta chir. scand. 138, 378-383 (1972).

Oi, M., Oshida, K., Sugimura, S.: The location of gastric ulcer. Gastroenterology 36, 45-56 (1959).

Okabe, H.: Growth of early gastric cancer. In: Early Gastric Cancer (*T. Murakami*, ed.), pp. 67-79. Baltimore–London–Tokyo: University Park Press 1971.

Oota, K.: Nippon Byori Gakkai 53, 3 (1964). Cited by *Nakamura* et al., Gann 58, 377-387 (1967).

Osmond, R.: A case of carcinoma "in situ" removed during gastric resections for chronic ulcer. Med. J. Aust. 40, 141-142 (1953).

Parturier-Lannegrace, Mme, Debeyre, J., Mariage, J.G.: Un cas de cancer de l'estomac "in situ". Arch. Mal. Appar. dig. 36, 445-451 (1947).

Pedersen, A.B.: Den endoskopiske undersögelse af ventriklen. Nord. med. 86, 827-829 (1971).

Planteydt, H.T., Willinghagen, R.G.J.: Enzyme histochemistry of gastric carcinoma. J. Path. Bact. 90, 393-398 (1965).

Prévôt, R.: Zur Frühdiagnose des Magenkrebs. II congrès de la Société International de Gastro-Entérologie. Bruxelles 1938.

Rubin, J.C.: Pathogenesis and further growth of carcinoma of the uterus in relation to clinical symptoms and early diagnosis. Amer. J. Obstet. Gynec. 78, 353 (1918).

Rubin, W., Ross, L.L., Sleisenger, M.H., Jeffries, G.H.: The normal human gastric epithelia. Lab. Invest. 19, 598-626 (1968).

Rösch, W.: Early carcinoma. Endoscopy 2, 64-70 (1970).

Rössle, R.: Über einen frühen Oberflächenkrebs der Magenschleimhaut. Zbl. allg. Path. path. Anat. 82, 165-170 (1944).

Sakita, T., Oguro, Y.: Routine gastrocamera examination. In: Early Gastric Cancer (*T. Murakami*, ed.), pp. 145-156. Baltimore–London–Tokyo: University Park Press 1971.

Sakito, T.: The role of gastrocamera for the detection of early stomach cancer. In: Epidemiological, experimental, and clinical studies on gastric cancer (*R. Kinosita* et al., eds.), pp. 181-183. Tokyo:Maruzen Co. 1968.

Sano, R.: Pathological analysis of 300 cases of early gastric cancer. In: Early Gastric Cancer (*T. Murakami*, ed.), pp. 81-89. Baltimore–London–Tokyo: University Park Press 1971.

Schade, R.: Pathologisch-anatomische Frühdiagnose des Magenkarzinoms. Chirurg 33, 93-197 (1962).

Schade, R.: Neuere Untersuchungen über das Magenkarzinom. Dtsch. med. Wschr. 88, 1125-1128 (1963).

Schauenstein, G.: Histologische Untersuchungen über atypisches Plattenepithel an der Portio und an der Cervix Uteri. Arch. Gynäk. 85, 576-616 (1908)

Serck-Hanssen, A., Marcussen, J., Liavag, L.: Endoscopic brush cytology in the diagnosis of gastric disease. Comparison with other diagnostic measures. In: Early Gastric Cancer. Current Status of Diagnoses (*E. Grundmann* et al., eds.), pp. 139-147. Berlin–Heidelberg–New York: Springer 1974.

Shida, S.: Biopsy smear cytology with the fiber gastroscope for direct observation. In: Early Gastric Cancer (*T. Murakami*, ed.), pp. 223-232. Baltimore–London–Tokyo: University Park Press 1971.

Shirakabe, H.: Early diagnosis of gastric cacner. In: Epidermiological, Experimental, and Clinical Studies on Gastric Cancer (*R. Kinosita* et al., eds.), pp. 169-176. Tokyo: Maruzen Co. 1968.

Shirakabe, H.: X-ray diagnosis of early gastric cancer. In: Early Gastric Cancer (*T. Murakami*, ed.), pp. 105-116. Baltimore–London–Tokyo: University Park Press 1971.

Silva, D.G.: The fine structure of multivesicular cells with large microvilli in the epithelium of the mouse colon. J. Ultrastruct. Res. 16, 693-705 (1966).

Stadelmann, O., Elster, K., Demling, L., Dayhle, P., Stolte, M., Ottenjann, R.: Histotopographic and functional investigation of the ulcer stomach. Advance abstracts p. 374. 4th World Congress of Gastroenterology. Copenhagen 1970.

Stevens, C.E., Leblond, C.P.: Renewal of the mucous cells in the gastric mucosa of the rat. Anat. Rec. 115, 231-243 (1953).

Stiller, D., Stiller, I.: Über die histochemischen Eigenschaften der Mucostoffe in Gallertkarzinomen des Magens. Virchows Arch. path. Anat. 337, 483-492 (1964).

Stout, A.P.: Superficial spreading type of carcinoma of the stomach. Arch. Surg. 44, 651-657 (1942).

Stout, A.P.: Tumors of the stomach. Atlas of Tumor Pathology fasc. 21. Armed Forces Institute of Pathology. Washington 1953.

Takagi, K.: Limit of detection of minute gastric cancer by endoscopy. In: Early Gastric Cancer (*T. Murakami*, ed.), pp. 177-183. Baltimore–London–Tokyo: Unversity Park Press 1971.

Takahashi, K.: Outline of gastric mass survey by X-ray. In: Early Gastric Cancer (*T. Murakami*, ed.), pp. 21-26. Baltimore–London–Tokyo: University Park Press 1971.

Takemoto, T., Ichioka, S., Suzuki, S., Nagasako, K.: The diagnosis of early gastric cancer through fiber gastroscopic biopsy. In: Early Gastric Cancer (*T. Murakami*, ed.), pp. 233-241. Baltimore–London–Tokyo: University Park Press 1971.

Teir, H., Räsänen, T.: A study of mitotic rate in renewal zones of non-diseased portions of gastric mucosa in cases of peptic ulcer and gastric carcinoma, with observation on differentiation and so-called "intestinalization" of gastric mucosa. J. nat. Cancer Inst. 27, 949-963 (1961).

Trier, J.S.: Studies on small intestinal crypt epithelium. I. The fine structure of the crypt epithelium of the proximal small intestine of fasting humans. J. Cell Biol. 18, 599-620 (1963).

Versé, M.: Die Histogenese der Schleimhautkarzinome. Diss. Leipzig 1903.

Versé, M.: Über die Entstehung, den Bau und das Wachstum der Polypen, Adenome und Karzinome des Magen-Darmkanals. In: Arbeiten aus dem pathologischen Institute zu Leipzig (*F. Marchand*, ed.), Vol. I, Heft 5, pp. 1-168. Leipzig: Hirzel 1908.

Walters, W., Gray, H.K., Priestley, J.T.: Carcinoma and other malignant lesions of the stomach. Philadelphia: W.B. Saunders Ltd. 1943.

Wanke, M.: Magen. In: Spezielle pathologische Anatomie (*W. Doerr* et al., eds.), Vol. II, Teil 1, pp. 666-678. Berlin–Heidelberg–New York: Springer 1971.

Wattenberg, L.W.: Histochemical study of aminopeptidase in metaplasia and carcinoma of the stomach. Arch. Path. 67, 281-286 (1959).

Whitehead, R.: Mucosal biopsy of the gastrointestinal tract. London–Philadelphia–Toronto: W.B. Saunders Ltd. 1973.

Wiendl, H.J., Piger, A.: Multizentrisches Frühkarzinom des Magens. Endoscopy 4, 210-211 (1971).

Willems, G.: Cell renewal in the gastric mucosa. Digestion 6, 46-63 (1972).

Yamagata, S., Masuda, O., Ooshiba, S., Gomi, T., Mochizuki, F., Kitagana, M., Hisamichi, S.: Early detection of stomach cancer in the mass survey. Advance abstracts p. 359. 4th World Congress of Gastroenterology. Cophenhagen 1970.

Yamagata, S., Masuda, H.: Magenkarzinom. In: Klinische Gastroenterologie (*L. Demling*, ed.), Vol. I. Stuttgart: Thieme 1973.

Zacho, A., Fischermann, K.: The results of surgical treatment of cancer of the stomach. Surg. Gynec. Obstet. 123, 73-84 (1966).

Zimmermann, K.W.: Beitrag zur Kenntnis des Baues und der Funktion der Fundusdrüsen in menschlichen Magen. Ergebn. Physiol. 24, 281-307 (1925).

Pathology of Coeliac Disease

H. THOMPSON

Coeliac disease is a malabsorption syndrome which is associated with subtotal villous atrophy in the jejunal mucosa due to the damaging effect of wheat gluten in susceptible members of the population. It occurs in children or adults in an overt symptomatic form or as an occult disorder which manifests itself through the development of complications. Introduction of a gluten free diet leads to restoration of a normal villous pattern in the jejunum and to an improvement in the patients general health although there is always a risk of relapse caused by failure to adhere to a strict gluten free diet or alternatively signalling the development of complications.

Children suffering from proven coeliac disease respond rapidly to a gluten free diet and it is rare to encounter an incomplete response or resistance to treatment. Adult subjects, however, respond more slowly to a gluten free diet and, in about 10% of the cases, there is an incomplete response or a total failure to respond to such treatment. Steroid therapy or elimination of milk from the diet may promote a satisfactory response in some patients. Failure to respond suggests the presence of serious complications of the disease. There is, however, disagreement regarding the recognition and classification of resistant cases of coeliac disease since they cannot be described as suffering from gluten sensitive enteropathy and this group requires further documentation and more detailed study.

The term "idiopathic" steatorrhoea is still useful to classify patients with the coeliac malabsorption syndrome who have not had a diagnostic jejunal biopsy. Certain patients refuse jejunal biopsy procedure or are unable to tolerate the tube and in other cases, the capsule fails to produce a diagnostic biopsy. If such patients are treated with a gluten free diet, it is desirable that further steps should be taken to substantiate the diagnosis "if the patients state of health" allows the reintroduction of gluten into the diet as a test procedure otherwise such patients will be condemned to a life long regime on inadequate grounds.

I. Interpretation of Jejunal Biopsies

A single jejunal biopsy can be obtained by the *Crosby* biopsy capsule or multiple biopsies can be obtained with the *Rubin* tube of other instruments. The biopsies should be spread out flat on single weight cardboard preferably black or dark in colour to provide contrast and immersed in 10% formal saline. Dissecting microscope examination should then be carried out, and if possible black and white photographs or colour transparencies should be taken of the biopsies. It is important that the histopathologist who is going to assess and report on the histological sections should observe the dissecting microscope appearances himself and not rely on the observations of others since there may be some variation in observer interpretation. The jejunal biopsies are then carefully processed, embedded in paraffin wax and cut in a vertical plane with the biopsy orientated so that the villous surface is uppermost. Oblique or tangential section cutting must be avoided or it will lead to misinterpretation. Step sections or serial sections are prepared, stained with haematoxylin and eosin and by a variety of other stains if necessary e.g., P.A.S. technique, *van Gieson* stain, *Perl*'s technique etc.

Jejunal biopsies for histochemical examination should be sent without fixative to the pathologist with a minimum of delay. Ice cooled containers can be made available for the purpose to minimise loss of enzymatic activity. Cryostat sections are prepared for such investigations.

Biopsies for electron microscope studies are placed in methacrylate or other suitable fixative and sent to the pathologist without delay.

Multiple biopsy procedure is preferable to single biopsy technique since it allows for patchy involvement of the mucosa and there is therefore less risk of misinterpreation or failure to diagnose coeliac disease.

Dissecting microscope photographs can be filed in the patients case notes and it is desirable that further biopsies should be taken after gluten withdrawal documenting the response to treatment.

II. Dissecting Microscope

Valuable information can be gained by examination at different magnifications. Normal digitate and leaf villi are immediately obvious and help to exclude a diagnosis of coeliac disease. Identification of digitate and leaf villi in a coeliac patient after introduction of a gluten free diet indicates a satisfactory response (Fig. 1).

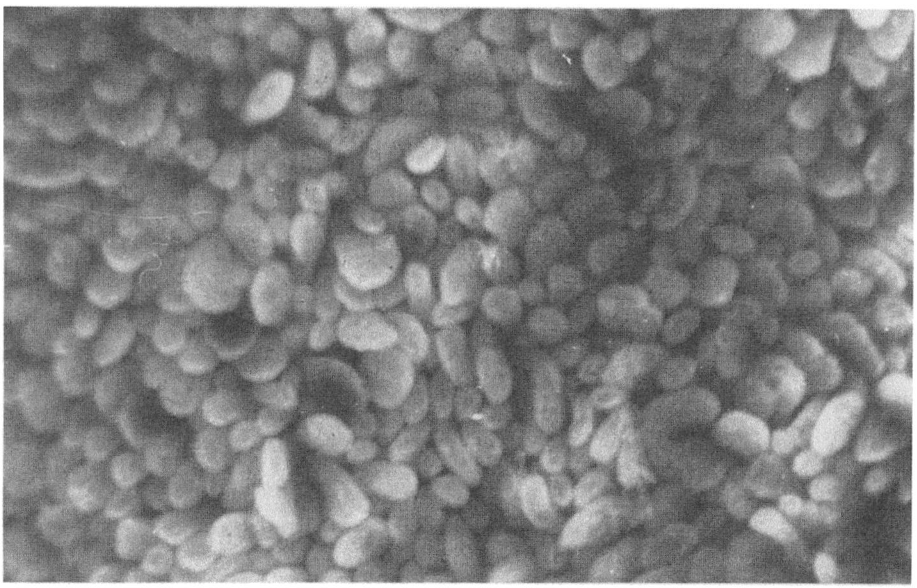

Fig. 1. Dissecting microscope view of digitate and leaf villi

The presence of ridges indicates mild abnormality of the mucosa since they are frequently found in immigrant subjects almost as a normal variation or in white subjects who have slight disease in other systems. Ridges usually coexist with digitate and leaf villi representing Grade 1 abnormality associated with minor morphological changes (Fig. 2).

Convolutions resembling the gyri of the cerebral cortex indicates an abnormal mucosa and suggest a differential diagnosis of various disease entities such as coeliac disease, Crohn's disease, tropical sprue, post gastrectomy syndrome, Zollinger-Ellison syndrome etc. The presence of convolutions indicate Grade 2 or Grade 3 abnormality corresponding with partial or subtotal villous atrophy. Convolutions may coexist with ridges, leaf or digitate villi or even with flat mucosa. Low convolutions are seen in adult coeliac disease and they may be complicated with a mosaic pattern (Figs. 3 and 4).

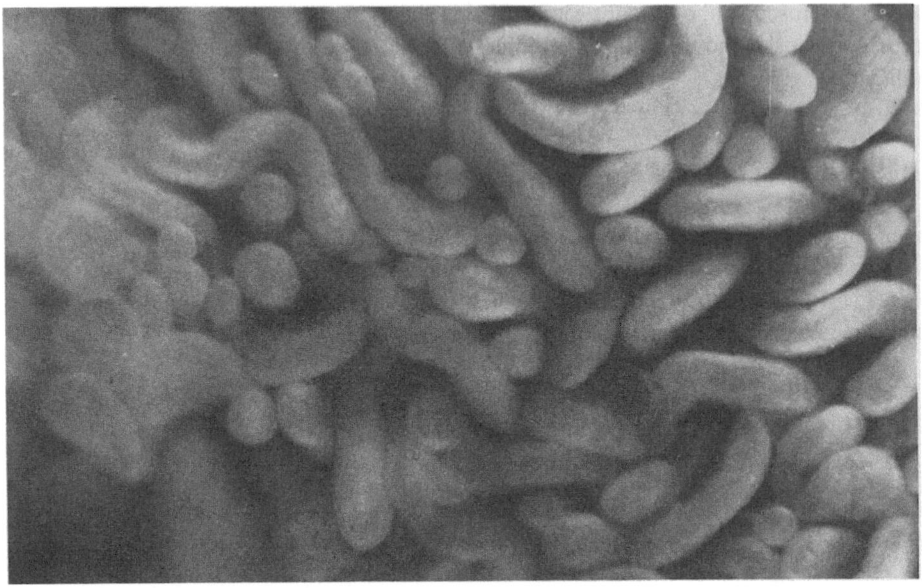

Fig. 2. Dissecting microscope view of Grade 1 abnormality with ridges, digitate and leaf villi

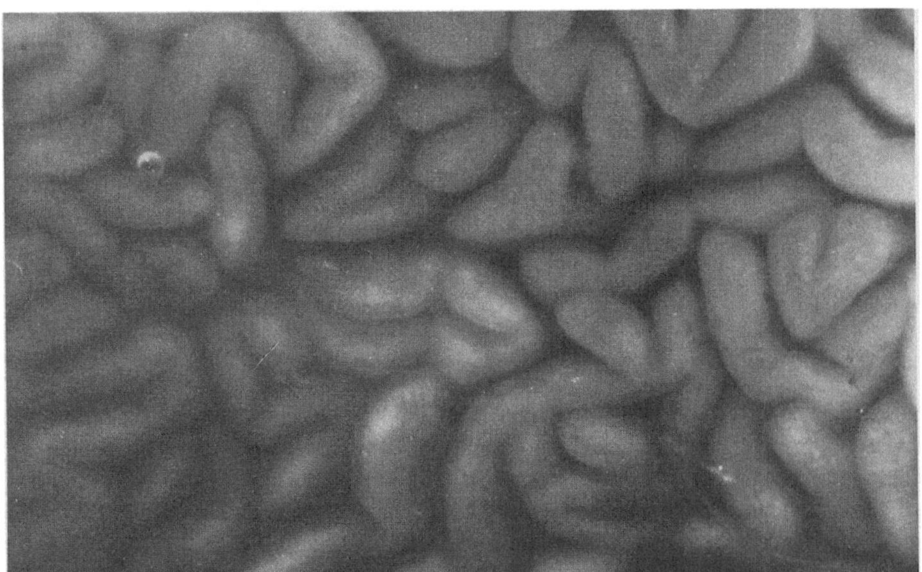

Fig. 3. Dissecting microscope view of convolutions

A flat mucosa (Fig. 5) with or without a mosaic pattern is characteristic of coeliac disease and such biopsies may also show low convolutions. Flat jejunal biopsies are rarely obtained in other disease entities such as tropical sprue, Crohn's disease, Whipple's disease etc.

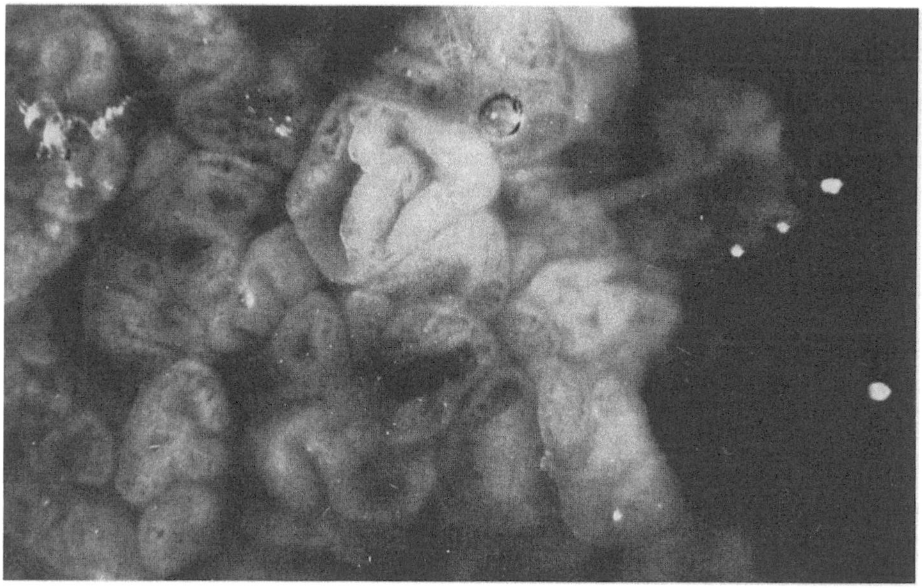

Fig. 4. Dissecting microscope view of convolutions with mosaic pattern

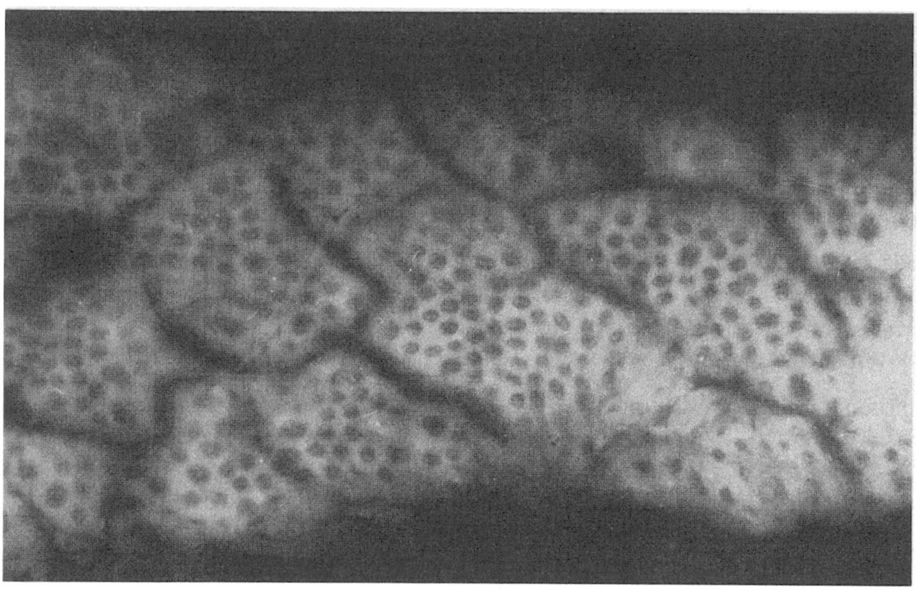

Fig. 5. Dissecting microscope view of flat mosaic jejunal biopsy, Grade 3 abnormality

Balloon villi are encountered in Whipple's disease, lymphangiectasia and Crohn's disease and immediately suggest a differential diagnosis at this stage of the investigation. Pedunculated lymph follicles occur in the mucosal surface in hypogammaglobulinaemia. Polypoid elevations are encountered in juvenile polyposis coli and in the Canada-Cronkhite syndrome.

It should be emphasised that there are certain problems of identification with jejunal biopsies which have undermined the confidence of occasional observers. Gastric biopsies often show a flat surface with or without mosaic elevations and they frequently show convolutions. Oesophageal biopsies may also appear flat or convoluted.

III. Histology

In our gastro-enterological unit, we have used a simple grading system which takes into account dissecting microscope appearances and histological changes (Table 1).

Table 1. Classification

Grading	Dissecting Microscopy	Histology
Normal	Digitate villi	Normal villous pattern
Grade 1 abnormality	Ridges, leaf and digitate villi. Occasional convolutions	Minor morphological abnormalities.
Grade 2 abnormality	Convolutions, ridges, leaf and digitate villi	Partial villous atrophy
Grade 3 abnormality	Flat or convoluted mucosa with or without mosaic pattern	Subtotal villous atrophy

Grade 1 represents minor morphological abnormality with slight alteration of the villous pattern.

Grade 2 represents partial villous atrophy and it is characterised by blunting and bridging of villi sometimes associated with abnormal surface epithelium and increased numbers of inflammatory cells in the lamina propria. Biopsies in this grade are not diagnostic of coeliac disease unless accompanied by the characteristic changes in the surface epithelium (Fig. 8).

Cell counts also assist in the interpretation of biopsies in this Grade. It, frequently, becomes necessary, however, to repeat the biopsy to resolve the diagnostic problem. I recall two cases in which the diagnosis remained uncertain. The first was a patient who presented with rapidly progressive malabsorption syndrome and marked weight loss. Two consecutive jejunal biopsies showed Grade 2 abnormality. A diagnosis of coeliac disease was not established. Death occurred 4 weeks later and revealed malignant lymphoma of the second part of the duodenum in the form of reticulum cell sarcoma. Careful examination of jejunal mucosa at necropsy revealed no evidence of flat or mosaic pattern and it was therefore concluded that this was not a case of adult coeliac disease. The second patient also had two separate jejunal biopsies which showed Grade 2 abnormality. Cell counts suggested that he had coeliac disease. He refused further jejunal biopsies and the physician started him on a gluten free diet which was followed by a good clinical response.

Grade 3 abnormality (Figs. 6 and 7) is diagnostic of coeliac disease corresponding to subtotal villous atrophy. Crypt hyperplasia is a prominent feature and the surface epithelium is more cuboidal than normal and also more cellular than normal with lymphocytes emigrating through the epithelium. There is an increased number of chronic inflammatory

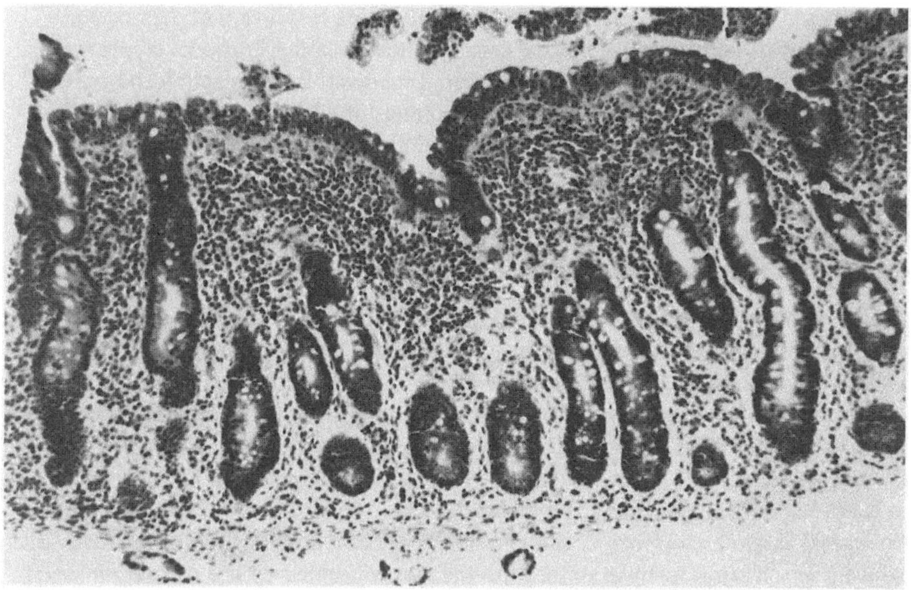

Fig. 6. Grade 3 abnormality representing subtotal villous abnormality

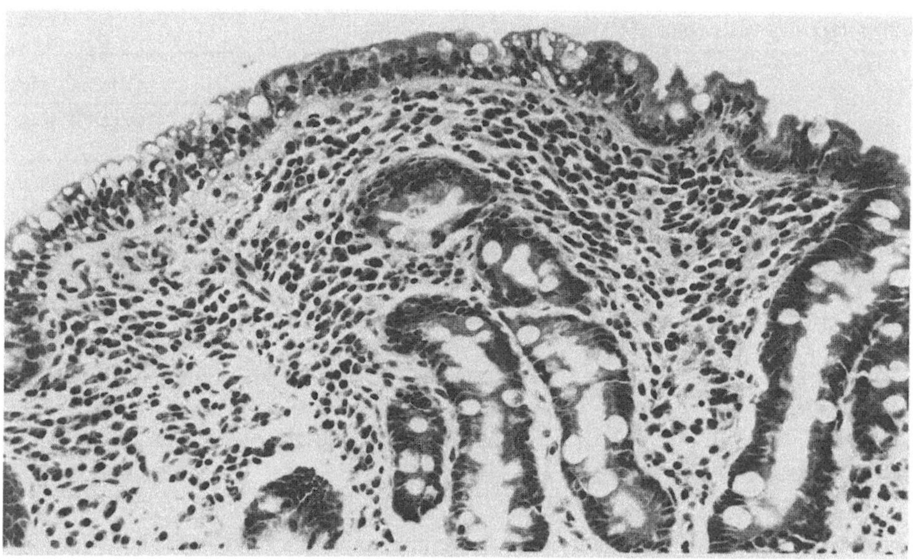

Fig. 7. Grade 3 abnormality showing abnormal surface epithelium which is more cellular than normal and also more cuboidal than normal

cells in the lamina propria including lymphocytes, plasma cells, eosinophils and histiocytes. In approximately one third of cases of untreated adult coeliac disease there is a narrow, eosinophilic subepithelial zone of hyalin which stains red like collagen with the *van Gieson* stain. This hyalin zone disappears with restoration of a normal villous pattern on a gluten free diet. The term "collagenous sprue" used for this variety by *Weinstein* et al. (1970) should be abandoned since there is no convincing evidence that presence of hyalin makes any difference to the natural course of the disease. Occasional crypts are encountered undergoing dissolution with a leucocytic inflammatory reaction and occasional inflammatory erosions occur on the surface. Lymphoid hyperplasia with lymph follicles bearing germ centres is occasionally seen and should not be confused with malignant lymphoma. Slight fibrosis is occasionally encountered in the lamina propria particularly in patients with a history of ulceration. *Paneth* cell granules are normally visible in the base of the crypts of *Lieberkuhn* but their absence makes no difference to the clinical course. Mitoses are more numerous than normal in the crypts of *Lieberkuhn*.

Histological measurements of jejunal mucosa using either a grid or linear occular micrometer calibrated against a stage micrometer provide useful formation for comparative studies. *Roy-Choudhury* et al. (1966) carried out a survey of these measurements in our gastro-enterological unit as outlined in Table 2. *Shiner* and *Doniach* (1960), *Rubin* et al. (1960), *Chako* et al. (1961), *Madanagopalan* et al. (1965), *Jos* (1962), *Sheehy* and *Floch* (1964), *Stewart* et al. (1967), and *Vogel* (1971) have also assessed these parameters. *Dunnill* and *Whitehead* (1972) have devised a method for quantitating the surface area to volume ratio in jejunal biopsies. *Chapman* et al. (1974) introduced a modification of the technique of colour television image analysis to measure the areas occupied by the surface and crypt epithelium respectively in histological sections of jejunal mucosa. *Meinhard* et al. (1975) introduced computer card morphometry.

Table 2. Histological measurements of jejunal mucosa

Category	Number of subjects	Number of villi	Height μ		Breadth μ		Mucosal thickness	
			Mean	Range	Mean	Range	Mean	Range
1. Normal controls	25	350	427±52	287-650	137±31	87-215	150	85-205
2. Grade 1	40	300	322	250-350	150	85-220	190	175-275
3. Grade II A.C.D.	23	175	250	100-300	190	150-250	265	250-320
4. Grade III A.C.D. (a)	29	–	120	100-150	–	–	375	300-480
(b)	35	–	–	–	–	–	447	375-590
5. R.E. jejunal	34	470	348±122	125-175	155±65	75-410	–	–
6. Post-gastrectomy	25	370	409±110	125-750	137±40	60-310	–	–
7. Pernicious anaemia	10	130	416	312-540	131	87-175	156	–
8. Folic deficiency	10	135	418	287-589	127	88-176	158	–
9. Pancreatitis	7	120	396	290-570	139	85-200	166	–

Cytokinetic studies have been carried out in the jejunal mucosa by *Wright* et al. (1972, 1973, 1974) and *Watson* and *Wright* (1974) by measuring the incidence of mitotic figures at each cell position in a statistically adequate number of crypts. Application of a stathmokinetic or metaphase direct technique with Vincristine in coeliac patients and control subjects revealed that the raised mitotic index was due to increased rate of cell division with a cell cycle time which is more than halved as compared with control values. The cytokinetic observations also apply to the coeliac situation in dermatitis herpetiformis.

Table 3. Cell counts

		Total cells	Plasma Cells	Lymphocytes	
				Lamina propria	Epithelium
Controls	Mean	5.702	1.974	1.948	42
	SD	1.068	620	526	12
Adult Coeliac Disease Normal diet	Mean	13.412	10.498	1.172	134
	SD	2.134	1.592	514	40
Gluten-free diet	Mean	9.584	6.148	2.004	94
	SD	1.072	1.840	846	39
Controls v Adult Coeliac Disease (normal diet)	p	<0.001	<0.001	<0.01	<0.001
Controls v Adult Coeliac Disease (Gluten free diet)	p	<0.001	<0.001	NS	<0.001
Adult Coeliac Disease (normal diet) v Adult Coeliac Disease (Gluten free diet)	p	<0.001	<0.001	<0.01	<0.05

Cell count studies in our gastroenterological unit carried out by *Holmes* (1973), *Stokes* et al. (1974), *Ferguson* et al. (1974) have yielded interesting information (Table 3). Chronic inflammatory cells including lymphocytes, plasma cells, eosinophils and histiocytes are increased in the lamina propria in untreated coeliac disease. The cell counts fall with the introduction of a gluten free diet. There was a statistically significant increased mean plasma cell count in jejunal biopsies from normal-diet coeliacs compared with controls $P < 0.001$ and although a significant fall occurred in the mean counts in patients after gluten withdrawal $P < 0.001$, the counts still remained above normal $P < 0.001$ in some instances even after 9 years on a gluten free diet. With reference to the mean lymphocyte counts there was a reduction in these cells compared with controls $P < 0.01$ but following gluten withdrawal the counts actually rose until there was no significant difference. The intra-epithelial lymphocytes were increased in normal-diet patients compared with controls $P < 0.001$ and fell after gluten withdrawal $P < 0.05$ but usually remained abnormal even though the patients had been on a gluten free diet for several years. *Lancaster-Smith* et al. (1975) have demonstrated an increase in jejunal plasma cells following gluten challenge in adult coeliac disease and dermatitis herpetiformis. Eosinophils also increase in lamina propria following gluten challenge. The jejunal cellular infiltrate in coeliac disease complicated by lymphoma differs from untreated coeliac disease in that there are lower plasma cell counts and higher lymphocyte counts in the lamina propria and lower lymphocyte counts in the epithelium for periods up to 5 years before the diagnosis of lymphoma is made. The counts are still abnormal compared to control cases.

Electron microscope abnormalities in coeliac disease have been documented by *Shiner* (1974) and scanning electron microscope changes have been described by *Asquith* et al. (1970) and *Marsh* (1972).

1. Surgical Specimens

Biopsies obtained during laparotomy should be treated in the same way as other jejunal biopsies. The mucosa often curls up due to retraction of the muscularis mucosae with rugosity of the mucosa and pinning out and stretching the mucosa may become necessary. The histological appearances of surgical biopsies appear different in the thickness and architecture from capsule biopsies.

Surgical specimens present similar problems. The specimen should be opened immediately after removal and pinned out on a flat surface to ensure adequate fixation of the mucosa. It is very important to examine surgical resection specimens of jejunum under the dissecting microscope since undiagnosed coeliac disease can be recognised in this way. This applies especially to carcinoma cases from surgical units. I have encountered 2 cases of carcinoma, one in the jejunum and the other in the ampullary region of the duodenum which were associated with flat mucosa in the jejunum. These patients had occult coeliac disease and both died from malignancy despite institution of a gluten free diet.

2. Necropsy Studies

These are important to confirm the clinical diagnosis of adult coeliac disease and assess the response to treatment, to exclude other possible causes of malabsorption and to inquire into the incidence of neoplasia, ulceration, strictures, diaphragms and other complications.

Two main techniques can be utilised for preserving the small intestine:

1. The intact small intestine is removed, filled and distended with 10% formalin solution and tied off at both ends. After fixation for 24 h, the specimen is opened and examined.
2. When adhesions or a perforation is present then it is necessary to open the small intestine immediately and immerse it in a large container filled with 10% formalin for 24 h.

The best preservation is obtained when necropsy is carried out within 2-4 h of death. Minimal autolysis occurs within this time and the dissecting microscope and histological changes have considerable clinico-pathological significance as shown by *Thompson* (1974) in studies from our gastro-enterological unit (Table 4).

The specimens provide an excellent opportunity to examine the entire mucosa from the pylorus to the ileo-caecal valve (Figs. 8-11). Unsuspected malignant disease is frequently brought to light particularly when detailed histological studies are carried out.

Table 4.

Case No.	Sex	Age	Duration of disease	Years follow-up	Diet	Duration	Response	Length of small intestine cm	Grade Percentage Gut Involvement 1 Leaf Dig	2 Conv	3 Flat	Cause of death
1	F	57	15	8	N.D.	–	Satis.	239	40	29	31	A.C.D. (*Wilding* et al.; 1964) Bronchopneumonia
2	M	58	16	2/52	N.D.	–	N.A.	395	2	30	68	Pulmonary embolus. Carcinoma stomach
3	M	38	30	2/52	N.D.	–	N.A.	415	38	32	30	Reticulum cell sarcoma
4	F	56	38	5	N.D.	–	Good	355	30	46	25	Reticulum cell sarcoma
5	F	49	22	19	N.D.	–	Good	565	33	53	114	Carcinoma of rectum
6	F	69	12	9	N.D.	–	Good	793	45	25	330	Cerebral thrombosis
7	F	63	17	12	G.F.	8/12	Satis.	584	65	25	10	Reticulum cell sarcoma
8	F	35	3	8/12	G.F.	3/12	N.A.	480	37	32	31	Reticulum cell sarcoma
9	F	54	50	16	G.F.	3	Poor	469	16	14	70	
10	M	50	47	1	G.F.	3	Poor	–	30	34	36	Neuropathy (*Cooke* and *Smith*, 1966) Bronchopneumonia
11	M	54	46	1	G.F.	1	Poor	244	30	17	5	Small intestinal ulcers. Bronchopneumonia
												Post-operation chest complications
12	M	46	40	5	G.F.	5	Good	452	66	35	9	Ca. oesophagus
13	M	47	5	6/12	G.F.	6/12	N.A.	631	13	32	55	Reticulum cell sarcoma
14	M	58	40	14	G.F.	12	Good	415	98	2	0	Renal and intestinal haemorrhage; Cor pulmonale
15	F	68	7	4	G.F.	4	Good	386	100	0	0	Reticulum cell sarcoma (*Cooke* et al., 1968)
16	M	56	11	9	G.F.	9	Good	270	26	68	6	Reticulum cell sarcoma
17	F	54	10	1/12	G.F.	3/12	N.A.	656	26	16	58	Reticulum cell sarcoma
18	F	78	32	9	G.F.	9	Good	510	94	6	0	Pulmonary embolus
19	F	55	4	2/12	G.F.	2/12	N.A.	760	28	13	59	Volvulus small intestine
20	F	59	30	30	G.F.	3	Good	415	68	20	12	Periarteritis nodosa
21	M	58	7	6	G.F.	6	Good	506	95	5	0	Coronary thrombosis
22	F	58	15	15	G.F.	15/12	Good	407	24	69	7	Aspergillosis pneumonia. Reticulum cell sarcoma
23	F	64	16	4	G.F.	4	Good	823	80	20	0	Post-operative aspiration pneumonia
24	F	81	70	17	G.F.	15	Good	327	39	61	0	Reticulum cell sarcoma

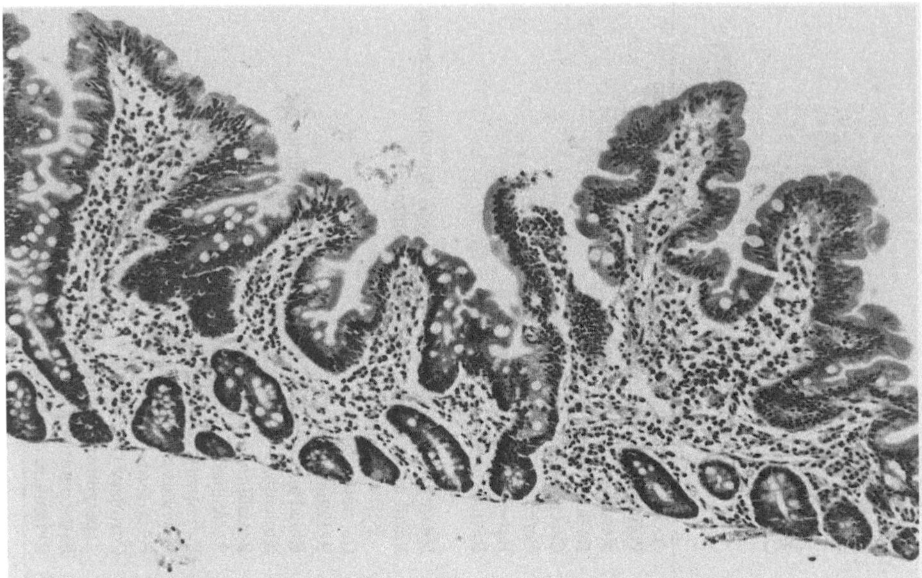

Fig. 8. Grade 2 abnormality with convolutions

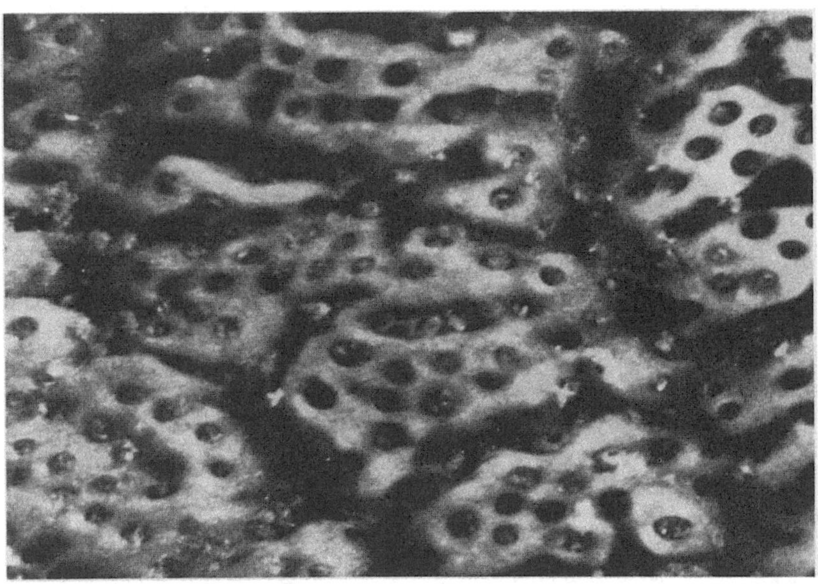

Fig. 9. Dissecting microscope view of flat mosaic mucosa in necropsy specimen

3. Mucosal Changes in Adult Coeliac Disease

In untreated coeliac disease, the upper third of the small intestine i.e., jejunum and duodenum, are covered by flat mucosa or low convolutions with or without a mosaic pattern.

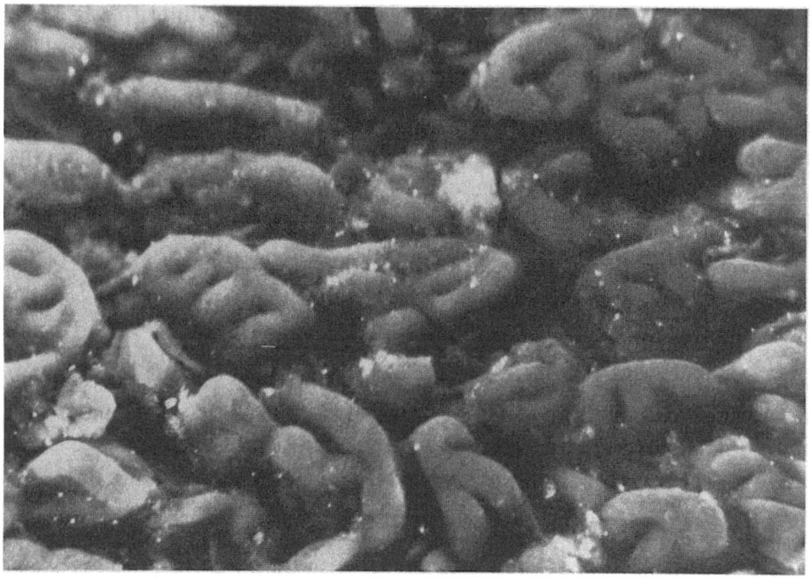

Fig. 10. Dissecting microscope view of convolutions in necropsy specimen

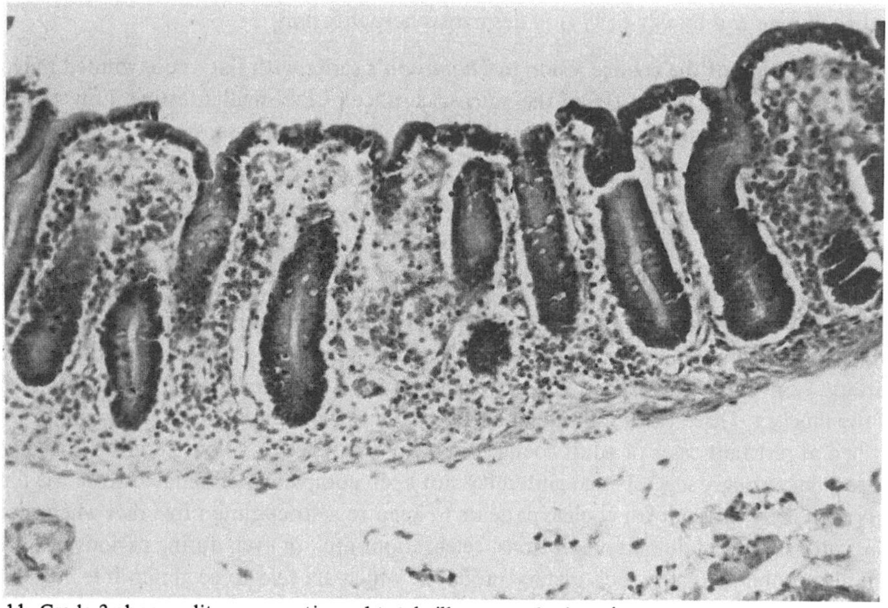

Fig. 11. Grade 3 abnormality representing subtotal villous atrophy in necropsy specimen

Histologically the appearances correspond to subtotal villous atrophy and partial villous atrophy i.e., Grade 3 and Grade 2 abnormality. Flat and convoluted mucosa may alternate particularly in transitional zones. The edges of the vulvulae conniventes usually show convolutions but sometimes the mucosa is flat. Digitate and leaf villi with ridges may occur in localised areas in the upper third of the small intestine even in untreated coeliac disease and this can be confusing in diagnosis.

The middle third of the small intestine in untreated coeliac disease usually shows convolutions merging into leaf villi and ridges at the lower end. Digitate villi may also be present appearing frequently half way along this segment. Flat mucosa may extend into the middle third and may alternate with convolutions.

The distal third of the small intestine usually shows digitate and leaf villi. Occasionally convolutions and even flat mucosa extends down to the ileocaecal valve. The villi in the terminal ileum tend to be smaller in size.

The occurrence of localised areas of digitate and leaf villi with ridges in the jejunum may cause diagnostic difficulties. *Roy-Choudhury* et al. (1967) in multiple biopsies encountered digitate villi in 3.4% of the biopsies. If only one biopsy is taken then there is a risk of missing a diagnosis of adult coeliac disease. In one of our cases of adult coeliac disease coming to necropsy, a random sample of jejunal mucosa revealed digitate and leaf villi but more detailed examination of the rest of the specimen after fixation revealed extensive distribution of flat and convoluted mucosa. If multiple biopsies are taken then there is less risk of missing the diagnosis since, even if digitate and leaf villi are sampled one of the other biopsies usually shows convolutions or flat mucosa indicating coeliac disease. The patchy distribution of the mucosal changes has also been confirmed by *Scott* and *Losowsky* (1975) in adult coeliac disease and by *Fry* (1974) in dermatitis herpetiformis.

The distribution of the coeliac lesion in *Thompson*'s series with flat or convoluted mucosa extended to involve up to 70% of the mucosal surface of the small intestine. Low convolutions were encountered in the terminal ileum in one untreated case.

The mucosal changes after institution of a gluten free diet are much less extensive. In some cases, the villous pattern returns to complete normality. In other cases Grade 1 abnormality or convolutions and flat areas persist. In a few cases the mucosa remains flat or convoluted indicating that there has been no response to a gluten free diet.

Out of 18 cases treated with a gluten free diet in *Thompson*'s series, only 6 showed no evidence of residual flat mucosa and only one had complete restoration of a normal villous pattern. Convolutions persisted in 5 cases with Grade 2 abnormality involving up to 69% of the mucosa. Three cases showed a poor response to a gluten free diet and could be described as resistant cases of adult coeliac disease. Persistance of villous abnormalities in these cases strongly suggests that gluten has not been completely eliminated from the diet. It is extremely difficult for coeliac patients to keep to a strict gluten free diet when socialising with friends at dinners, receptions, celebrations etc., or even during periods of illness. It is also probable that certain dietary products, which are said to be gluten free, may contain small amounts of gluten. Moreover it is possible that gliadin in other cereals may damage the intestinal mucosa. The development of serious complications can also lead to a relapse.

Cytokinetic studies on the jejunal mucosa indicate that enteroblastic hyperplasia occurs in coeliac disease with a more rapid turnover of cells than in the normal subject. *Pink, Croft* and *Creamer* (1972) assessed the rate of cell loss by measurement of DNA in the washings from perfused segments of small bowel and concluded that patients with untreated coeliac disease showed a sixfold increase over the normal rate. According to *Watson* and *Wright* (1974) the large increase in the rate of cell production in untreated coeliac disease is attributable to a three fold increase in the number of proliferating cells and to a doubling of the rate of cell division.

Pink and *Creamer* (1967) have described a group of patients with coeliac disease who showed low mitotic indices and *Barry, Morris* and *Read* (1970) have also reported a similar case. Crypt hypoplastic villous atrophy has also been described in association with untreated pernicious anaemia by *Pena* et al. (1972).

Documentation of cases of crypt hypoplasia is still not completely convincing and there is insufficient evidence that it constitutes a significant subgroup.

Introduction of a gluten free diet leads to restoration of a relatively normal villous pattern. The response is more rapid in children than in adults. *McNeish* and *Anderson* (1974) have seen complete reversal of all histological abnormalities within 3 months of gluten withdrawal. However at the discussion of the ESPGA (*Meeuweisse*, 1970) several workers stated that normalisation of the jejunal mucosa might take 1 or 2 years. I have also seen rapid response in adults with normal biopsies becoming available within 3-6 months. *Stewart* (1965), however, comments that adults on a really strict diet usually achieve normal leafy villi within 2 or 3 years, often sooner. Generally, however, response occurs within one year. The mucosa frequently becomes convoluted during the normalisation process but villi can appear without a preceeding convoluted stage. Further studies on the response to a gluten free diet are clearly desirable taking into account clinical parameters, enzyme histochemistry, cell counts, dissecting microscope appearances on follow-up biopsies and necropsy studies. Gluten challenge studies should also be taken into account and assessment of immunological depression with lymphoreticular atrophy requires consideration.

Resistant cases of coeliac disease require intensive study to elucidate the aetiology of the disease. The possibility of irreversibility of the mucosal changes must be considered. Steroid therapy, elimination of milk or eggs as described by *Cooke* (1968), treatment of complications such as strictures by surgical resection or surgical treatment of malignant disease may be needed. The time factor in assessing failure of response can perhaps only be decided by the observation of progressive clinical deterioration. The possibility of hypersensitivity to other cereal proteins should also be considered in such cases.

IV. Complications

1. Malignancy

Malignant lymphoma was demonstrated in 13 of our 31 necropsy cases and has been described by *Harris* et al. (1967) and *Cooke* (1968). The incidence in the clinical series was approximately 7% and in the necropsy series approximately 42%. Many of these patients have had coeliac disease for more than 20 years and some have been treated with a gluten free diet. Other patients have had a short history of adult coeliac disease and it is probable that coeliac disease had been present for many years in an occult or latent form.

The tumour occurs as a multicentric lesion (Fig. 12) with circumferential ulcerating lesions, nodular ulcerating lesions, small ulcers or nodules in the mucosa. Occasional more diffuse infiltration occurs over short segments or the lesions may present as strictures. The tumour may also present as a solitary lesion. In some cases there is no evidence of intestinal involvement although malignant lymphoma was identified in the mesenteric lymph nodes, liver, peritoneum or other lymph nodes. Occasionally the stomach is the site of malignant lymphoma.

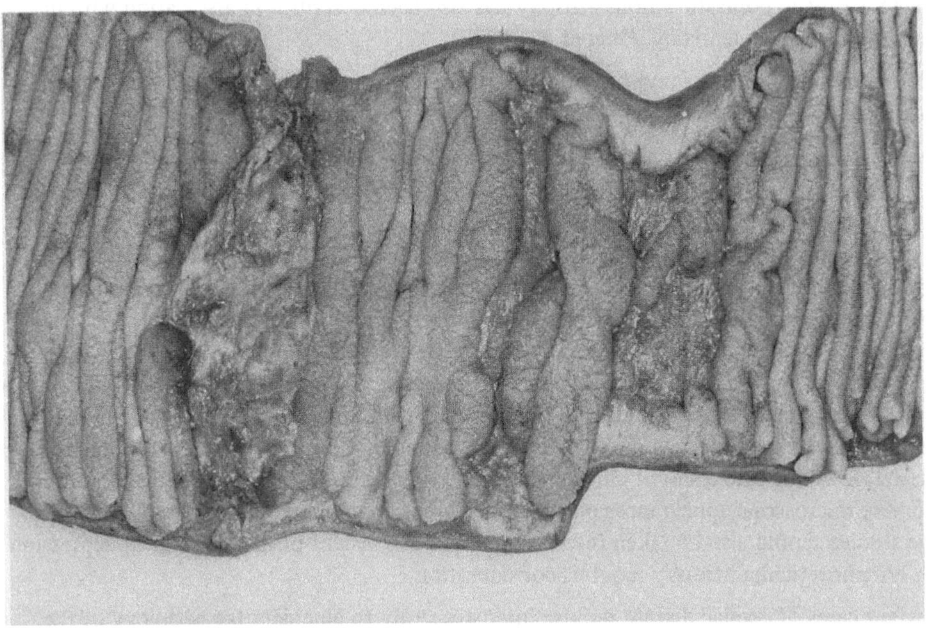

Fig. 12. Ulcerated lesions of reticulum cell sarcoma

Ulceration and perforation of intestinal lesions is a serious hazard. Perforating lesions may be difficult to differentiate from simple ulceration but the appearances of neoplastic reticulum cells infiltrating the muscularis propria at the edge of the perforation is a characteristic feature although no solid tumour may be recognisable. Perforation may lead to generalised peritonitis or to local abscess formation. Some of our cases of malignant lymphoma could not have been detected without a postmortem examination.

In our series the primary site was identified as small intestine in 7 cases (jejunum 2, mid ileum 4, terminal ileum 1) stomach in one case and lymph nodes in 5 cases. Multiple lesions were present in the gastrointestinal tract in 7 cases. Metastases were found in 10 cases. It is particularly interesting that perforation occurred in 4 cases, in the necropsy series.

Clinical diagnosis of malignant lymphoma during life in our unit has been established on lymph node biopsies, intestinal resection, partial gastrectomy, liver biopsy, diagnostic cytology of peritoneal and pleural fluid, peritoneal biopsy and skin biopsy. Unexplained clinical deterioration, relapse on a gluten free diet or failure to respond to a gluten free diet stimulates a search for enlarged or palpable lymph nodes and lymph node biopsy is usually carried out as a preliminary step. Absence of enlarged glands and progressive deterioration with an abnormal barium follow through may lead to exploratory laparotomy. Liver biopsy is performed if there is hepatomegaly and effusions are examined for malignant cells if detected. There is a general awareness in our unit of the risk of lymphoma and all patients in the clinical series are carefully followed up and reviewed at intervals.

Patients with malignant lymphoma who have had a surgical resection or who have been treated with cytotoxic drugs or radiation therapy may have no residual evidence of lymphoma at necropsy.

In 2 of our cases, there was persistent ulceration of the small intestine and it seems probable that the neoplastic cells had been destroyed.

Histological studies show that the lymphoma is a reticulum cell sarcoma or histiocytic lymphoma (Fig. 13). *Gough,Reed* and *Naish* (1962) and *Austad* (1967) however classified some of their cases as Hodgkin's disease; *Harris* et al. (1967) described 10 cases as reticulum cell sarcoma and 4 cases as Hodgkin's disease with Reed Sternberg giant cells (Fig. 14). There is therefore, some confusion in terminology. It should be emphasised that the natural history of this type of lymphoma is more in keeping with that of reticulum cell sarcoma.

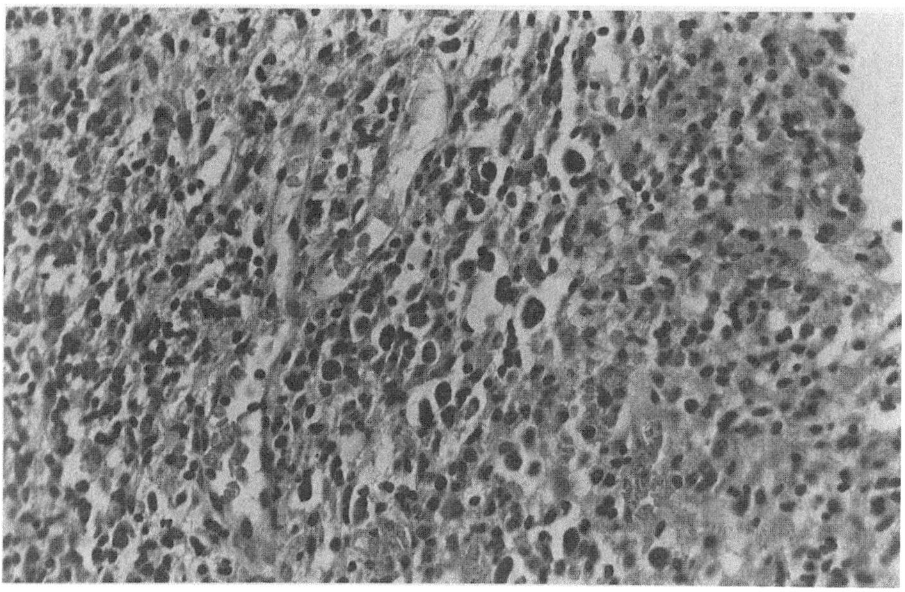

Fig. 13. Reticulum cell sarcoma

Most of the patients die from malignancy within 6 months to 2 years. The histological picture may resemble Hodgkin's disease with Reed Sternberg giant cells, eosinophils and fibrosis but if we were encountering true Hodgkin's disease then we would expect the same kind of 5, 10, 15 and 20 year survival figures, which are found in that disease. We have only one survivor in our series and in that case lymphoma in glands in one side of the neck was treated with excision and radiation therapy. This patient is still alive and well 14 years later with no evidence of residual lymphoma.

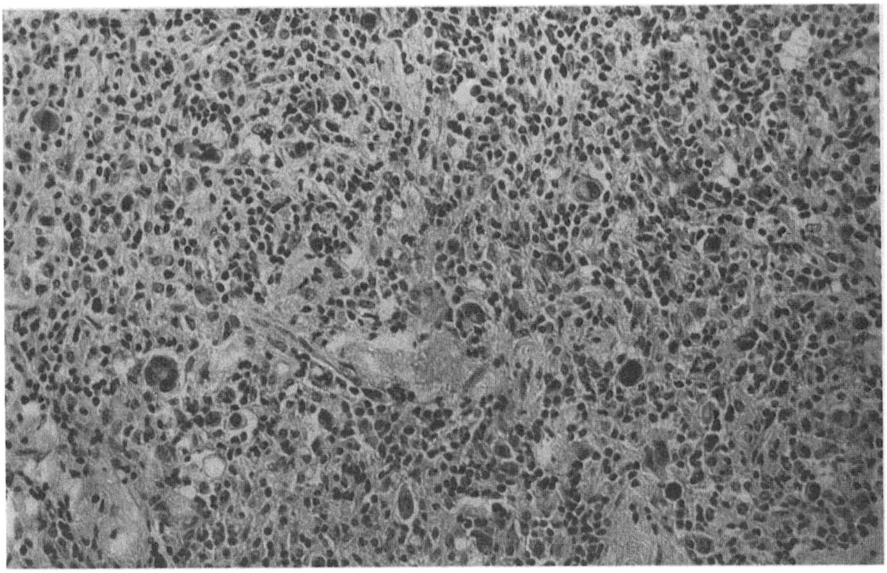

Fig. 14. Pleomorphic reticulum cell sarcoma in lymph nodes resembling Hodgkin's disease

It is known that Reed Sternberg cells can occur in other lymphomas such as reticulum cell sarcoma, Burkitt's lymphoma, mycosis fungoides, lymphosarcoma and even follicular lymphoma. It seems advisable therefore to regard these tumours as reticulum cell sarcoma unless further proof of Hodgkin's disease is forthcoming.

Reticulum cell sarcoma usually shows evidence of reticulin production and occasionally slight or moderate fibrosis. In some cases, there may be no evidence of reticulin formation but the degree of nuclear pleomorphism enables one to classify the tumour as reticulum cell sarcoma. Plasma cell differentiation is noteworthy in some of these lymphomas and it is of particular interest that *Brunt, Sircus* and *MacLean* (1969) have reported two cases of adult coeliac disease complicated by plasmacytosis of the small intestine. Plasma cells normally develop from lymphocytes or from plasma cell precursors and it is of great interest that plasma cell differentiation can occur in this variety of neoplasia since it provides a link with the 1gA and 1g M plasma cells in the lamina propria in adult coeliac disease. Malignancy may be associated with alteration in the serum immunoglobulin levels. I have also seen one case of plasmacytoma associated with coeliac disease outside the present series.

The nature of plasma cell differentiation is still undetermined since we are still uncertain whether the reticulum cell sarcoma is derived from histiocytic cell origin – histiocytic lymphoma or whether the reticulum cells represent activated lymphocytes undergoing blast transformation, which could of course develop into plasma cells if they are of B cell origin. It is still uncertain whether any of these lymphomas show evidence of T or B cell differentiation or whether a mixture of cells could be present. It is also significant that reticulum cell sarcoma can emerge as a complication of α chain disease as reported by *Rambaud.* We are considering these unresolved problems and hope to study each new lymphoma with electron microscopy and immunological procedures.

With reference to clinical syndromes in relation to lymphoma it is interesting that one patient showed the clinical features of mycosis fungoides d'emblee, one developed Raynaud's phenomenon and digital gangrene (fingers) and one patient presented with lymphoma of the thyroid gland.

In one of our cases of untreated adult coeliac disease, I discovered a microscopic focus of reticulum cell hyperplasia in the mucosa of the small intestine. The features suggested that this was an early microscopic reticulum cell sarcoma. This particular patient also had early carcinoma of the pyloric region of the stomach.

So far, I have not been impressed by premalignant changes in the lymph nodes and with reference to pleomorphic reactive changes seen in lymph nodes in diverse clinical disorders, e.g. rheumatoid arthritis, toxoplasmosis, measles and hydantoin therapy I would regard prelymphomatous changes as extremely dubious. It is true that certain lymphomas have a long natural history e.g. mycosis fungoides, giant follicle lymphoma and Hodgkin's disease but at the moment there is no evidence that this applies to lymphoma complicating adult coeliac disease.

Non-coeliac lymphoma cases coming to necropsy in our Department have been considered from the coeliac point of view and a sample of jejunal mucosa has been studied in each case provided that postmortem autolysis was not too far advanced. None of these cases have displayed any evidence of subtotal villous atrophy with Grade 3 abnormality and a flat villous surface or low convolutions. Occasional lymphoma patients representing clinically with lymphadenopathy have had a flat jejunal biopsy typical of coeliac disease. We prefer to regard these cases as examples of occult adult coeliac disease complicated by lymphoma.

Some of our lymphoma patients have demonstrated a satisfactory response to a gluten free diet. *Cooke* et al. (1969) describe a patient with adult coeliac disease who responded to a gluten free diet and then developed reticulum cell sarcoma of the stomach (malignant granuloma). Surgical jejunal biopsy and necropsy studies of the intestinal mucosa revealed no evidence of residual flat mucosa or Grade 3 abnormality when she died 4 years later. The histological appearances ranged from normal to Grade 1 abnormality with occasional small areas of Grade 2 abnormality. Two recent cases of adult coeliac disease complicated by lymphoma have also shown a good histological response with a gluten free diet. A few of our coeliac patients who were satisfactorily controlled with a gluten free diet showed clinical deterioration and relapse when they developed malignant lymphoma and their jejunal biopsy showed Grade 2 and Grade 3 abnormality. Strict attention to their gluten free diet led to improvement in the villous pattern although Grade 1 abnormality and patches of Grade 2 abnormality persisted in some patients. Since most of the lymphoma patients died within 6-12 months there has not been sufficient time to study the response to a gluten free diet to our satisfaction. Radiation therapy and cytotoxic drug therapy, moreover, have been used in treatment and it appears probable that therapy alone could have been responsible for persistence of Grade 1 and Grade 2 abnormality in some of these cases.

Squamous carcinoma of the oesophagus is a recognised complication and we have confirmed this in one of our necropsy cases. We have also encountered carcinoma of the stomach, colon, rectum, palate and tongue and also cancers of other sites. There were 5 carcinoma cases in the series of 31 necropsy cases. *Harris* et al. (1967) found that the incidence of carcinoma of the gastrointestinal tract in a series of 202 cases of coeliac disease was 6.4%. Carcinoma in other systems were also encountered.

The total incidence of malignancy reported by *Harris* was 31 cases in a series of 202 patients i.e., approximately 15%. The incidence of malignancy in the necropsy series is 18 out of 31 cases, i.e., approximately 58%. The high necropsy incidence is probably due to the fact that coeliac patients developing complications are intensively studied in our gastro-enterological unit while well controlled coeliac patients may die outside hospital from heart attacks etc., and do not become available for necropsy examination. The factor of selection is therefore important since if all coeliac patients were routinely subjected to necropsy the total incidence of malignancy would probably be much lower.

Institution of a gluten free diet has reduced the incidence of carcinoma but malignant lymphoma remains a problem. Reticulum cell sarcoma developed in four patients who had been on a gluten free diet, for 4, 7, 9 and 15 years respectively with a good clinical and histological response.

Creamer (1964) suggested that coeliac disease was a complication of malignancy but there is little evidence to support this contention. Many of our patients had a long history of adult coeliac disease before developing malignancy. With reference to those patients with a short history of adult coeliac disease and malignancy, it seems more likely to us that they represent occult or unrecognised cases of adult coeliac disease. Observations in dermatitis herpetiformis by *Marks, Shuster* and *Watson* (1966) show that the flat mucosal lesion can exist in an occult manner and it is probable that adult coeliac disease is more common in the community than most of us realise. The high incidence of malignancy suggests a defect in immune surveillance or viral oncogenesis.

2. Ulceration and Strictures

Bayless et al. (1967) and *Goulston* (1965) have drawn attention to ulceration as a dangerous complication of adult coeliac disease with a risk of perforation, haemorrhage, intestinal obstruction, relapse and clinical deterioration. I have studied 4 cases of ulceration and strictures in patients with adult coeliac disease who presented with the features of subacute intestinal obstruction and clinical deterioration (Figs. 15 and 16). Surgical resection was carried out in 3 of the 4 cases and led to a dramatic improvement in their clinical state and a satisfactory response to a gluten free diet. Another of our patients developed intestinal ulceration due to polyarteritis nodosa which resulted in fatal gastro-intestinal haemorrhage. Small ulcers were encountered at necropsy in 5 out of 24 necropsy cases as an incidental finding. Ischaemic ulceration of small intestine is responsible for some of these ulcers found at autopsy.

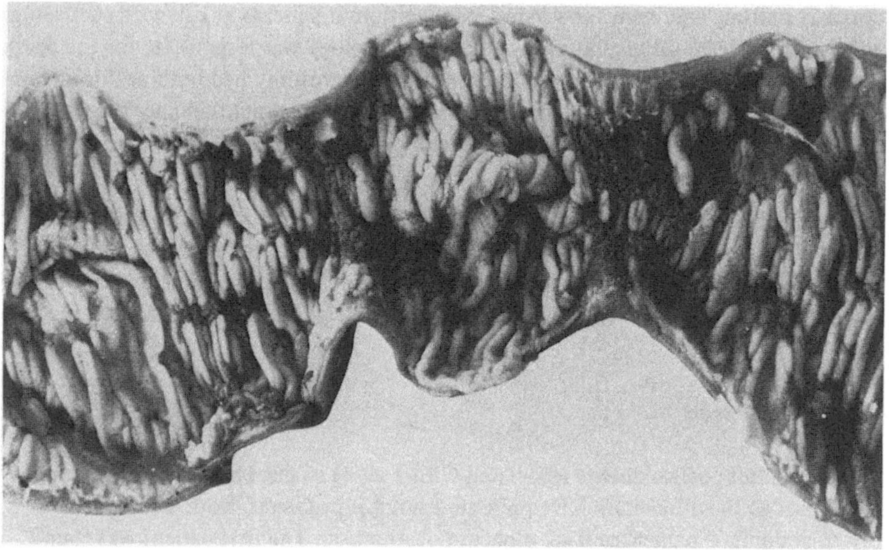

Fig. 15. Resected surgical specimen with ulceration in a patient with adult coeliac disease

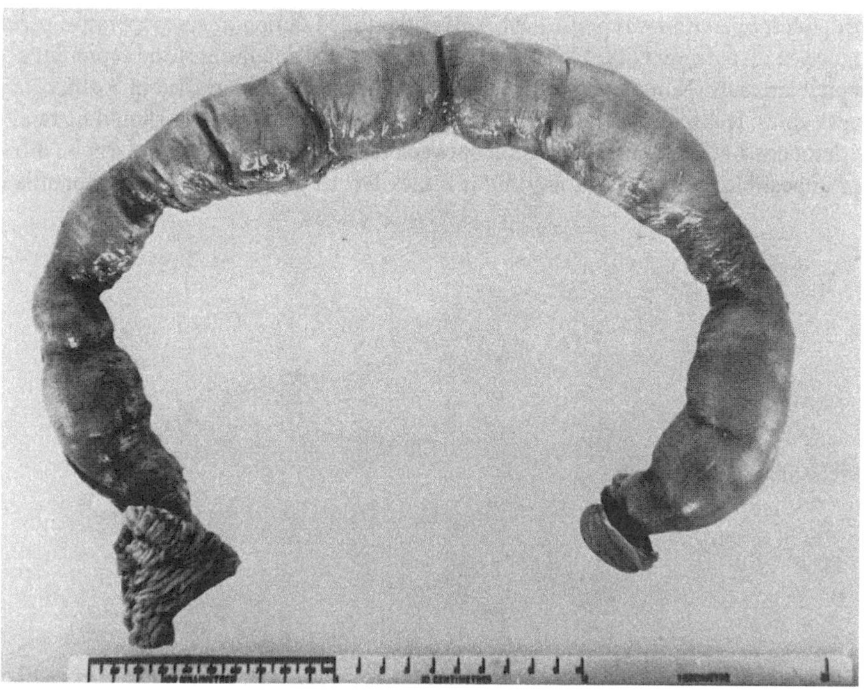

Fig. 16. Multiple strictures associated with ulceration in patients with adult coeliac disease

Although the incidence of ulceration and strictures is low, *Bayless* (1967) and *Goultson* (1965) recorded a high mortality rate of 75%. Our experience with 3 successful surgical resections is a strong argument for surgical intervention in patients at risk with such a high mortality rate. Widespread ulceration of unknown aetiology was responsible for the death of one of our coeliac patients in the necropsy series. Laparotomy had been performed on this patient but resection was not carried out. Radiological examination may suggest the presence of ulceration and strictures and jejunal biopsy occasionally shows erosion of the mucosa.

All our surgically treated cases responded to a gluten free diet and there is indisputable proof that they represent adult coeliac disease. The fatal case in the necropsy series failed to respond to a gluten free diet over a period of one year during which there was progressive clinical deterioration. This, therefore, was a resistant case of adult coeliac disease.

3. Mucosal Diaphragms

Two cases of adult coeliac disease associated with a series of diaphragms in the jejunum and third part of the duodenum have presented surgical problems. Both patients had a history of abdominal pain suggesting subacute obstruction. The first patient was found to have an early carcinoma of the stomach. During the operation the obstructing diaphragms were discovered and surgical resection was performed. The second patient also had diaphragms discovered during laparotomy, and although no resection was carried out, a short circuit operation was performed. This patient died during the postoperative period. The mucosal diaphragms (Fig. 17) are exaggerated valvulae conniventes and represent a congenital anomaly. Non-obstructing mucosal diaphragms were identified in 3 other necropsy cases. It is important that surgeons operating on these patients should be familiar with mucosal diaphragms. Distinction between diaphragms and strictures can be difficult or impossible during laparotomy and it is then left to the pathologist to differentiate

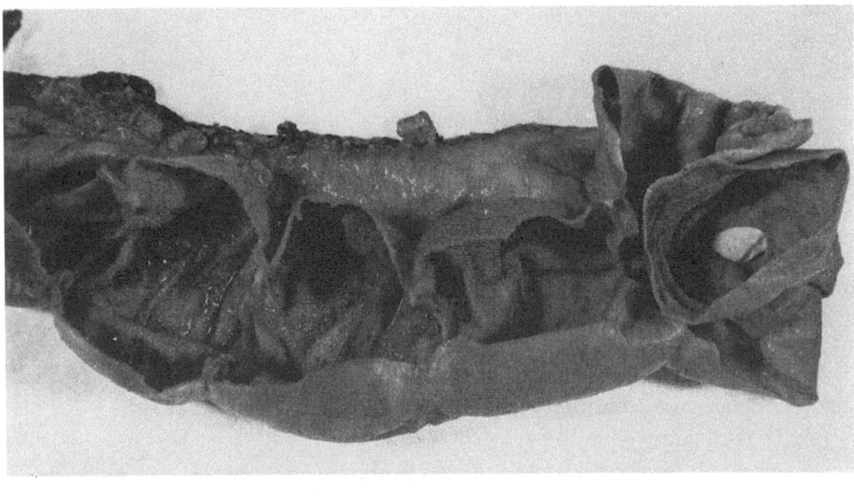

Fig. 17. Mucosal diaphragms in adult coeliac disease

between these two possibilities. Surgical resection specimens require to be opened very carefully for identification of diaphragms in order to demonstrate the curtain-like fold with definite evidence of narrowing of the lumen. Sacculation of the small intestine may occur in the segments between diaphragms and strictures. The diaphragms may be distributed in pairs in such specimens.

4. Pigmentation

Brownish pigmentation of the small intestine is a prominent feature in untreated cases and it may also be encountered in patients who have been on a gluten free diet. It was a feature in 9 out of 24 of the necropsy cases. Histological study reveals brownish black lipofuscin granules in the muscle cells of the muscularis propria particularly the external coat. The pigmentation is due to Vitamin E deficiency and this can be treated and reversed by α-tocopherol therapy. This type of "brown bowel" is not specific for coeliac disease since it may be encountered in other malabsorption states such as Crohn's disease or postgastrectomy syndrome. Special stains such as P.A.S. technique show up the pigment. In these cases, it is probable that muscle atrophy may also be present as in brown atrophy of the heart and the role of autonomic neuropathy as described by *Smith* (1972) has still to be assessed.

5. Lymphoreticular Atrophy

Lymphoreticular atrophy with a small spleen weighing under 100 g was noted in 13 out of 31 necropsies. It is noteworthy that 4 patients with lymphoreticular atrophy developed malignant lymphoma. Lymphoreticular atrophy has been documented as a complication of adult coeliac disease by *Martin* and *Bell* (1965), *McCarthy* et al. (1966), *Ferguson* et al. (1970) and by *Marsh* and *Stewart* (1970) and also as a complication of dermatitis herpetiformis by *Pettit* et al. (1972). It seems probable that there could be altered immunological reactions in such patients. Small spleens weighing less than 100 g, however, are not uncommonly encountered at necropsy in elderly subjects who have neither coeliac disease nor malignancy.

6. Associated Gastro-Intestinal Disease

Two cases of coincident ulcerative colitis and adult coeliac disease have been encountered in the clinical series. One of these is included in the necropsy series. I have seen one case of coincident Crohn's disease and coeliac disease. A more recent case presented as inflammatory bowel disease with colonoscopic evidence of proctocolitis supported by multiple biopsies. This patient was found to have adult coeliac disease complicated by malignant lymphoma confirmed by jejunal biopsy and lymph node biopsy. The colonoscopic features favoured a diagnosis of Crohn's disease in the colon and the biopsies showed no evidence of malignant disease. This patient died at home and autopsy studies were not carried out.

7. Skin Eruptions

A significant proportion of patients with dermatitis herpetiformis have occult adult coeliac disease. A number of patients in the clinical series have developed non-specific skin eruptions. One patient had eczematous skin lesions resembling mycosis fungoides d'emblee which proved to be metastatic reticulum cell sarcoma.

8. Infection

Bronchopneumonia was a common terminal complication and was present at necropsy in 15 out of 31 cases. The incidence of viral infections in association with lymphoreticular atrophy would be of interest to us.

9. Volvulus

Two fatal cases have occurred in our necropsy series. In one patient the sigmoid colon had undergone volvulus and in the other several loops of small intestine were involved. Death occurred in both cases before surgery could be undertaken.

10. Metabolic Bone Disease

Osteomalacia is a recognised complication of coeliac disease with bone pain, bone tenderness and liability to develop fractures. *Harris* et al. (1970) reported on 47 case studies of adult coeliac disease. Undecalcified sections of bone biopsies from the iliac crest are assessed by measurement of osteoid seams and a point counting technique.

11. Neuropathy

Peripheral neuropathy, paraesthesia, epileptic-form attacks, depression and psychiatric disorders occur in association with coeliac disease and have been documented by *Cooke* and *Smith* (1966), Binder et al. (1967) and *Hall* (1968). *Morris* et al. (1970) indicate that they may be the presenting features of coeliac disease and that they are not influenced by gluten withdrawal and are not related to pyridoxine deficiency.

12. Fibrosing Alveolitis

An association between bird fancier's lung and coeliac disease has recently been described by *Berril* et al. (1975).

13. Anaemia

Iron deficiency anaemia and folate deficiency with megaloblastic anaemia may be presenting features of coeliac disease. Vit. B12 deficiency with megaloblastic anaemia is rare.

14. Aphthous Ulcers in the Mouth

Ferguson et al. (1975) described the detection of adult coeliac disease in patients attending the Dental Hospital with aphthous ulceration in the mouth. Cell count studies have been carried out on jejunal biopsies and on biopsies of the ulcers.

References

Asquith, P., Johnson, A.G., Cooke, W.T.: Scanning electron microscopy of normal and coeliac jejunal mucosa. Am. J. dig. Dis. 15, 511-521 (1970).

Austad, W.I., Cornes, J.C., Gough, K.R., McCarthy, C.F., Read, A.E.: Steatorrhoea and malignant lymphoma. The relationship of malignant tumours of lymphoid tissues and coeliac disease. Amer. J. dig. Dis. 12, 475-490 (1967).

Barry, R.E., Morris, J.S., Read, A.E.A.: A case of small intestinal mucosal atrophy. Gut 11, 743-747 (1970).

Berrill, W.T., Fitzpatrick, P. F., MacLeod, W.M., Eade, O.E., Hyde, I., Wright, R.: Bird Fancier's lung and jejunal villous atrophy. Lancet 1975 II, 1006.

Binder, H.J., Solitare, G.B., Spiro, H.M.: Neuromuscular disease in patients with steatorrhoea. Gut 8, 605-611 (1967).

Brunt, P.W., Sircus, W., MacLean, N.: Neoplasia and the coeliac syndrome in adults. Lancet 1969 I, 180-186.

Chapman, B.L., Henry, K., Paice, F., Coghill, N.F., Stewart, J.S.: Measuring the response of the jejunal mucosa in adult coeliac disease to treatment with a gluten free diet. Gut 15, 870-874 (1974).

Chako, C.J., Job, C.K., Johnson, S., Baker, S.J.: Histopathological changes in the upper jejunum in tropical malabsorption studied by peroral biopsy. Indian J. Path. Bact. 4, 203 (1961).

Cooke, W.T.: Adult coeliac disease. Prog. Gastroent. 1, 299-338 (1968).

Cooke, W.T., Smith, W.T.: Neurological disorders associated with adult coeliac disease. Brain 89, 638-722 (1966).

Cooke, W.T., Thompson, H., Williams, J.A.: Malignancy and adult coeliac disease. Gut 10, 108-111 (1969).

Creamer, B.: Malignancy and the small-intestinal mucosa. Brit. Med. J. 1964 II, 1435-1436.

Dunnill, M.S., Whitehead, R.: A method for the quantitation of small intestinal biopsy specimens. J. clin. Path. 25, 243-246 (1972).

Ferguson, R., Asquith, P., Cooke, W.T.: The jejunal cellular infiltrate in coeliac disease complicated lymphoma. Gut 15, 458-461 (1974).

Ferguson, R., Basu, M.K., Asquith, P., Cooke, W.T.: Regional mucosal abnormalities in patients with recurrent aphthous ulceration. Brit. Med. J. 1976 I, 11-13.

Ferguson, A., Hutton, M.M., Maxwell, J.D., Murray, D.: Adult coeliac in hyposplenic patients. Lancet 1970 I, 163-164.

Fry, L., Seah, P.P., Harper, P.G., Hoffbrand, A. V., McMinn, R.A.H.: The small intestine in dermatitis herpetiformis. J. clin. Path. 27, 817-824 (1974).

Gough, K.R., Read, A.E., Naish, J.M.: Intestinal reticulosis as a complication of idiopathic steatorrhoea. Gut 3, 232-239 (1962).

Goulston, K.J., Skyring, A.P., McGovern, V.J.: Ulcerative jejunitis associated with malabsorption. Austral. Ann. Med. 14, 57-64 (1965).

Hall, W.H.: Proximal muscle atrophy in adult coeliac disease. Am. J. dig. Dis. 13, 697-704 (1968).

Harris, O.D., Cooke, W.T., Thompson, H., Waterhouse, J.A.H.: Malignancy in adult coeliac disease and idiopathic steatorrhoea. Amer. J. Med. 42, 899-912 (1967).

Harris, O.D., Philip, H.M., Cooke, W.T., Pover, N.F.R.: 47 Ca. studies in adult coeliac disease and other gastrointestinal conditions with particular reference to osteomalacia. Scand. J. Gastroent. 5, 169-175 (1970).

Holmes, G.K.T., Asquith, P., Stokes, P.J., Cooke, W.T.: Cellular infiltrate of jejunal biopsies in adult coeliac disease (A.C.D.) in relation to gluten withdrawal. Gut 14, 429 (1973).

Jos., J.: La biopsie de la muquese intestinale chez l'enfant. In: Etude des syndromes de malabsorption. Paris: R. Foulon et cie. 1962.

Lancaster-Smith, M., Kumar, Parveen, J., Dawson, A.M.: The cellular infiltrate of the jejunum in adult coeliac disease and dermatitis herpetiformis following the reintroduction of dietry gluten. Gut 16, 683-688 (1975).

Madanagopalan, N., Shiner, M., Rowe, B.: Measurements of small intestinal mucosa obtained by peroral biopsy. Amer. J. Med. 38, 42-53 (1965).

Marks, J., Shuster, S., Watson, A.J.: Small-bowel changes in dermatitis herpetiformis. Lancet 1966 II, 1280-1282.

Marks, J., Shuster, S.: Intestinal malabsorption and the skin. Gut 12, 938-947 (1971).

Marsh, G.W., Stewart, J.S.: Splenic function in adult coeliac disease. Brit. J. Haemat. 19, 445-457 (1970).

Martin, J.B., Bell, H.E.: The association of splenic atrophy and intestinal malabsorption. Canad. med. Ass. J. 92, 875-878 (1965).

McCarthy, C.F., Fraser, I.D., Evans, K.T., Read, A.E.: Lymphoreticular dysfunction in idiopathic steatorrhoea. Gut 7, 140-148 (1966).

Meeuwisse, G.W.: Diagnostic criteria in coeliac disease (Round Table Discussion, European Society of Paediatric Gastroenterology). Acta paediat. Scand. 59, 461-463 (1970).

Meinhard, E.A., Wadbrook, D.G., Risdon, R.A.: Computer card morphometry of jejunal biopsies in childhood coeliac disease. J. Clin. Path. 28, 85-93 (1975).

McNeish, A.S., Anderson, C.M.: Chapter on the disorder in childhood in clinics in Gastroenterology. Vol. 3, No. 1, 127-144 (1974).

Morris, J.S., Ajdukiewicz, A.B., Read, A.E.: Neurological disorders and adult coeliac disease. Gut 11, 549-553 (1970).

Pena, A.S., Truelove, S.C., Whitehead, R.: Small intestinal mucosal abnormalities and disacchasidase activity in pernicious anaemia. Brit. J. Haemat. 23, 313-321 (1972).

Pettit, J.E., Hoffbrand, A.V., Seah, P.P., Lionel Fry: Splenic atrophy in dermatitis herpetiformis. Brit. Med. J. 1972 II, 438-440.

Pink, I.J., Creamer, B.: Response to a gluten free diet of patients with the coeliac syndrome. Lancet 1967 I, 300-304.

Pink, I.J., Croft, D.N., Creamer, B.: Cell loss from small intestinal mucosa; a morphological study. Gut 11, 217-222 (1970).

Rambaud, S.C., Matuchawsky, C.: Alpha chain disease. Pathogenesis and relation to Mediterranean lymphomas. Lancet 1973 I, 1430.

Roy-Choudhury, D., Cooke, W.T., Tan, D.T., Banwell, J.G., Smits, B.J.: Jejunal biopsy: Criteria and significance. Scand. J. Gastroent. 1, 57-64 (1966).

Roy-Choudhury, D.C., Cooke, W.T., Bannell, J.G., Smits, B.J.: Multiple jejunal biopsies in adult coeliac disease. Amer. J. dig. Dis. 12, 657-663 (1967).

Rubin, C.E., Brandborg, L.L., Phelps, P.C., Taylor, H.C., Jr.: Studies of coeliac disease 1. The apparent identical and specific nature of the duodenal and proximal jejunal lesion in coeliac disease and idiopathic steatorrhoea. Gastroent. 38, 28-49 (1960).

Scott, B.B., Losowsky, M.S.: Patchiness of the mucosal abnormality in coeliac disease and dermatitis herpetiformis. Gut 16, 393 (1975).

Sheehy, T.N., Flock, M.H.: The small intestine. Its function and disease. New York: Harper and Row 1964.

Shiner, M., Doniach, I.: Histopathological studies in steatorrhoea. Gastroent. 38, 419-440 (1960).

Shiner, M.: Electron Microscopy of Jejunal Mucosa in Coeliac Disease. Clinics in Gastroent. Vol. 3, No. 1, p. 33-53 (1974).

Stewart, J.S.: Chapter on Clinical and Morphological Response to Gluten Withdrawal in Clinics in Gastroenterology. Vol. 3, No. 1, p. 109-126 (1974).

Stewart, J.S., Pollock, D.J., Hoffbrand, A. V., Mollin, D.L., Booth, C.C.: A study of proximal and distal intestinal structure and absorptive function in idiopathic steatorrhoea. Quart. J. Medicine 36, 425-444 (1967).

Stokes, P.L., Holmes, G.K.T.: Chapter on Malignancy in Coeliac Disease. Clinics in Gastroent. Vol. 3, No. 1, p. 159-170 (1974).

Thompson, H.: Necropsy studies on adult coeliac disease. J. Clin. Path. 27, 710-721 (1974).

Vogel, A.: Vergleichende Untersuchungen zur Morphologie der Dünndarmschleimhaut bei verschiedenen Formen des Malabsorptionssyndromes sowie bei anderen Erkrankungen im Kindesalter. Virchows Arch. Path. Anat. 352, 226-245 (1971).

Watson, A.J., Wright, W.A.: Morphology and cell kinetics of the jejunal mucosa in untreated patients. Coeliac Disease. Clinics in Gastroent. Vol. 3, No. 1, p. 11 (1974).

Weinstein, W.M., Saunders, D.R., Tygat, G.N., Rubin, C.E.: Collagenous sprue an unrecognised type of malabsorption. New Engl. J. of Medicine 283, 1297-1301 (1970).

Wright, N.A., Morley, A.R., Appleton, D.: Variation in the duration of mitosis in the crypts of Lieberkuhn of the rat: a cytokinetic study using vincristine. Cell and Tissue. Kinetics 5, 351-364 (1972).

Wright, N., Watson, A., Morley, A., Appleton, D., Marks, J., Douglas, A.: Cell kinetics in flat (avillous) mucosa of the human small intestine. Gut 14, 701-710 (1973).

Wright, N., Watson, A., Morley, A., Appleton, D., Marks, J., Douglas, A.: The cell cycle time in flat (avillous) mucosa of the human small intestine. Gut 14, 603-606 (1973).

Wright, N.A., Watson, A.J., Morley, A.R., Appleton, D.R., Marks, J.M., Douglas, A.P.: The measurement of cell production rate in the small bowel: a clinical and experimental study (1973) (unpublished).

Wright, N.A., Watson, A.J., Appleton, D.R., Marks, J.M., Bell, D.: Cytokinetic diversity in coeliac disease. Gut 14, 363 (1973).

Histologic Classification of Gastric Polyps

K. ELSTER

In all papers dealing with polyps of the gastro-intestinal tract the term polyp is defined in the introductory remarks. Mucosal prominences of different size and shape are called polyps. Therefore this word can only be used as a preliminary clinical "working diagnosis." When *Morson* (1972) complains that the uncritical use of the term polyp is the cause of our poor knowledge of benign neoplasias of the stomach, this is due to the fact that even pathologists use the word polyp as a diagnostic term or at least as part of one. The histologic findings often remain subordinate as descriptive adjectives. This misinterpretation can be counteracted if the histologic structure and the pathogenesis are the basis for the nomenclature of gastric polyps. This is not new because it corresponds with *Morson*'s (1962) criteria for the histologic classification of colonic polyps. Actually in making histologic classifications this analogous thinking may lead to uncertainty (*Elster*, 1974). Gastric polyps have a different histogenesis compared with large bowel polyps so that one cannot expect mucosal polyps in the stomach to grow the same way as in the colon. Neglect of this fact has, in my opinion, not only led to confusion in terminology but also to clinical misinterpretation (*Monaco* et al., 1962; *Nakamura*, 1970; *Jansen*, 1974; *Nagayo*, 1975).

The following histologic classification is based on these considerations and is oriented primarily to problems in clinical gastroenterology. It is not necessary to reject the term polyp, only to restrict it to its clinical meaning.

I. Criteria for Classification

1. Size and Shape

The macroscopic pattern, which means the size and shape of the polyp, has played and still plays an important role (*Nakamura*, 1970; *Kawai* et al., 1970). With the introduction of endoscopic polypectomy these criteria only have significance with regard to the technical problems of the therapeutic procedures. For example, the stalked polyp may be removed by snare during endoscopy and will not pose any problems whereas the larger broad-based polypoid lesion has to be treated surgically. Subtle measurements of the diameter of a polyp, which are supposedly informative of possible "malignant degeneration", are irrelevant.

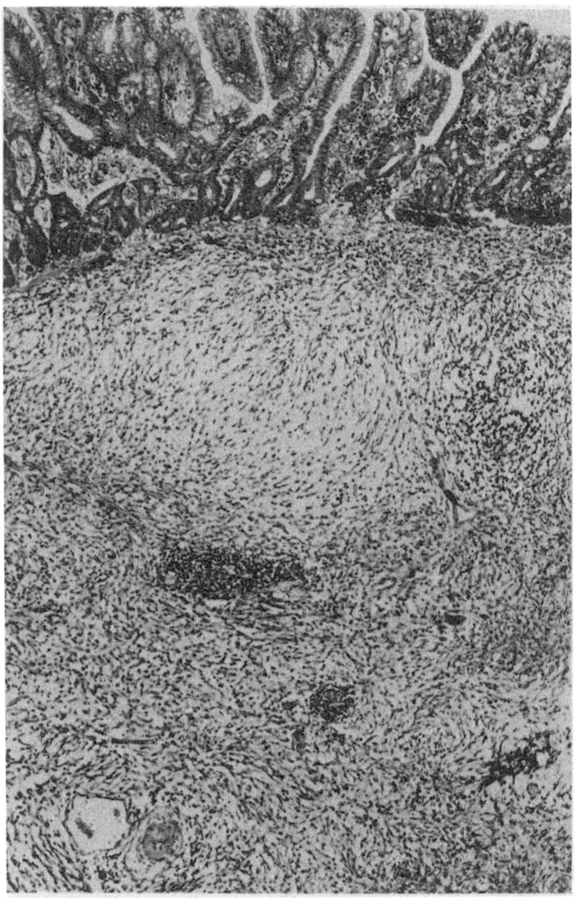

Fig. 1. Socalled inflammatory fibroid polyp: spiraling and layered ordering of the cell structure with small spindle-like nuclei, localized mainly in basal part of mucosa and submucosa. H&E x 45

2. Pathogenesis

A grouping of colon polyps in the light of their pathogenesis has proved suitable for the study of malignant transformation and this should also be tried for gastric polypoid lesions. It is necessary to separate hyperplasia from true neoplasia, which means that the hyperplastic polypoid lesion must be differentiated from benign epithelial growths of the gastric mucosa. The significance of polypoid hamartomas of the stomach will be discussed below.

3. Histologic Structure

Classification of the histologic structure and cellular pattern should also include the non-epithelial polyps. However, the connective tissue of the gastric mucosa has no special features and gastric polyps of this kind can therefore be excluded in this paper.

An exception in regard to mesenchymal polyps is the so-called inflammatory fibroid polyp. It is only seen in the stomach and is a connective tissue nonneoplastic process. It has been suggested that it may have a neurogenic origin (*Goldman* et al., 1967); in addition, a pathogenetic relationship to eosinophilic granuloma of the stomach has been considered (*Wanke*, 1971) (Fig. 1).

When epithelial polyps, independent of their hyperplastic or neoplastic origin, are defined as proliferation of gastric mucosal epithelium, the question of the type of epithelium and thereby their histogenesis has to be considered for purposes of classification. Here the decisive difference emerges in contrast to the classification of colonic polyps. The manifold structure of the gastric mucosa not only depends on the different topography of the cardiac, fundic, antral, and pyloric mucosa but also on the different mucosal layers. The tissue of origin of a polyp can be the surface epithelium, the glandular neck (foveolar) region, the gastric glands, or combinations of several types of epithelia.

II. Practical Application of the Theoretical Basis for Histologic Classification

1. Foveolar (Focal) Hyperplasia

If an epithelial proliferative process originates from the foveolae or the surface of the gastric crests, the pattern of foveolar hyperplasia results. The pits are elongated and the crests adopt a papillary structure (Fig. 2). Endoscopically a small, at most a bean-sized, broad-based polyp is seen. Sometimes, especially in the antrum, the histologic equivalent of this polyp is the inflammatory reactive foveolar hyperplasia of chronic or "complete" erosions (Fig. 3). The type II polyp of *Nakamura* (1970) corresponds to this pattern. Also the regenerative process of healing ulcers and erosions is often accompanied by foveolar hyperplasia and a variety of circumstances can thus lead to the development of these polyps. When the cellular inflammatory reaction has completely subsided the focal hyperplasia may persist forming a "polyp". The "inflammatory reactive" or "inflammatory hyperplastic" polyp and the pseudopolyp of the older literature can be grouped to-

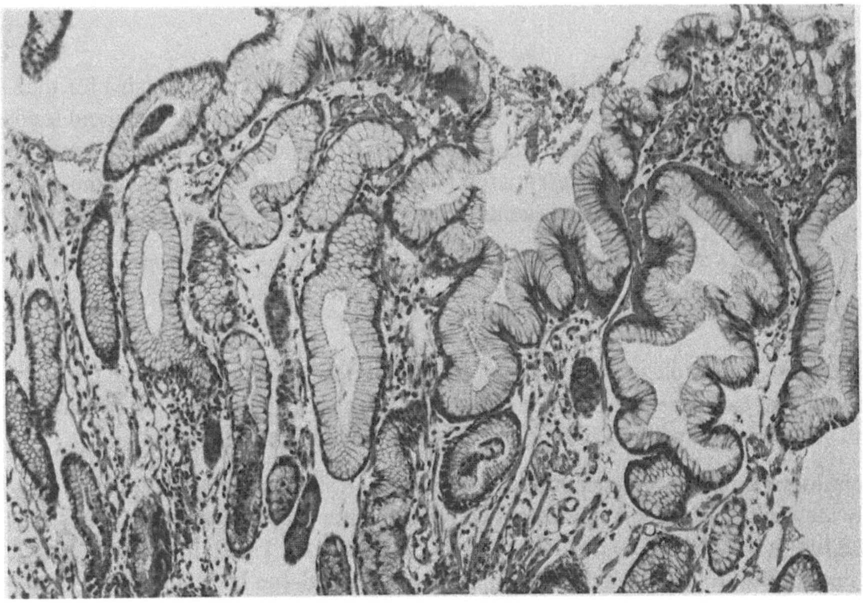

Fig. 2. Foveolar (focal) hyperplasia; deep elongated winding and branching pits; high cylindric epithelium, no inflammatory infiltration. H&E x 150

gether here. The excessive foveolar proliferation seen in Ménétrier's disease is more than an "inflammatory reaction." In the neighbourhood of tumors, especially of submucosal lesions, foveolar hyperplasia is not an unusual finding (Fig. 4). It is here in a pure form because the tunica propria is not infiltrated by inflammatory cells; no epithelial alteration is seen. This may be the reason why this lesion has commonly been called "hyperplastic polyp." The term could lead to misinterpretation, since the same name has been applied to a colonic polyp. The hyperplastic polyp of the large bowel is however organotypical and shows a characteristic histologic pattern which is determined by altered cell kinetics (*Wiebecke* et al., 1969; *Hayashi* et al., 1974). The term focal foveolar hyperplasia, as a descriptive finding, is therefore more suitable for the definition of this type of gastric polyp. In the classification of benign epithelial polyps of *Ming* (1973) this polyp is not included. This can be explained by the fact that we are dealing with a reactive process and not with a "true gastric polyp." However, the clinical discovery of a polyp, whatever it may be histologically, has to be defined by the pathologist. The presence of an epithelial proliferation justifies the grouping under epithelial polyps.

2. The Hyperplasiogenous Polyp

If one classifies the various polyps by the type of epithelium from which they were generated, it is important to know the origin. It is conceivable that either epithelium of the surface, of the foveolae, or of the glandular body may proliferate. Indeed this pattern of devel-

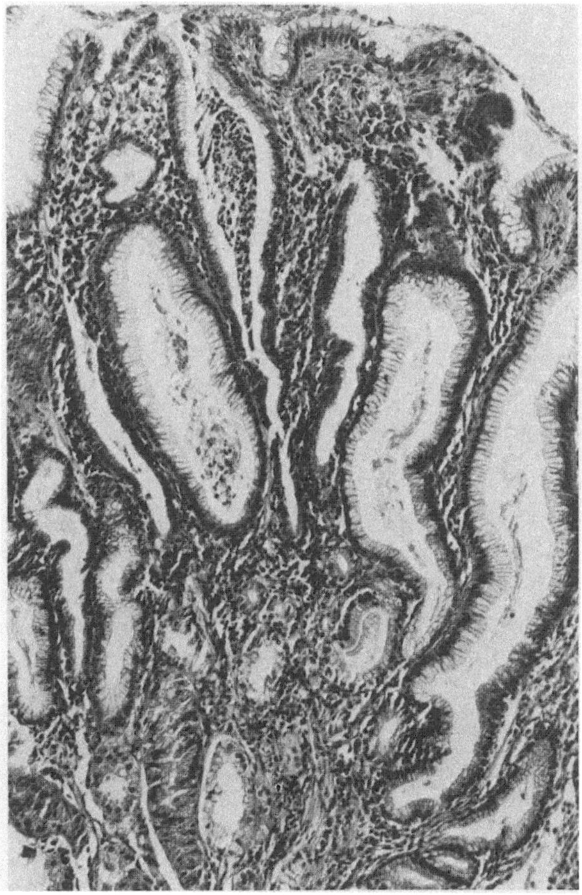

Fig. 3. Foveolar (focal) hyperplasia with inflammatory cellular infiltration in lamina propria. Leukocytic exudate within pit. Characteristic finding for border of chronic (complete) erosion. H&E x 150

opment is seen in the most common type of gastric polyps (*Ming*, 1973; *Seifert* and *Elster*, 1975) (Figs. 5 and 6). Histologically they are characterized by an irregular broadened contour of pits and crests as is also seen in focal hyperplasia. The epithelium is strikingly cylindrical; the nuclei are small and situated at the base. The elongated pits communicate with glandular formations. They have epithelium of the foveolar type and are of variable width. One should not assume that these glandular components develop from the gastric glands (Fig. 7). Although between these groups of glands, which are commonly cystic, cells of the gastric glands may be seen – depending on the topography – they show no tendency to proliferate. The tunica propria is often edematous and loosened, and exhibits, especially in the area close to the surface, profuse capillarization, occasionally resembling an angioma. In addition, bundles of smooth muscle fibers are seen which are terminations of a splintering and branching muscularis mucosae (*Muto* and *Oota*, 1970). In varying density plasma cells with Russel bodies are demonstrable near the surface within the tunica propria. The type of epithelium in the area of the hyperplastic foveolae can, however, vary,

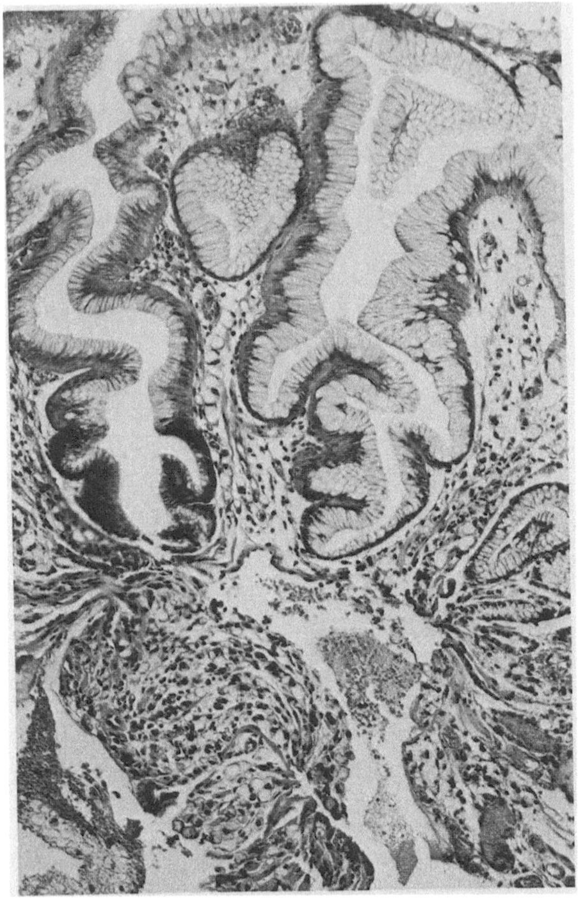

Fig. 4. Foveolar (focal) hyperplasia overlying small signet ring cell carcinoma. H&E x 180

so that occasional goblet cells are found; but the full pattern of intestinal metaplasia with Paneth cells is not seen in this type of polyp (Fig. 8). Epithelial dedifferentiation with flattened epithelium, intensive staining of the cytoplasm, and to a certain degree nuclear pleomorphism is occasionally observed in the vicinity of erosive lesions with a marked inflammatory reaction. However, these changes never reach the intensity of a borderline lesion.

This complex pattern resembles a hamartoma, but the classical definition of a faulty compostion or organ-specific tissue does not apply completely. The picture is determined by the hyperplastic foveolae. The "adenomatous" formations also exhibit the basic structure of foveolae, especially in regard to the type of epithelium. The cells of the gastric glands are largely displaced and play no part in the histogenesis of the polyp. Under these circumstances, with the preponderance of hyperplastic components, we prefer to call this polyp "hyperplasiogenous" (H.P.G.) (*Elster*, 1973). The terms hyperplastic-adenomatous polyp

(*Ming*, 1973) or adenomatous polyp (*Muto* and *Oota*, 1970) do not indicate that this polyp is very different from the "true" adenoma.

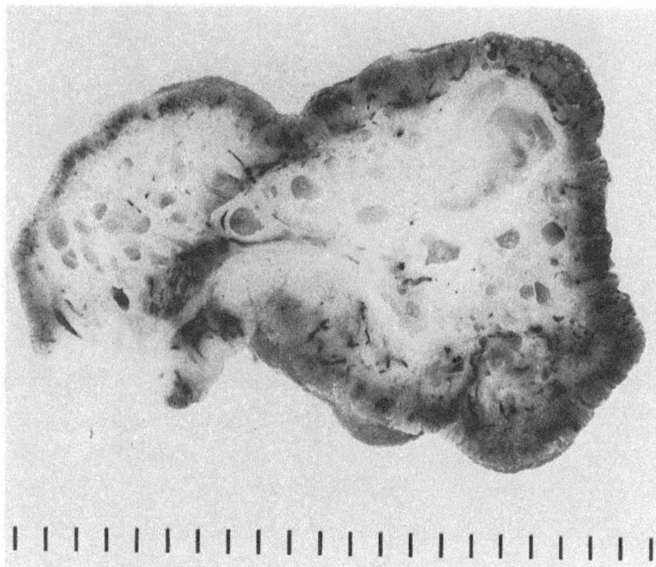

Fig. 5. Hyperplasiogenous polyp: macroscopic section. Dark border is hyperplastic component of foveolar region, lighter center is cystic region. H&E x 10

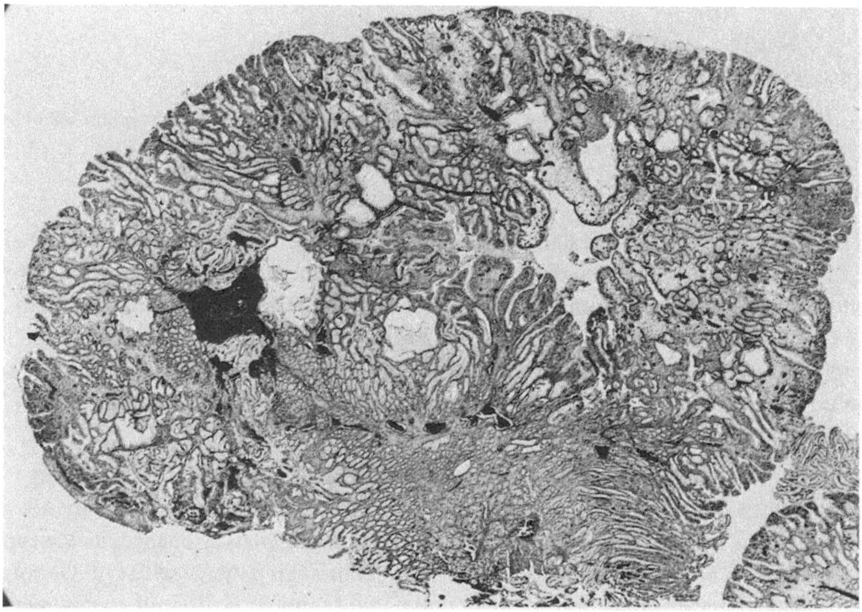

Fig. 6. Hyperplasiogenous polyp section: smooth transition from superficial hyperplastic foveolae to deeper glandlike formations. H&E x 10

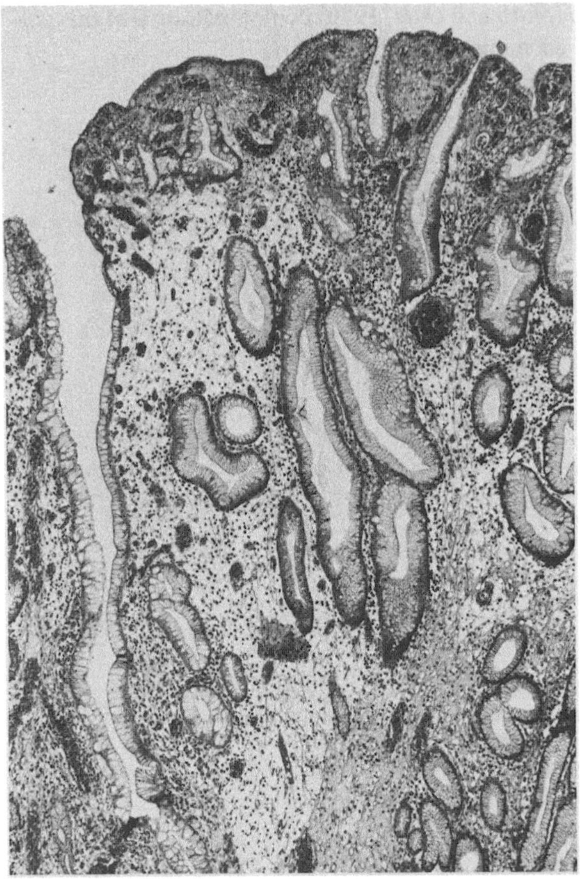

Fig. 7. Hyperplasiogenous polyp; superficial section with irregular deep pits, epithelium tall cylindrical. In deeper layer occasional glands with similar epithelium. H&E x 120

In addition it must be emphasized that the H.P.G.-polyp has no counterpart in other parts of the gastrointestinal tract and is thereby organotypical for the stomach. No comparison can be made with the adenomatous polyp of the colon. This is especially important because the H.P.G.-polyp of the stomach has no potential for malignant degeneration. If cellular atypia caused by surface necrosis with attempted regeneration occurs, this has to be interpreted differently from the cellular atypia chracteristic of the adenomatous polyp of the colon.

The intermediate position of the H.P.G.-polyp between hyperplasia and neoplasia is expressed by the fact that a tendency toward malignant degeneration is generally not observed (excluding, of course, secundary erosive and inflammatory changes at the surface). But there is an increased incidence of gastric carcinoma in patients with H.P.G.-polyps, with no anatomical connection between polyp and tumor. It is difficult to comment on this unusual "blastomatous potency" of the polyp-bearing stomach because only a few cases have been reported (*Bötticher* et al., 1975). However, *Roesch* (1976) reported an

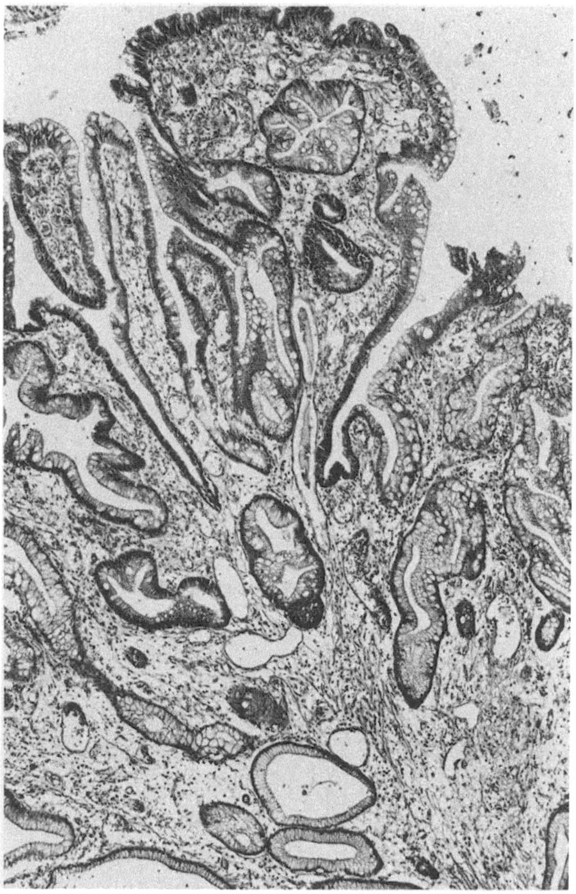

Fig. 8. Hyperplasiogenous polyp with goblet cells in epithelium. Intense capillarization of lamina propria; small disordered smooth muscle bundles are seen. H&E x 120

incidence of 18% H.P.G.-polyps in stomachs with an early gastric carcinoma and of 10% in advanced carcinoma.

In summarizing, it has to be stressed that this common type of gastric polyp is characterized by special structural, cellular, and pathogenetic criteria. Ignorance of the pecularities has not only led to misunderstandings in terminology of gastric polyps but also to misinterpretation.

3. The Adenomas

Two basic formations of the mucosa come under consideration with regard to the origin of adenomas: the gastric glands and the regenerative zone of the glandular neck region. Thus adenomas of different grades of differentiation can be expected. Proliferation of the gastric glands in the fundic region is known in its diffuse form as the Zollinger-Ellison syndrome.

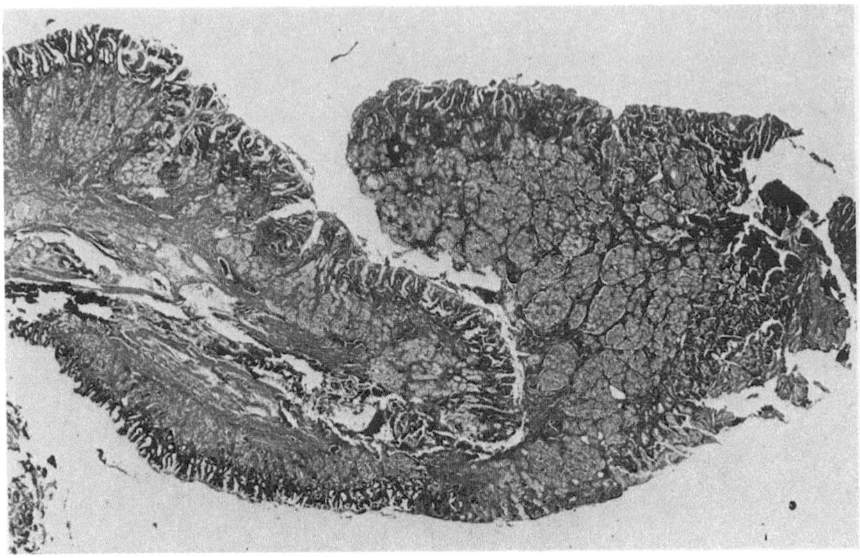

Fig. 9. Adenoma-like lesion of pyloric glands, possibly only glandular hyperplasia. H&E x 8

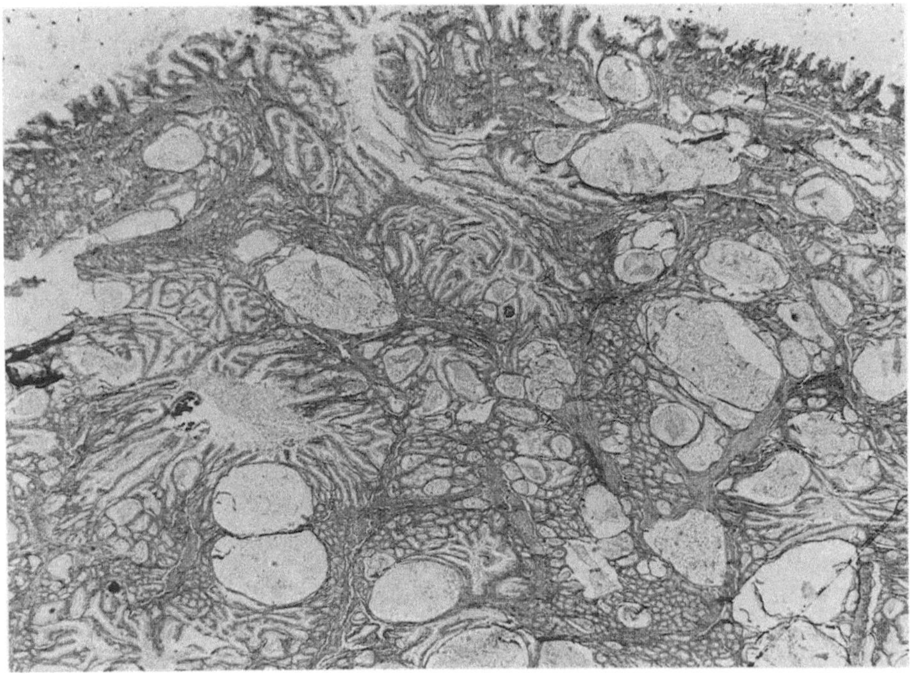

Fig. 10. Adenoma of cardiac glands: basic glandular structure is intact. Papillary proliferation of epithelium in glandular cysts. H&E x 10

Within the antrum, however, and especially in the prepyloric region, a proliferation of mucoid glands with lobule formation is occasionally seen resulting in an adenoma-like lesion. Applying critical standards one has to confess that this could also be called hyperplasia, especially when encapsulation is lacking (Fig. 9). This is underlined by a complete absence of dedifferentiation of the epithelium. One should, therefore, be very reluctant to make a diagnosis of a highly dedifferentiated adenoma of the antral or pyloric region. The same is true of the cardiac region (Fig. 10).

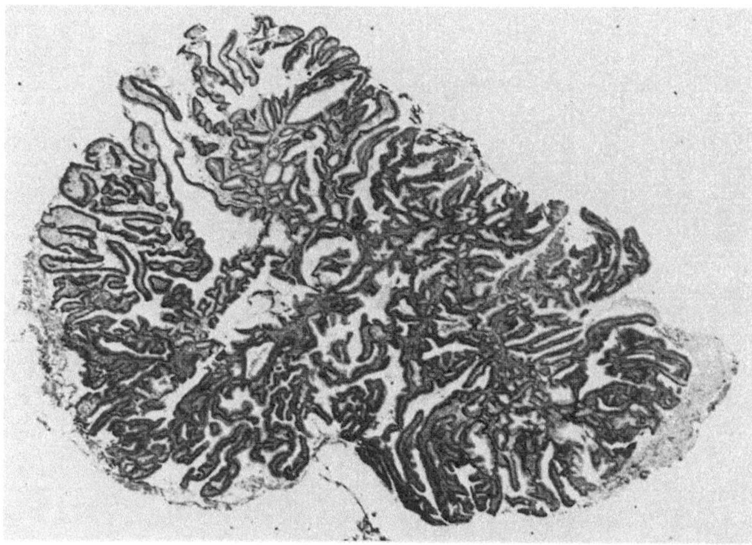

Fig. 11. Adenoma with predominant papillary formations with "indifferent" flat-cuboid epithelium (papillary adenoma). H&E x 10

The neoplastic proliferation of the neck cells without atypia results usually in papillary-adenomatous formations. The epithelium covering the papillae and the glands is flat-cuboid and shows homogeneously formed round nuclei corresponding to the glandular neck cells (Fig. 11). Under these circumstances the evaluation must cause problems since the old problem of differentiation between "reactive dysplasia" and "neoplastic dysplasia" arises. The judgment is made more difficult by the fact that such papillary adenomas are usually situated in the cardiac regions with all its difficult therapeutic implications and consequences. These "true" adenomas are a very rare finding, however (*Ming*, 1973; *Seifert* and *Elster*, 1975).

4. Proliferation with Cellular Atypia (Borderline Lesion: Protruded Type)

From the pathogenetic aspect the borderline lesion is also caused by proliferation of neck cells. However, in contrast to the above-mentioned adenoma, we are concerned here with a primary cellular atpypia. This atypia may be of differing intensity and severity as described by various authors (*Sugano* et al., 1971; *Grundmann*, 1975; *Nagayo*, 1975). In the development of these proliferations toward a "polyp" the cellular atypia reaches a stage which leads to the classification of "borderline lesion" (Fig. 12). Use of this term means that the cellular pattern alone does not allow a decision as to whether we are dealing with a hyperplastic or with a neoplastic process. Recently, these changes have also been called a subtype – IIa (*Fukuchi* et al., 1975). This term, too, indicates developmental direction toward an early gastric carcinoma (Fig. 13). Clinically, the picture of a flat broad-based polyp is seen.

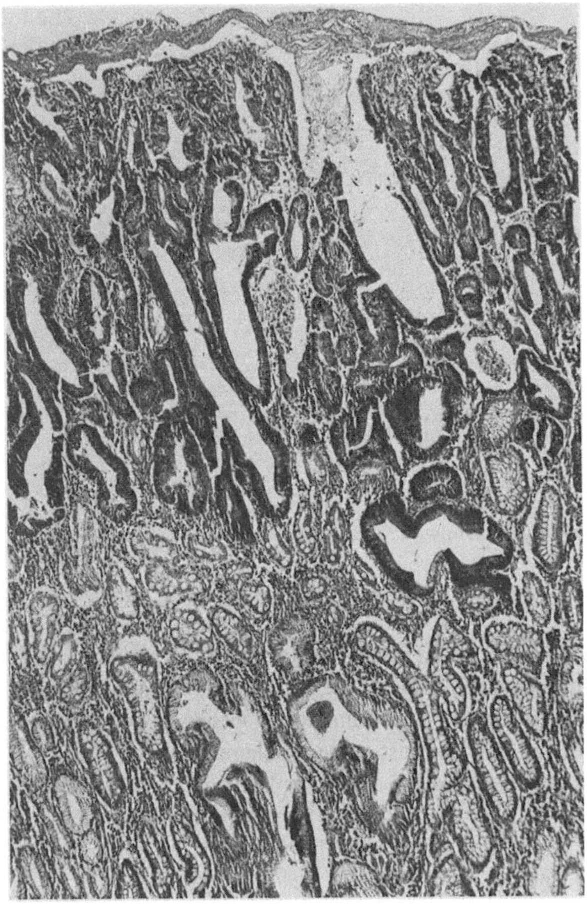

Fig. 12. Glandular-neck proliferation with cell atypia (borderline lesion) in form of polyp. H&E x 120

The criterion for classification as an early gastric carcinoma type I is merely a greater degree of exophytic proliferation. With respect to the pathogenesis the term polypoid carcinoma is preferable to carcinomatous polyp. The precursor of the early gastric cancer type IIa and I is usually the borderline lesion, whereas the "malignant degeneration" of a H.P.G.-polyp is extremely rare if it exists at all. More likely this transformation occurs in the rare case of a true adenoma.

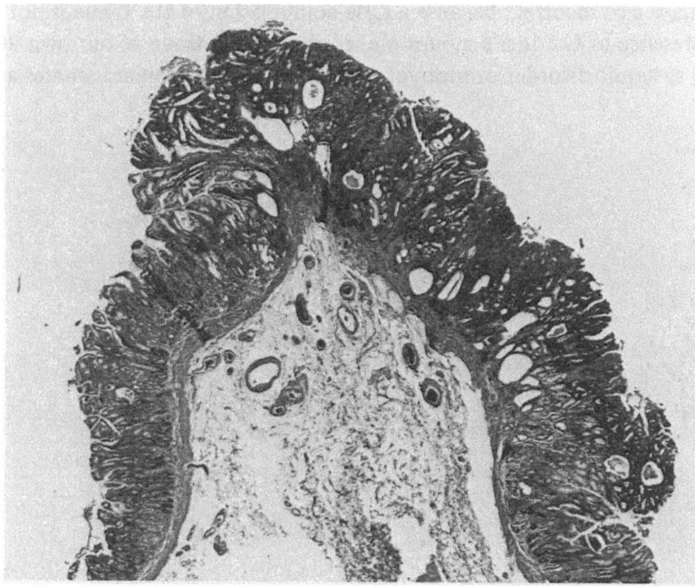

Fig. 13. Early carcinoma type IIa in form of polyp. H&E x 8

5. Gastric Polyposis

Theoretically all the above mentioned types of polyps may be multiple and in sufficient number to justify the term polyposis. However, this applies essentially to the focal hyperplasias and the H.P.G.-polyps. Multiple bean-sized polyps, arranged in rows, which are usually found in the antrum, are caused by chronic or complete erosions in the healing stage or in scar formation.

A true polyposis of H.P.G.-polyps seldom occurs, and its location may be different from that described in the literature. In one of our more than 50 cases, polyps of up to cherry-size were located exclusively in the fundic mucosa allowing a sharp demarcation from the antrum.

Multiple, but usually minute, polyps characterize a polypoid process which can not be classified according to pathogenesis nor by structure as are the above mentioned polyps. Grossly the polyps have a glassy appearance and show histologically a flat, uniform contour or short gastric pits. The tunica propria exhibits no cellular infiltration. Within the gastric glands – this finding is limited to the fundic mucosa and the intermediate zone – cysts of variable size can be seen which are usually lined by epithelium. Although this epithelial border may be flattened, chief cells and parietal cells are easily recognized.

Only occasionally is a cyst with gastric pit epithelium found in segments near the surface. The glandular body is remarkably intact; no reactive changes are seen (Fig. 14). The term gastritis cystica superficialis is obsolete since inflammatory cells are lacking. A neoplastic process can be ruled out in the absence of epithelial proliferation. The definition of hamartoma is also incorrect because a false composition of the tissue is not present. Whether the presence of Gardner's syndrome, as observed in three of our own 90 cases, indicates some systemic disorder cannot yet be decided since follow-up studies are not complete.

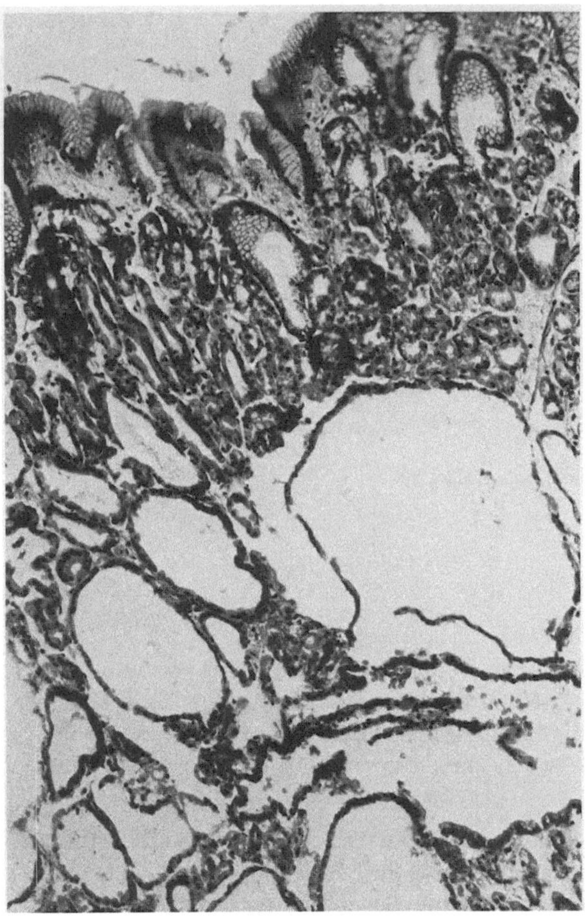

Fig. 14. Cysts of gastric glands; cysts of varying size, lined by flattened glandular epithelium. No alteration of surface. H&E x 150

The uncertainty in the pathogenesis and histologic evaluation of this finding was the reason why we prefer the descriptive diagnosis "cysts of the gastric glands". The term "gastric cystic polyposis" (*Chakravorty* and *Schatzki*, 1975) as an anatomical diagnosis is not acceptable because there may be single or multiple polyps.

Gastric polyps in the Cronkhite-Canada-Syndrome show a cystic pattern similar to the above mentioned cysts of the gastric glands. However, here an inflammatory cellular reaction is usually seen. The cysts are lined with pit epithelium and usually a local connection to the pits is seen (Fig. 15). According to our definition this polypoid lesion cannot be called an epithelial polyp.

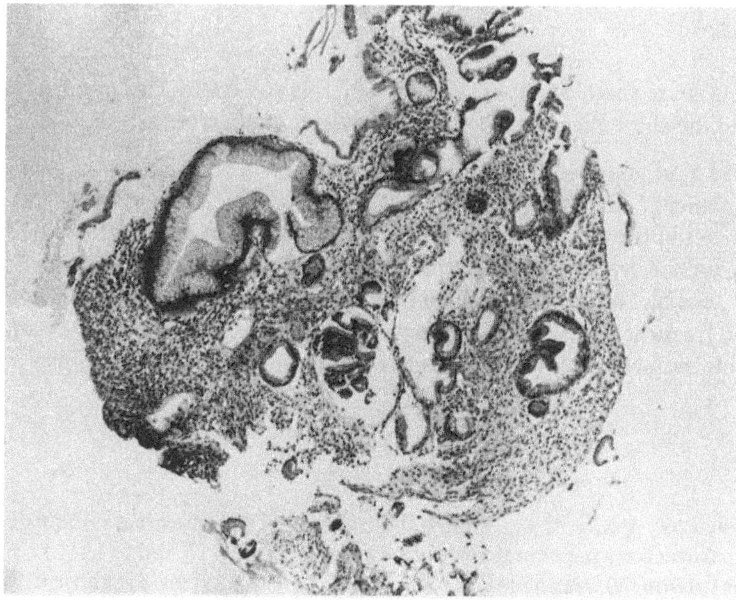

Fig. 15. Biopsy of polyp (Cronkhite-Canada-Syndrome). Cysts with foveolar epithelium, lamina propria with cellular infiltration. H&E x 120

The hamartomatous Peutz-Jeghers polyp, which is a manifestation of an inherited disorder is said to occur in the stomach in 24% of patients with this syndrome (*Bartholomew* et al., 1962). The histologic pattern resembles in general the intestinal polyps with prominent "hypertrophic foveolar cells" whereas the gastric glands are inconspicuous. Branches of the muscularis mucosae growing towards the mucosal surface are characteristic.

Returning to the discussion of surface structure one of our cases can be used as an example. We received a biopsy from the tip of a polyp which we diagnosed as focal hyperplasia. Later the excised specimen proved, however, to be a hamartomatous polyp. This finding emphasizes the multiple possible causes of focal hyperplasia.

6. Summary

The following classification of epithelial gastric polyps is suggested: *(Footnote see p. 92)

Term	Tissue of origin	Pathogenesis	Localization
Focal hyperplasia	Foveolar epithelium	Hyperplasia	anywhere
Hyperplasiogenous polyp	Foveolar epithelium	Hyperplasia + glandular component	anywhere
Adenoma, high differentiation	Gastric glands (of pyloric type)	Blastoma (neoplasia)	antrum-pylorus-cardia
Adenoma, moderate differentiation	Neck cells	Blastoma (neoplasia)	Predominantly cardia
Borderline lesion-protruded type (subtype IIa)	Neck cells	Hyperplasia with atypia – blastoma	anywhere
Early carcinoma type IIa + I	Neck cells	Blastoma (neoplasia)	anywhere

III. Conclusions

It is our intention to forgo a historical review of terms and classifications of gastric polyps so as to avoid the above mentioned confusion in the literature.

Data from the literature reporting a malignancy rate of gastric polyps between 4 and 80% are "pathognomonic" for the old classifications or for the omission of a clear-cut differentiation between histologic types. This classification does not pretend to be final; it should be used as a working hypothesis. With the development and increased use of endoscopic polypectomy the fact has emerged that gastric polyps are by no means rarities. Because of the increased frequency of excision of gastric polyps for examination by the pathologist it is our aim to evaluate the clinical usefulness of this proposed classification.

References

Bartholomew, L.G., Moore, C.E., Dahlin, D.C., Waugh, J.M.: Intestinal polyposis associated with mucocutaneous pigmentation. Surg. Gynec. Obstet. 115, 1-11 (1962).

Bötticher, R., Bünte, H., Hermanek, P., Rösch, W.: Magenpolypen. Prognose u. Therapie. Dtsch. med. Wschr. 100, 167-170 (1975).

Chakravorty, R.C., Schatzki, P.F.: Gastric cystic polyposis. Digestive Diseases 20, 981-989 (1975).

Elster, K.: Morphologie der Polypen des oberen Verdauungstraktes. In: Endoskopische Polypektomie im Gastrointestinaltrakt. Stuttgart: Thieme 1973.

Elster, K.: A new approach to the classification of gastric polyps. Endoscopy 6, 44-47 (1974).

Fukuchi, S., Hiyama, M., Mochizuki, T.: Endoscopic diagnosis of IIa-subtype of polypoid lesions which belong to borderline lesions between benignancy and malignancy. Stomach and Intest. 10, 1487-1493 (1975).

Goldman, R.L., Friedman, N.B.: Neurogenic nature of so-called inflammatory fibroid polyps of the stomach. Cancer (Philad.) 20, 134-143 (1967).

Grundmann, E.: Histologic types and possible initial stages in early gastric carcinoma. Beitr. Path. 154, 256-280 (1975).

Hayashi, T., Yatani, R., Apostol, J., Stemmermann, G.N.: Pathogenesis of hyperplastic polyps of the colon: A hypothesis based on ultrastructure and in vitro cell kinetics. Gastroent. 347-356 (1974).

Jansen, H.H.: Magen. In: Organpathologie, *W. Doerr* (ed.). Stuttgart: Thieme 1974, Vol. II.

Kawai, K., Akasaka, Y., Shimamoto, K., Kohli, Y., Murakami, K., Kobayashi, A., Misaki, F.: Differential Diagnosis of Polypoid Lesion of Stomach. Gastroenterologia Japonica 5, 215-221 (1970).

Ming, S.Ch.: Benign epithelial polyps. In: Tumors of the Esophagus and Stomach. Atlas of Tumor Pathology. Washington, D.C.: Armed Forces Institute of Pathology 1973.

---

* Footnote to page 91

The various types of polyps such as those found in Peutz-Jeghers-Syndrome, Cronkhite-Canada-Syndrome and Gardner's syndrome are not listed here, since they are not only polypoid gastric lesions but are part of generalized disorders.

Monaco, A., Roth, S.J., Castleman, B., Welch, C.E.: Adenomatous polyps of the stomach. Cancer (Phila.) 15, 456-467 (1962).

Morson, B.C.: Some pecularities in the histology of intestinal polyps. Dis. Colon Rectum 5, 337-344 (1962).

Morson, B.C., Dawson, I.M.P.: Gastrointestinal Pathology. Oxford–London: Blackwell 1972.

Muto, T., Oota, K.: Polypogenesis of gastric mucosa. GANN. 61, 435-442 (1970).

Nagayo, T.: Histological Criteria of Malignant Transformation of Gastric Polyp and its Results. Stomach and Intest. 10, 301-308 (1975).

Nakamura, T.: Pathohistologische Einteilung der Magenpolypen mit spezifischer Betrachtung ihrer malignen Entartung. Chirurg 41, 122-130 (1970).

Rösch, W.: Magenfrühkarzinom –Makroskopie und Biopsie. Erfahrungen bei 50 Fällen. Akt. Gastrologie 1976 (in press).

Seifert, E., Elster, K.: Gastric polypectomy. Amer. J. Gastroent. 63, 451-456 (1975).

Sugano, H., Nakamura, K., Takayi, K.: An atypical epithelium of the stomach. Gann Monograph on Cancer Research 11, 257-263 (1971).

Wanke, M.: Magen. In: Spezielle Pathologische Anatomie, *W.Doer, G. Seifert, E. Uehlinger* (eds.). Berlin–Heidelberg–New York: Springer 1971, Vol. II/1.

Wiebecke, B., Löhrs, U., Brandts, A., Eder, M.: Vergleichende tierexperimentelle und bioptische Untersuchungen zur Morphogenese der Dickdarmpolypen. Verh. dtsch. Ges. Path. 53, 239-243 (1969).

Polyps and Cancer of the Large Bowel

H.T. ENTERLINE

The title of this chapter bears within it a major reason for both our delay in understanding the adenoma-carcinoma relationship and for mismanagement of some patients presenting with one or more polypoid lesions of the colon and rectum. "Polyp" is a nonspecific term to which any lesion is entitled that has the characteristic of being a circumscribed protuber-

Table 1. Classification of Colonic Polyps

Single or multiple polyp	Polyposes
A. Reactive	
Inflammatory (inflammatory pseudopolyp)	Inflammatory polyposis
Colitis cystica profunda	
Lymphoid	Lymphoid polyposis
B. Nonneoplastic growth disorder	
Peutz-Jeghers	Peutz-Jeghers polyposis
Juvenile (retention)	Juvenile polyposis
Metaplastic (hyperplastic)	
C. Of uncertain nature	
Inflammatory fibroid polyp (eosinophilic granuloma, localized)	Cronkhite-Canada syndrome Juvenile polyposis of infancy
D. Neoplastic other than adenomatous	
Lipoma	Lipomatous polyposis
Leiomyoma	Lymphosarcomatous polyposis
Carcinoid	Leukemic polyposis
Polypoid carcinoma	
Other (by predominant component)	Other (by predominant component)
E. Neoplastic – adenomatous	
Tubular (glandular adenoma, adenoma)	Adenomatosis (familial adenomatous polyposis, multiple polyposis coli)
Tubulo-villous (mixed, villoglandular)	Adenomatous variants
Villous (papillary adenoma)	Gardner's syndrome
	Other (named by associated lesions)

ance into the bowel lumen. This is a trite statement, but all too frequently the term is equated as synonymous with adenoma. An adenoma is not of necessity polypoid and certainly not all polyps are adenoma. There are, of course, a wide variety of polypoid lesions of widely varying histology and significance. In the first table (Table 1) I have suggested a classification of polyps and polyposes and have placed in parentheses synonyms which are often used but to the author's mind are less preferable. Unfortunately there is not yet complete agreement on terminology.

In the following pages the various types of polyps and polyposes which may involve the large bowel are described and our present understanding of their relationship to cancer of various types is discussed.

I. Inflammatory Polyps (Inflammatory Pseudopolyp)

Colitis cystica profunda, juvenile polyps, lymphoid polyps, and others have been considered, with varying degrees of justification, to be inflammatory. Since this is a debatable assumption, they will be discussed separately.

I see no justification for the term "inflammatory pseudopolyp" since polyps arising in the course of ulcerative or granulomatous colitis meet the previously criteria for polyp.

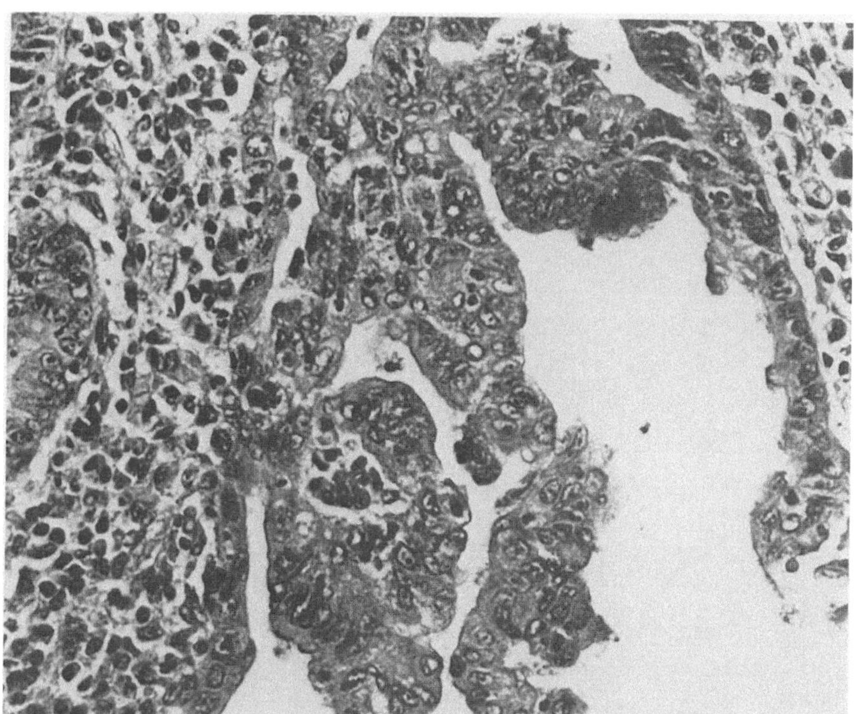

Fig. 1. Regeneration atypia near edge of ulcer in inflammatory polyp. Note loss of polarity and nuclear variation. X 300

Isolated, usually small, inflammatory polyps unassociated with colitis are rather frequent in the rectum. They show little but edema, hyperemia, and variable degrees of lymphocytic or polymorphonuclear infiltrate. Focal ulceration may be present. The crypt epithelium is unremarkable except for occasional cytoplasmic and nuclear irregularities of regenerative nature (Fig. 1). Care should be taken not to consider focal lymphoid aggregates, which are a normal feature of colonic mucosa, as evidence of colitis.

II. Inflammatory Polyps Associated with Colitis

These vary in size from small mucosal tags to large elaborate polypoid masses which, when pedunculated, may have bifid or trifid stalks. Their histology varies depending on the severity of the basic colitis. In remission phases the polyp mucosal epithelium will often form distorted or branched crypts or small mucus filled cysts. In any event, as in the solitary inflammatory polyp, the nuclei do not have the crowded appearance of adenoma. The stroma is not as relatively abundant as in the juvenile polyp and they lack the smooth muscle bands of the Peutz-Jeghers polyp. Again, a certain degree of surface atypia may be disregarded as regenerative and should not be confused with carcinoma in situ. They arise from a concurrent undermining of mucosa by ulceration and by regeneration.

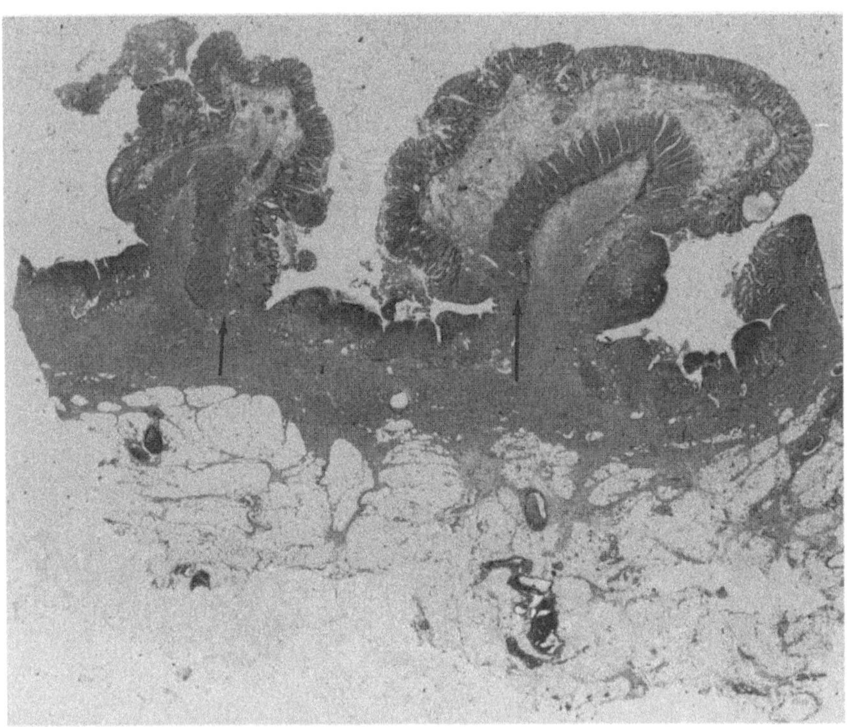

Fig. 2. "Pseudo" polyp in toxic megacolon of ulcerative colitis. Area between arrows has undergone complete loss of muscularis. X 4

Inflammatory polyposis is commonly diffuse, involving all or much of the colon and rectum. Such cases may be confused, both by X-ray and on gross examination, with familial adenomatous polyposis. The polyps on the other hand, may be only occasional or, especially in granulomatous colitis, present as groups of closely appressed polyps in a narrow segment or segments. We have seen polyps produced by another mechanism in toxic megacolon. In the case of ulcerative colitis illustrated, ulceration had essentially destroyed all coats. Much of the colonic wall consisted only of serosa and fibrous reaction. The polyps consisted of residual islands of preserved mucosa and muscularis (Fig. 2).

The increased risk of adenocarcinoma in longstanding ulcerative colitis is well accepted. It does not appear that inflammatory polyps are important in the pathogenesis of the carcinomas which may occur. Most such carcinomas in our experience and others have been rather diffuse. Precancerous changes have been described by *Morson* and *Dawson* (1972). *Dawson* and *Pryse-Davies* (1959) warn that one cannot assume that polyps occurring in patients with ulcerative colitis are inflammatory but may be adenomas or carcinoma. In 9 of 17 cases, in their series, of ulcerative colitis in which carcinoma had developed, adenomatous polyps were also present. They describe what they interpret as transition from polyps of inflammatory to adenomatous type. Their illustrations do not permit judging this point.

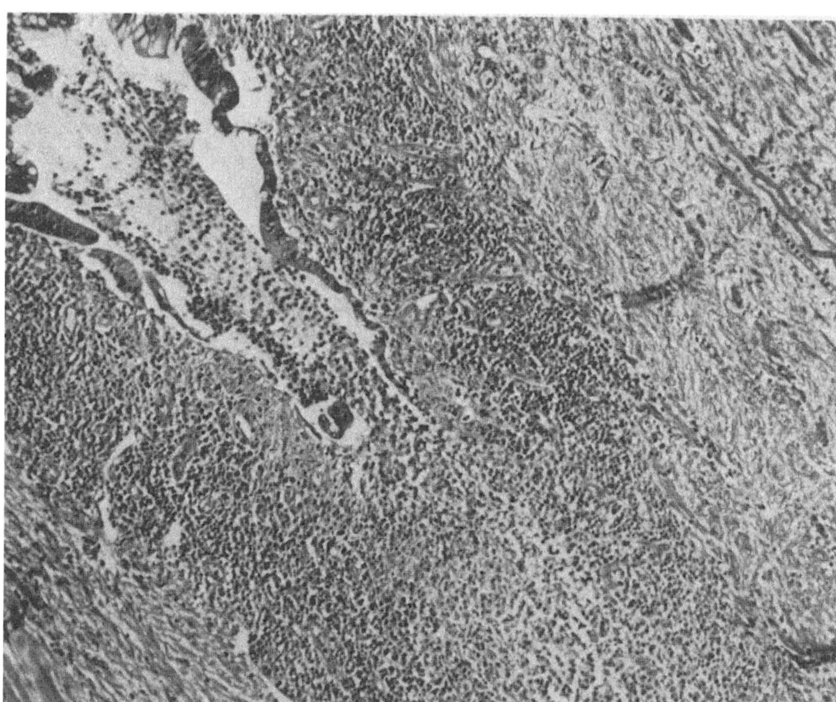

Fig. 3. Epithelization of fissure ulcer in granulomatous enteritis. X 60

III. Colitis Cystica Profunda

This condition, first described by *Virchow* (1863), exists in both diffuse and localized forms. In both it consists of mucus-filled cysts within the submucosa. The descrete form

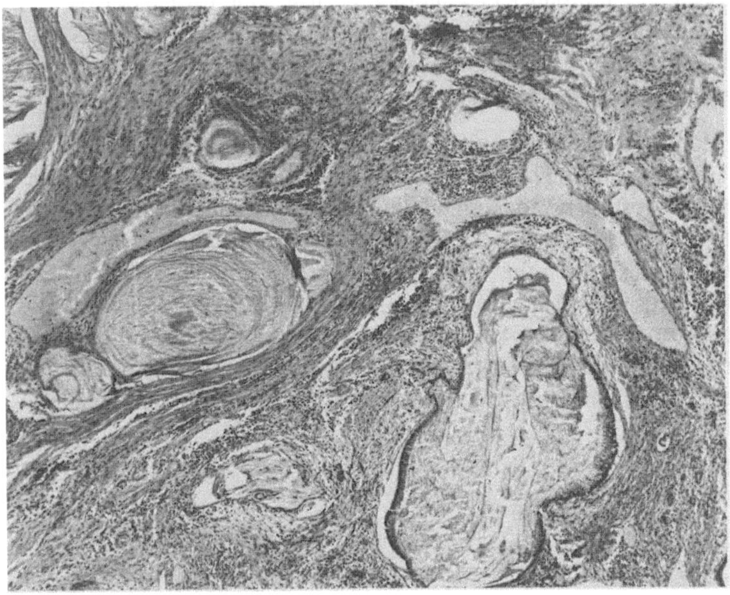

Fig. 4. Colitis cystica profunda. Rectal polyp near anus showing submucosal mucin-filled cysts. X 40

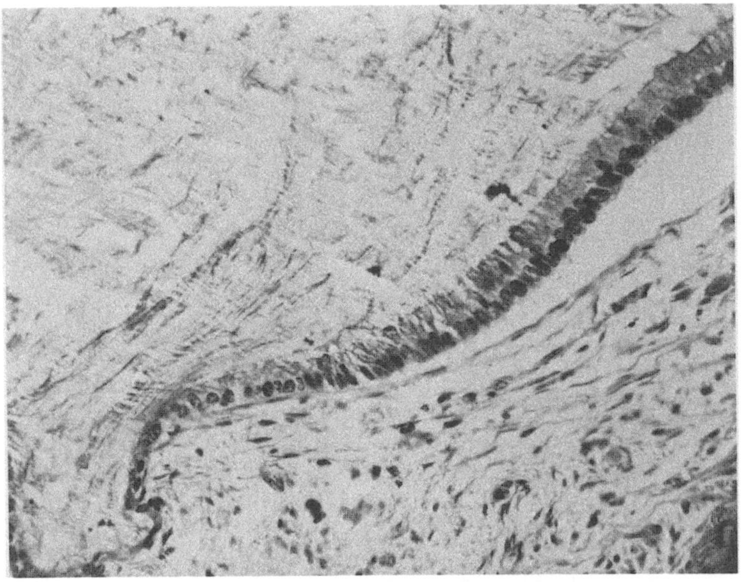

Fig. 5. Colitis cystica profunda. Detail of cyst lining from Figure 4 epithelium. Note lack of nuclear crowding, abundant goblet cells. X 250

occurs chiefly in the rectum and presents as polyps, masses or plaques. According to *Wayte* and *Helwig* (1967) the patients usually present with rectal bleeding, prolapse or tenesmus. These lesions are probably of inflammatory origin, i.e. sequelae of colitis or trauma. A hamartomatous origin has also been proposed by *Allen* (1966). *Buckwalter* and *Kent* (1972) have described submucosal glands without cysts in a patient with diverticulitis and suggests defects of the muscularis mucosa as important in pathogenesis.

The author has seen one case of Crohn's disease with similar glands and cysts extending into the muscularis of the terminal ileum. Some of these foci suggest epithelization of fissure ulcers as a pathogenetic mechanism (Fig. 3).

There is no evidence to suggest that these peculiar lesions are precancerous. The problem is rather in mistaking them for carcinoma. The cysts may lack epithelium in whole or part. Where present, the epithelium is well differentiated, well polarized, rich in goblet cells, and does not show either the crowded nuclei of adenoma or the hyperchromatism, loss of polarity, and pleomorphism of most carcinomas (Figs. 4 and 5). Signet cells or cell clusters are not present. The patients are distinctly younger on average than those with carcinoma. Diagnostic error will be minimal if one considers the younger age of the patient, insists on adequate biopsy, and does not consider ectopic epithelium or mucin pools as of necessity malignant by virtue of location. Rare adenocarcinomas are focally so well differentiated that confusion is possible, but the crowded nuclei suggest adenoma rather than colitis cystica (Fig. 6).

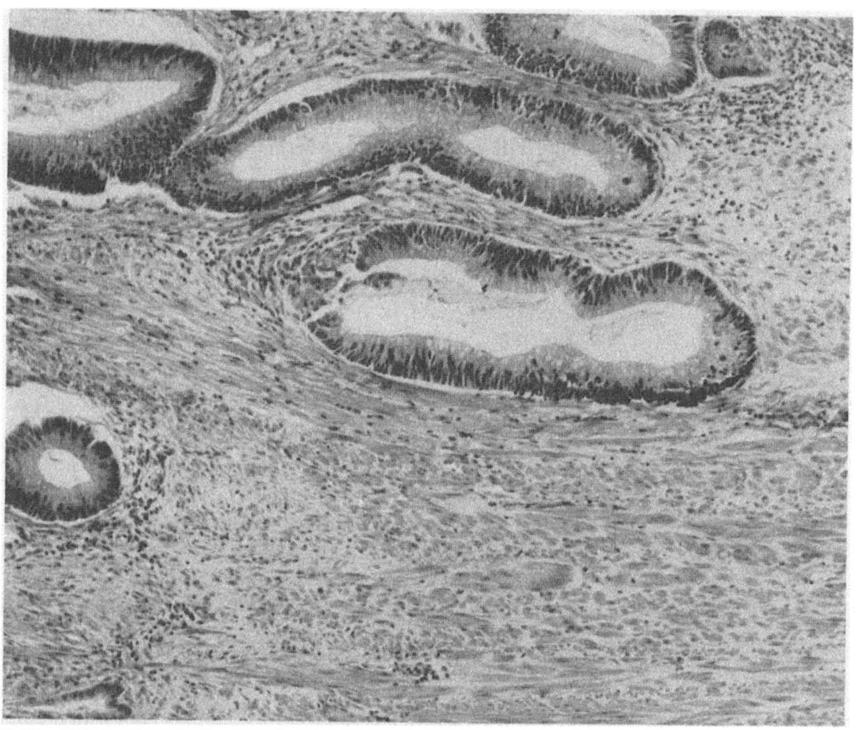

Fig. 6. Highly differentiated adenocarcinoma in muscularis. This area indistinguishable from adenoma except by position deep in muscularis. Less differentiated elsewhere with no adenomatous remnant. x 150

IV. Lymphoid Polyps and Lymphoid Polyposis

Several forms of polypoid lymphoid infiltrates are now fairly well recognized. Two of these are localized lesions. The first, lymphoid hyperplasia of the terminal ileum, consists of a polypoid or cobblestone thickening of terminal ileum in children and may act as a site for intussusception into the caecum (*Danis*, 1974). The cause is unknown. Lymphoid polyps in the adult are usually restricted to the anal verge and lower rectum. These may be up to 5 cm in size and may be multiple. They were first clearly separated by *Helwig* and *Hansen* (1951) from nodular (follicular) lymphosarcoma by virtue of their primarily submucosal position, lack of free infiltration of mucosa, and especially by the presence of well defined germinal centers.

Diffuse lymphoid polyposis of the G.I. tract exists in several differing settings though histologically indistinguishable. The first of these is lymphoid polyposis associated with IgA deficiency and often with girardiasis. According to *Ajdukiewicz* et al. (1966) this form is chiefly, if not entirely, restricted to the small intestine. A similar lymphoid polyposis involving the colon of children without protein deficiencies has been described by *Capitanio* and *Kirkpatrick* (1970) and by *Robinson* et al. (1973). In this condition all or much of the colon and often the distal ileum is studded with small polyps which tend to be larger and more numerous as the rectum is approached. They are notable for gross umbilication producing a distinctive pattern on air contrast films.

Lymphoid polypoid hyperplasia of ileum and colon may occur associated with familial adenomatous polyposis or with Gardner's syndrome (*Shull* and *Fitts*, 1974). Involvement of the terminal ileum in such cases may lead to unnecessary partial ileectomy. At least three cases of needless colectomy have been reported in kindred of adenomatous polyposis families in which the colon was later found to be diffusely involved with lymphoid rather than adenomatous polyps. The importance of adequate biopsy samples of polyps before extensive surgery is obvious.

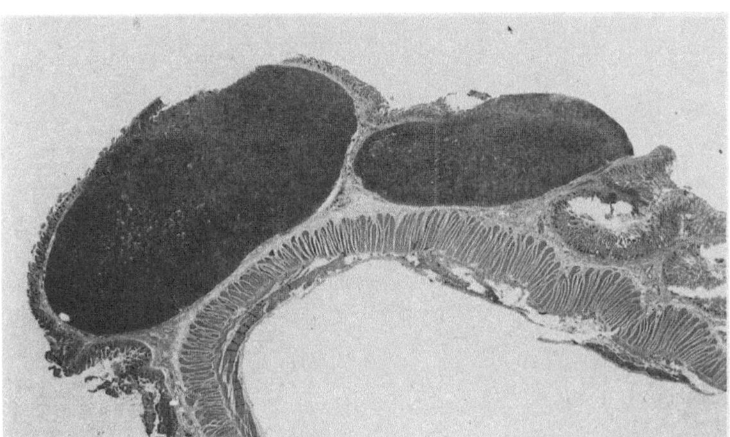

Fig. 7. Polypoid lymphosarcoma. Section from ileocecal region in a 75 year old man with multiple polyps of ileum, cecum and ascending colon. Polyps covered with normal mucosa. Apparent ulcer is sectioning artifact. X 5

All of these various polyposes are usually considered reactive to various infections or possibly other stimuli. All show well defined germinal centers. Lymphoid follicles are normal in the colon and should not be mistaken for polyposis.

Primary lymphosarcomas of various types of colon and rectum are usually bulky solitary tumors. Rarely, however, they may present, as may leukemia, as polyposis of small or large bowel. The term pseudoleukemia has in the past been applied to some of these. An example (see Fig. 7) was a 75 year old male who, at operation for sigmoid adenocarcinoma, was also found to have numerous grapelike, freely movable, mucosal polyps of terminal ileum and caecum. The histology was that of a lymphoblastic lymphosarcoma. The diagnosis of malignant lymphoid polyposis is not usually difficult if one bears in mind the lack of reaction centers, the monomorphic character of the infiltrate, and the free infiltration of mucosa by the lymphosarcomas. I know of no evidence to implicate benign lymphoid polyps and polyposes as predecessors of the malignant lymphoid disesases except for the indirect relationship of those associated with dysproteinemias which are largely of small intestine and need not concern us here.

V. Inflammatory Fibroid Polyp (Eosinophilic Granuloma)

These peculiar rare tumors are most common in the stomach and small bowel and will not be considered here. They have no known relationship to carcinoma.

VI. Peutz-Jeghers Polyposis

Peutz-Jeghers syndrome with its polyps and rather distinctive skin and oral mucosal pigmentation was described by *Peutz* in 1921 and became more widely recognized after the article by *Jeghers* and coworkers in 1949. It is usually thought of in connection with the small intestine since at this site the polyps more readily cause intussusception. The polyps, however, are distributed throughout the GI tract. In the recent review of *Utsunomiya* et al. (1975), 189 of their 222 patients developed polyps, at some stage, in the colon or rectum. The polyps apparently continue to appear and may either grow or remain static for long periods.

The gross appearance of these peculiar polyps is that of a firm lobulated or cerebriform mass, sessile or stalked. The histology is distinctive, consisting of (1) a variety of mature epithelial cells, typical of their site of origin (such as parietal cells, chief cells and goblet cells in Peutz-Jeghers gastric polyps); (2) strands of smooth muscle which course through and divide the polyp into sectors; and (3) orientation of the epithelium to the smooth muscle bands as they would to muscularis mucosae (Fig. 8). Mucin-filled cysts may occur and may involve the muscularis. Anaplasia and nuclear crowding are not a feature. These polyps are best thought of as being growth anomalies rather than neoplastic.

Though the syndrome is known to be familial, polyps and abnormal pigmentation may be independent of each other. *Gannon* et al. (1962) pointed out that solitary polyps, identical in structure, occur which lack both associated pigmentary changes or familial histories.

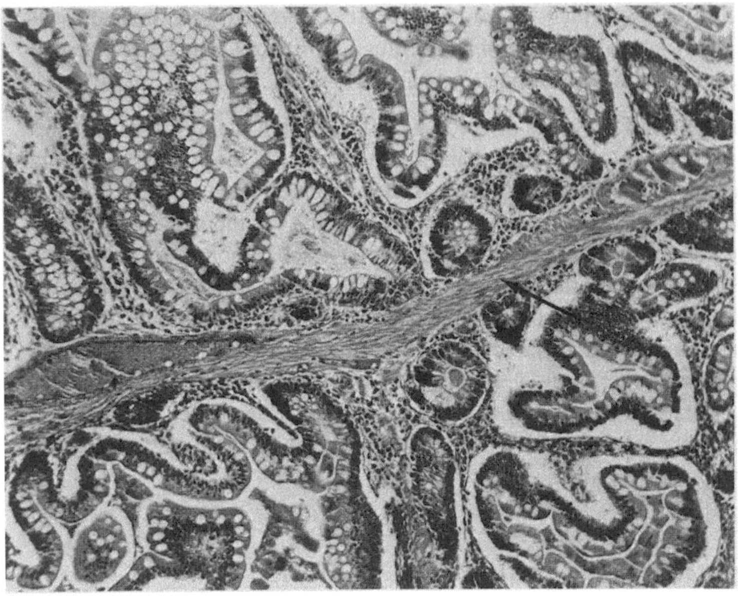

Fig. 8. Peutz-Jeghers polyp. Arrow points to one of many bands of smooth muscle dividing polyp into sectors. Note orientation of glands to smooth muscle as if muscularis mucosa. X 100

Because the pecular relationship to proliferated smooth muscle was mistaken for invasion, as were mucinous pools which may occur, earlier opinions held that a considerable percentage of these polyps was malignant. This view was corrected by the Mayo Clinic group (*Bartholomew* et al., 1962; *Dozois* et al., 1969). Following these reports the general opinion has been that these polyps have little or no precancerous disposition, see *Williams* (1965). This position seems too extreme.

Proof of origin of invasive carcinoma directly from Peutz-Jeghers polyps is rare although several polyps have been reported with foci of anaplasia justifying the term "in situ carcinoma." There are nonetheless a scattering of case reports of cancer in the upper gastrointestinal tract in young people who have the Peutz-Jeghers syndrome. In *Utsunomiya* et al.'s 1974 series of 222 cases from Japan the cause of death in four patients under the age of 30 was carcinoma (colon – 2, stomach – 1, and duodenum – 1). A total of 17 of the 36 deaths in the series of 222 patients were from cancer – chiefly of the colon. They reviewed reports of three deaths from adenocarcinoma of the stomach in teen age patients with this condition. Carcinoma of the colon is such a common neoplasm in the western world that proof by association is open to question.

Scully (1970) described and reported on a rare form of ovarian tumor which he termed "sex cord tumor with annular tubules." Six of the 13 cases were in patients with Peutz-Jeghers syndrome and only one of the seven other cases had been studied to adequately rule out the syndrome.

It seems reasonable to conclude at this time that (1) patients with the Peutz-Jeghers syndrome have an increased propensity to neoplasia, at least of the upper GI tract; (2) the order of magnitude of such associated malignancy is much less than that of the adenomatous polyposes; and (3) the exact definition of such risk needs further study.

VII. Juvenile Polyps and Polyposis

Juvenile polyps, sometimes called retention polyps, are another distinctive polyp which nonetheless has been only clearly separated from adenomatous polyps in the past 15 years (*Horrilleno* et al., 1959; *Morson*, 1962; *Roth* and *Helwig*, 1963). These polyps are most common in the rectum or sigmoid, but may occur at any site in the colon. Bleeding or prolapse of the polyp are the common presentations.

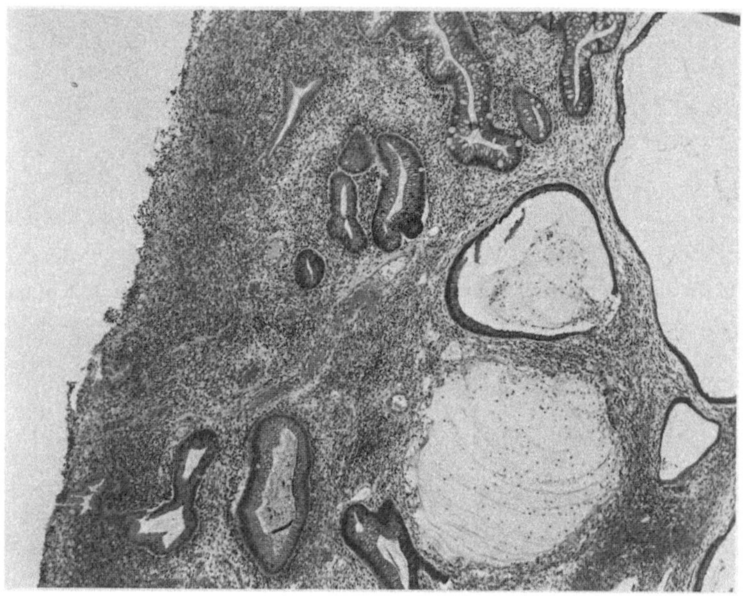

Fig. 9. Juvenile (retention) polyp. Patient aged 6 years. Note abundance of lamina propria, cystically dilated glands and irregular, slightly branched non-cystic glands. Note inflammatory infiltrate. X 40

These present as sessile or, more commonly, pedunculated rounded masses. Under the microscope they are composed of glands, usually cystic and often with some branching, whose epithelial cells show no evidence of crowding or anaplasia. The lamina propria is abundant and widely separates adjacent epithelial structures. The surface is usually, though not always, ulcerated. The cysts are mucin-filled and both cysts and stroma often show polymorphonuclear leukocyte infiltrates. Lymphoid aggregates may also occur. Evidence of hemorrhage in the form of hemosiderin-ladenmacrophages in these polyps is frequent. Eosinophils may also be present (Figs. 9 and 10).

About 15% of the patients have more than one such polyp either at the same time or developing later.

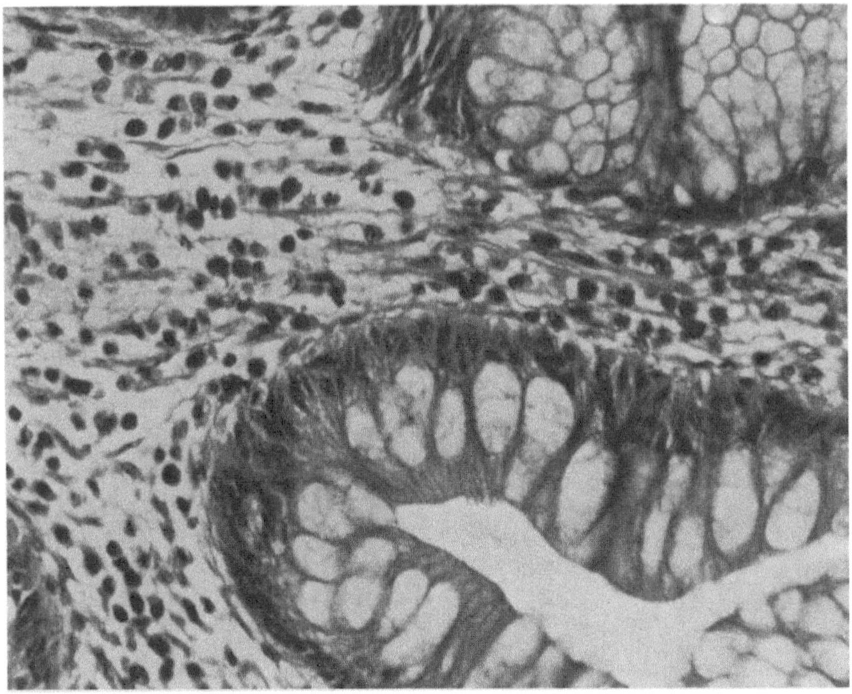

Fig. 10. Juvenile polyp. Detail from Fig. 8. Note abundant goblet cells, lack of nuclear crowding. X 300

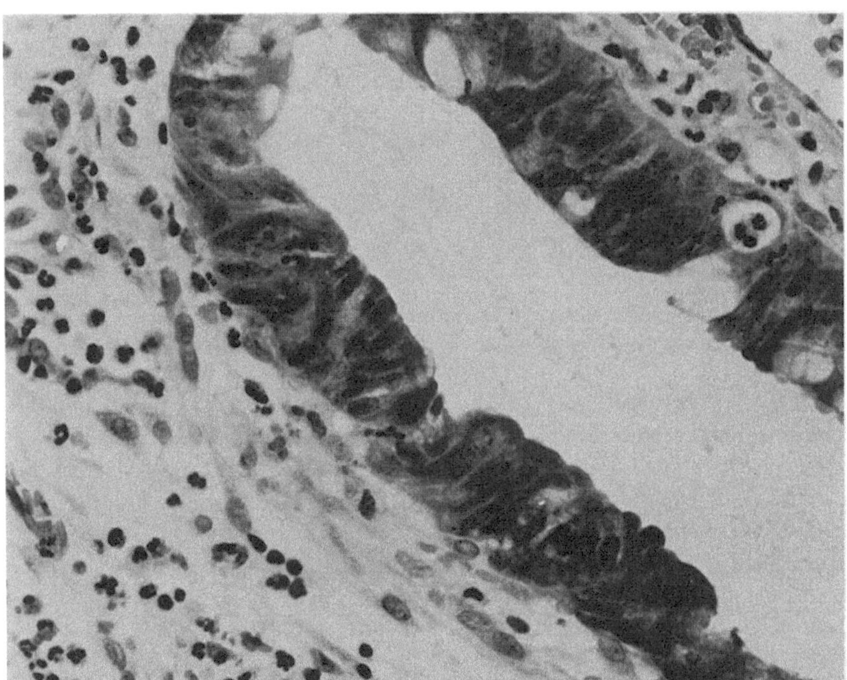

Fig. 11. Area of atypia in juvenile polyp. Unique case showing detail of gland with crowding and loss of nuclear polarity in polyp of sigmoid from a 21 year old woman. Polyp elsewhere typical of juvenile type. (Courtesy of Drs. Steele, Simpson and Associates, Denison, Texas.) X 300

The term "juvenile" has been used since three-quarters of these polyps occur in the first decade of life with a peak incidence at age 6 (*Holgerson* et al., 1971). They do, however, occur at all ages. For this reason some prefer the term retention polyp because of the characteristic mucus-filled cysts. There is no evidence that these are predecessor lesions of adenoma or that they are precancerous. *Shermata* et al. (1969) could find no examples of relationship to malignancy in 800 cases surveyed. I have seen one juvenile polyp in which areas were in part replaced by highly atypical glandular epithelium approaching carcinoma in situ in character (Fig. 11). I have seen no references to this nor other examples and at the moment consider it a chance association.

Their etiology has variously been considered inflammatory (*Horrilleno* et al., 1959; *Roth* and *Helwig*, 1963), hamartomatous (*Morson*, 1962), and allergic (*Alexander* et al., 1970). A simple inflammatory origin seems difficult to reconcile with the peculiar age distribution, relative rarity, and disparity in structure from polyps known to be of inflammatory origin such as those in ulcerative colitis. *Haggitt* (1970) suggests that the earliest polyps of this type may be due to stromal proliferation.

VIII. Juvenile Polyposis

McColl et al. in 1964 described a condition of diffuse polyposis of the colon in which the polyps resembled juvenile polyps rather than adenomas. Eleven cases in eight families were

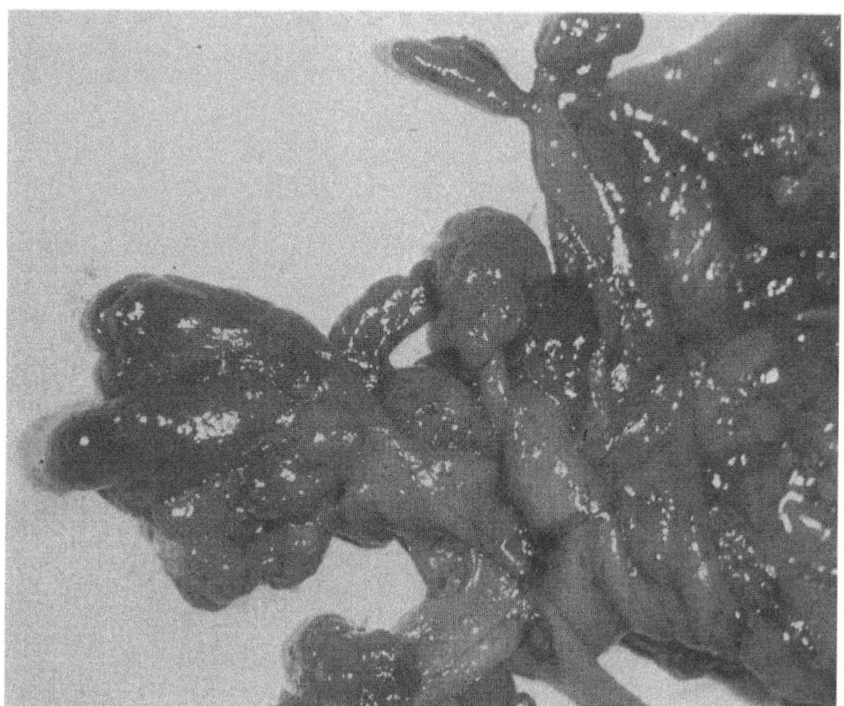

Fig. 12. Juvenile polyposis. Gross photograph of one of polyp clusters of colon. Note branching and frond-like character. Petient is a 16 year old black female. X 4

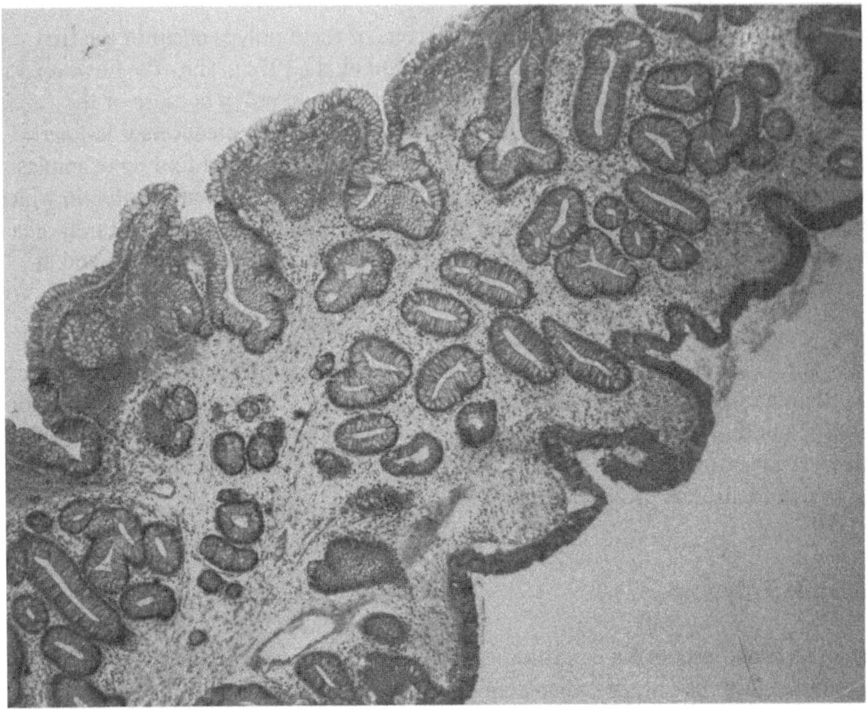

Fig. 13. Juvenile polyposis. Low power view of section of one of polyps from Figure 11. Note non-crowded nuclei, rather abundant lamina propria. X 30

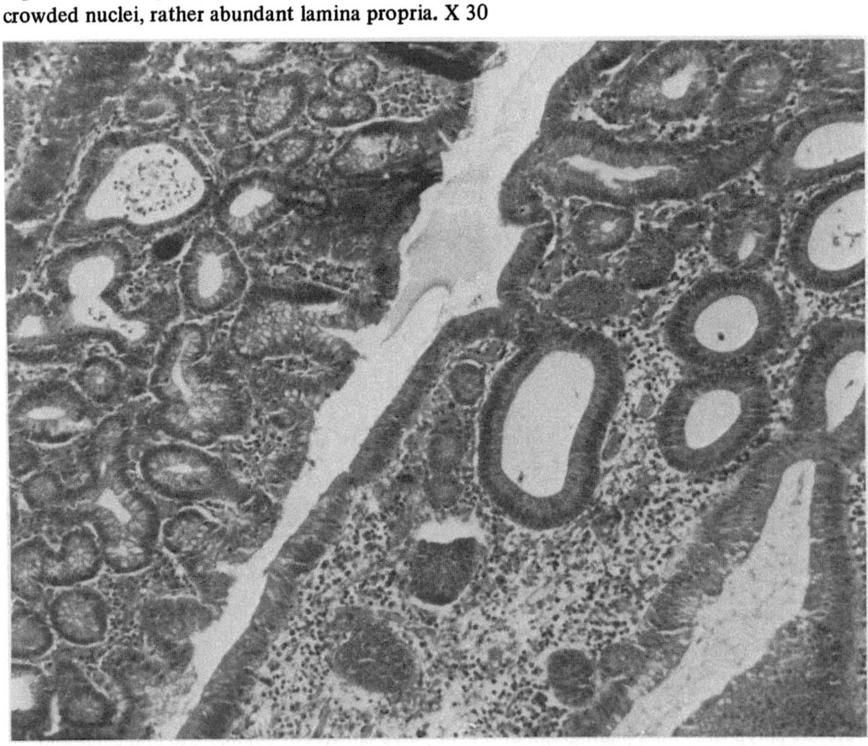

Fig. 14. Juvenile polyposis. Area of another polyp in same case as Figures 11 and 12. Note glands with nuclear crowding suggestive of adenomatous polyp. Other areas in same polyp lacked this feature. X 100

reported. Since then very similar polyposes have been described with involvement of stomach and small intestine as well as colon.

Both familial and nonfamilial forms of juvenile polyposis have been described. The genetics are in need of further work.

Sachatello (1972) believes three subgroups exist. (1) Juvenile polyposis of infancy, (2) juvenile polyposis coli, and (3) generalized juvenile gastrointestinal polyposis. To the author it is not clear that the infantile form of juvenile polyposis associated with cachexia and hyperproteinemia belongs in this group. It may be closer to the changes described in the mucosa of Cronkhite-Canada syndrome (to be discussed later).

The polyps in this condition (or conditions) tend to be more irregular in shape with irregular branching of glands and often with less stroma than is true of the isolated juvenile polyps. They may contain Paneth cells (*McColl* et al., 1964).

No direct relationship between the polyps of juvenile polyposis and adenocarcinoma is known. However, patients with juvenile polyposis have been reported in families with adenomatous polyposis (*Haggitt* and *Pitcock*, 1970; *Horrelleno* et al., 1959; *Veale*, 1966). They have also been reported in families with cases of carcinoma of the colon occurring at a young age (*Haggitt* and *Pitcock*, 1970). A kindred with single or multiple juvenile polyps and also with a high incidence of carcinoma of the stomach, duodenum, pancreas, and proximal colon has been studied by *Stemper* et al. (1975). *Veale* (1966) postulates the condition as being due to a modfier gene which when present with the gene for adenomatosis results in polyposis of the juvenile rather than the adenomatous type. Further study is necessary before complete understanding of these various genetic linkages is reached.

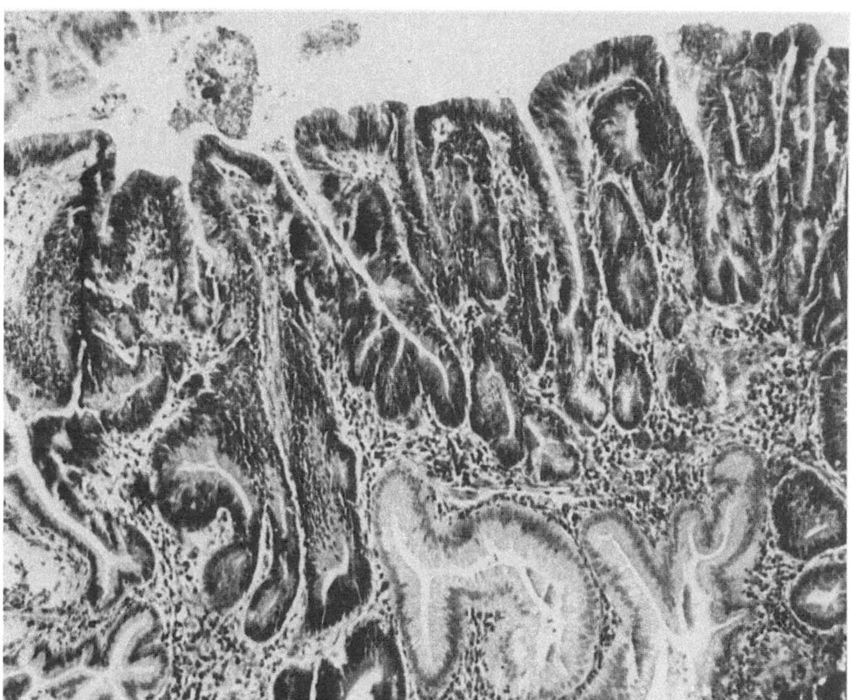

Fig. 15. Juvenile polyposis. Polyp of adenomatous type from stomach in same patient as Figures 11 to 13. X 100

We have encountered a case which illustrates the possible relationship of juvenile polyposis to true adenomatous neoplasia. The patient was found at age 12 to have multiple polyps of the colon, some of which were excised on several occasions, the last being a subtotal colectomy. The polyps showed gross branching (Fig. 12). Some resembled juvenile polyps though with more crowding of glands and branching than typical (Fig. 13). Areas in some polyps were suggestive of adenoma (Fig. 14). A gastric polyp was removed which was clearly adenomatous (Fig. 15) and age 21 and 22, two small purely adenomatous polyps were excised from her rectum. The patient's family could not be traced. A similar case was reported by *Kashula* (1971). Obviously more work needs doing to define this relationship.

Juvenile polyposis is not simply a case of a patient with multiple juvenile polyps, but rather a distinct condition. The polyps are not identical to juvenile polyps and a relationship to adenomatous polyposis is known in some cases. Whether patients with juvenile polyposis are themselves at higher risk of ultimately developing carcinoma of the colon remains to be determined, but long-term careful followup is indicated.

IX. Cronkhite-Canada Syndrome

This very rare syndrome consists of a polyposis of stomach, small intestine and colon associated with a diffuse pigmentation of the skin, alopecia, atrophy of the nails, and hypo-

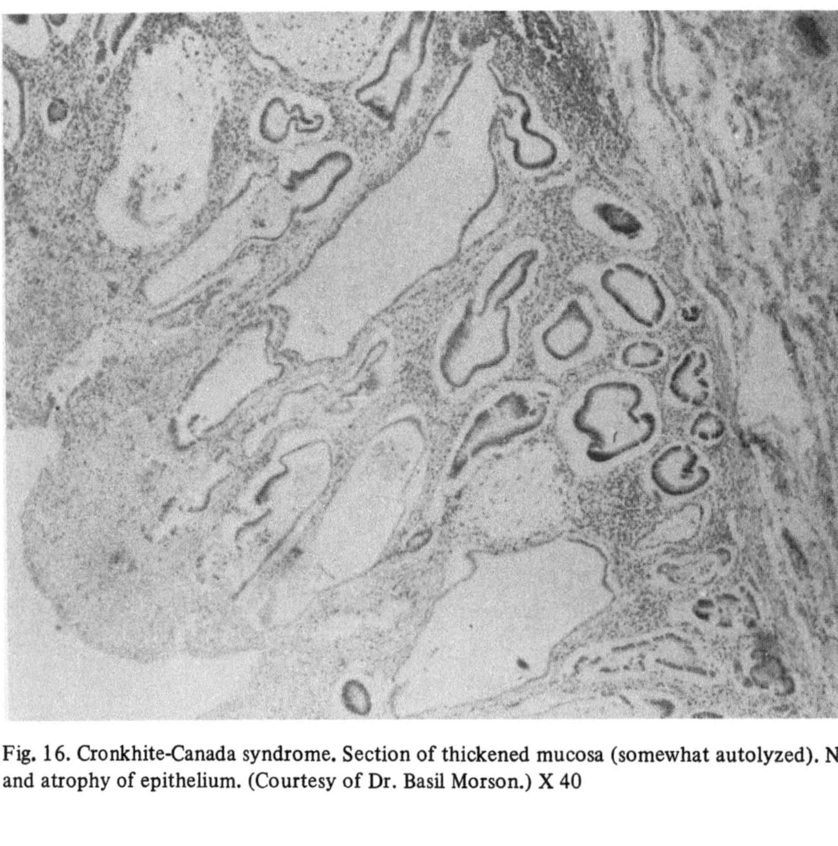

Fig. 16. Cronkhite-Canada syndrome. Section of thickened mucosa (somewhat autolyzed). Note cysts and atrophy of epithelium. (Courtesy of Dr. Basil Morson.) X 40

proteinemia (*Cronkhite* and *Canada*, 1955). The cases reported have been in adults and have been nonfamilial (*Orime* et al., 1969). The mucosa is thickened and diffusely polypoid and has been likened to juvenile polyps. In the single case I have seen (courtesy of Dr. B.C. Morson), the mucosa appears to show a combination of epithelial atrophy and cystic dilation (Fig. 16) and would, to me, appear closer to the changes described in Menetrier's disease. There is no known relationship to malignancy.

X. Metaplastic (Hyperplastic) Polyps

It is interesting that, despite the frequency of these little polyps, most observers, until the early 1960's, have confused them with adenomas. *Morson* (1962) in England, and *Lane* and *Lev* (1963) in the United States carefully described and differentiated them from adenoma. *Morson* used the term "metaplastic" for these lesions and *Lane* and *Lev* used "hyperplastic." The terms "hyperplastic" and "focal mucosal hyperplasia" have been used in a different sense by others (*Crocker* and *Veith*, 1964). In addition, it is questionable whether these lesions are produced by excessive cell proliferation as much as by delay in shedding (*Hayashi* et al., 1974). For these reasons the term metaplastic seems preferable, implying only a change in appearance and structure of the cells concerned.

These polyps are almost always sessile, dome-shaped lesions, 5 mm or less in diameter, sharply demarcated from and paler than the normal mucosa. Very rarely pedunculated variants or large en placque changes in the mucosa of this type are encountered.

Histologically metaplastic polyps differ sharply from adenomas. The cytoplasm is distinctly eosinophilic, the lining of the crypts and surface has a serrated appearance due to inequality of height of adjacent cells (Fig. 17). The nuclei are basal and lack the crowding

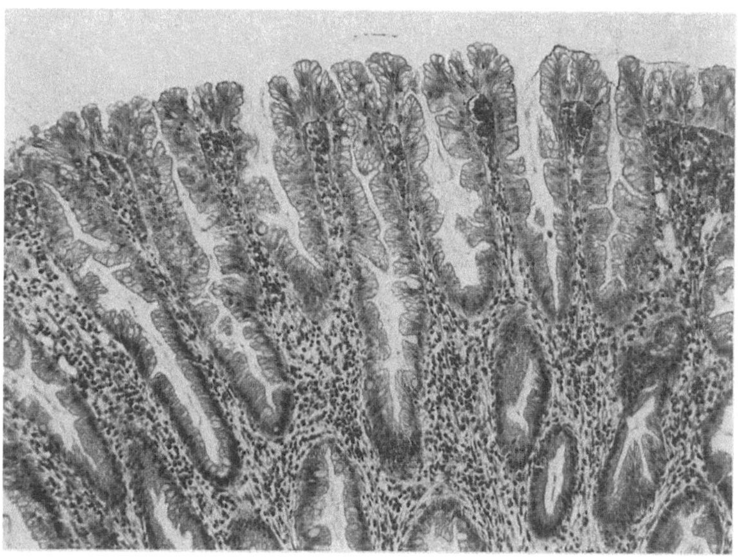

Fig. 17. Metaplastic polyp. Note "tufted" effect due to irregular height of cells. Note lack of nuclear crowding. Cells tend to be more eosinophilic than normal. X 100

of the adenoma. Mucin production is present and uniformly distributed. At a finer level, *Lane* et al. (1971), the basement membrane and associated PAS positive material between it and the epithelium is thicker than normal rather than thinner as is true of adenoma. Mitoses are restricted to the crypts rather than being present on the surface as may be seen in adenoma. The deeper portion of the crypts appear normal as compared to the uniform involvement of the entire gland, at least in the more central portion, of adenoma.

Metaplastic polyps are extremely common, at least in the rectum. They have been reported to be an aging phenomenum by *Arthur* (1968). He found one or more metaplastic polyps in 40% of rectums examined at autopsy in patients under the age of 40, in 75% of those in the over 40 category and in 95% of the rectums removed surgically for carcinoma. *Lane* et al. (1971) report that 92% of polyps, 3 mm or less, in their study were of this type.

At times metaplastic glands may be found in adenoma (Fig. 18) or in villous adenoma. There is, however, no evidence that the metaplastic polyp is a predecessor of the adenoma, villous or otherwise. Extremely minute adenomas much more commonly do not contain metaplastic areas. Metaplastic areas may also be seen in inflammatory polyps and near carcinomas. The ubiquity of these lesions in the average age group of patients with carcinoma and the fact that they are found in about the same incidence in colons with and without carcinoma (*Arthur*, 1968) is against an etiologic relationship of metaplastic polyps to carcinoma. I have seen only one metaplastic polyp (in the en plaque form) which contained markedly atypical cells. A large number of studies on the frequency and distribution of adenomas are worth-

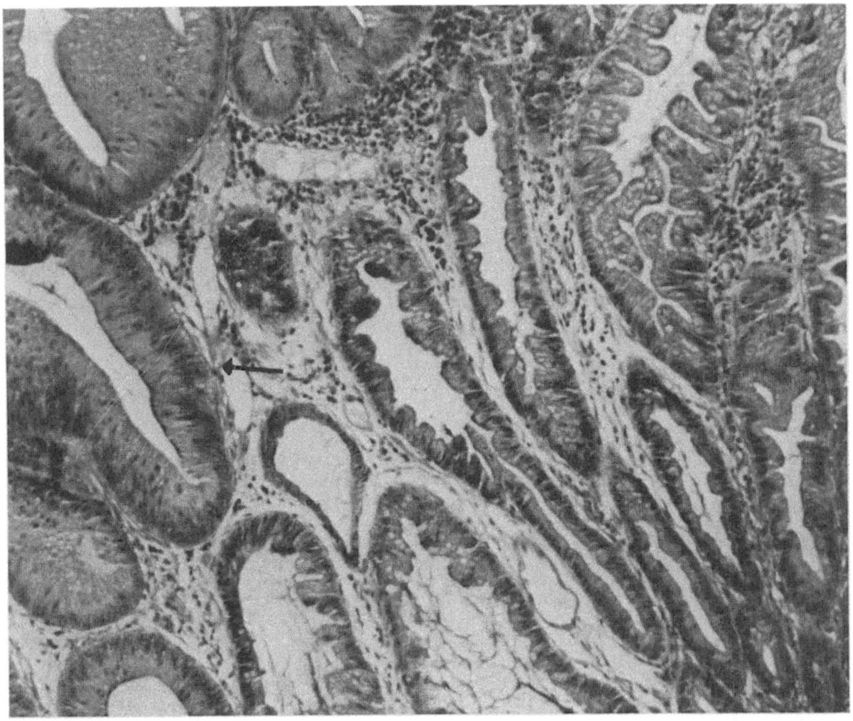

Fig. 18. Metaplastic area in adenomatous polyp. Note contrast between adenomatous gland (arrow) and metaplastic glands. X 150

less since the authors have failed to make the distinction between adenomatous and metaplastic polyps.

1. Lipomas

Submucosal adipose tissue of the colon is seldom remarked on in the literature, but does occur. Lipomas are usually submucosal and bulge out the overlying mucosa in a polypoid fashion. *Long* et al. (1949) in 13,000 necropsies reported such lipomas in 69 instances (0.5%). They may occasionally cause bleeding or intussusception. They occur at any site with perhaps some predilection of the larger lipomas for the caecum and ascending colon. Large lipomas may ulcerate and may mimic carcinoma on X-ray. Two such cases in our hospital had hemicolectomies performed on the assumption they were carcinoma. Liposarcoma, though theoretically possible, must be extremely rare if it exists at all. A case of lipomatous polyposis of the colon in a 2 year old child associated with hypertrophy of the appendices epiploicae has been reported by *Swain* et al. (1969).

2. Leiomyomas

Leiomyomas are common gastrointestinal neoplasms, especially in the stomach and small bowel. Most leiomyomas in the large bowel present as small asymptomatic polyps of the rectum removed incidentally during routine proctoscopies. They presumably arise from the muscularis mucosa. I have not encountered reports of a leiomyomatous form of polyposis though multiple leiomyomas certainly occur in the colon and rectum. Larger lipomas and leiomyomas as a rule do not present as polyps.

3. Neurofibromas and Ganglioneuromas

There is some confusion between leiomyoma and neurofibroma in the literature and gastrointestinal leiomyomas have in addition been reported in cases of neurofibromatosis (*Lukash* et al., 1966). Submucosal neurofibromas and ganglioneuromas both benign and malignant may occur with or without von Recklinghausen's disease as stated by *Lukash* et al. (1966). *Donnelly* et al. (1969) report a case in a nine year old boy without neurofibromatosis and with multiple ganglioneurofibromatous polyps of the colon as well as, interestingly, multiple polyps of the juvenile type.

4. Carcinoids

Colonic carcinoids, though relatively uncommon compared to those of the ileum, present as polypoid lesions in colon and rectum. In the last few years considerable information has accumulated as to their biology and management.

Large bowel carcinoids are rare before 30 and occur in a distinctly older age group than those of appendiceal origin. They occur throughout the colon and rectum, but in the colon are more common in the caecum than elsewhere according to *Berardi* (1972). In the rectum, the relative incidence compared to colon is distorted because small asymptomatic rectal carcinoids are frequently discovered in the course of routine proctoscopic examinations as incidental findings. This is reflected in the average size – those in the colon averaging 4.9 cm [in the excellent review by *Berardi* (1972)], while those in the rectum average much smaller. In *Ponka* and *Walke*'s (1971) report, 35 of 46 rectal carcinoids were 1 cm or less in diameter.

Carcinoids present as firm nodules with or without ulceration. On section they are distinctly yellow, ill defined, tumors. The histology is of rather uniform small cells in sheets or festoons subdivided by variable amounts of fibrous tissue (in contrast to the microacinar pattern of those in the midgut). Only a small percentage (5-10%) is positive by argentaffin or argyrophil staining techniques and as expected, therefore, are usually not active endocrinologically. *Berardi* (1972) reports that only four of 136 cases of carcinoid syndrome originated in colonic carcinoids. Statements that hindgut carcinoids are never reactive with silver stains or hormonally active are thus generally, but not strictly, correct.

There have been scattered reports of examples of tumors with both carcinoid and adenocarcinomatous structure. We have seen two such examples. In these one area of a tumor will appear typical of adenocarcinoma, sometimes well differentiated, while another will be equally typical of carcinoid. If one recalls that argentaffin positive cells may be found in some colonic adenocarcinomas, this need not be too surprising.

Histologic features are of no help in predicting behavior. All carcinoids are infiltrative tumors. Malignant behavior is predictable on size, and to some degree, on depth of invasion. Four hundred and seventy-five cases of rectal carcinoids were reviewed by *Greenwood* et al. (1974). Of those less than 2 cm in size, 85% were benign and of 89 over 2 cm, only 12% were benign. Carcinoids under 1 cm may for practical purposes be considered benign. This means that the small incidental carcinoid polyp of the rectum may be treated conservatively. Larger tumors are best treated as carcinoma. Size may reflect aggressiveness of tumor rather than chronology of discovery since some small carcinoids have been observed to remain static for long periods.

Greenwood et al. (1974) have carefully analyzed the association of carcinoids with other tumors. As reported in the literature, they conclude that one of eight patients with rectal carcinoids may be expected to harbor a coexistant significant benign or malignant neoplasm at any site, but most likely in the gastrointestinal tract. One of 12 patients may be expected to have an adenocarcinoma or adenoma of colon or rectum. They believe that association with non-gastrointestinal tract tumors is not significant, but that a real association between rectal carcinoids and adenocarcinoma and adenoma does exist. Reports by *Brown* and *Smith* (1973) have reported even higher percentages of associated GI neoplasms. Thus, patients with rectal carcinoids, however small, are at high risk of other tumors and deserve a careful assessment of the GI tract and particularly of the colon.

5. Adenomas of Colon

Adenomas of the colon, with the exception of metaplastic polyps, are the most common type of polyp encountered. While they may on occasion be the cause of bleeding or even intussusception, their clinical importance rests upon their much debated potential as a seedbed for colonic adenocarcinoma. This will be discussed in detail. Since much of the debate has been clouded by misidentification of other polyps (especially metaplastic polyps as adenomas), it is first necessary to clearly define what is meant by adenoma in its variant forms.

Adenomas may be sessile or pedunculated, large or of microscopic dimensions, villous or non-villous. Their common denominator is to be found in the nuclei. These are more hyperchromatic than the nuclei of normal mucosal epithelium, somewhat enlarged and elongated. They are more crowded than normal mucosal nuclei and occupy a greater fraction of the total cell height (Fig. 19). Mucin production is sharply reduced as compared to the normal. An exception to this last statement is seen in certain villous adenomas and very rarely in non-villous (tubular) adenomas. In addition, histochemical changes in the type of mucin have been described by *Filipe* (1969). The histochemistry of adenomas has also been shown to differ both from that of normal mucosa and from metaplastic polyps in the activity of a variety of enzymes (*Czernobilsky* and *Tsou*, 1968; *Wattenberg*, 1959).

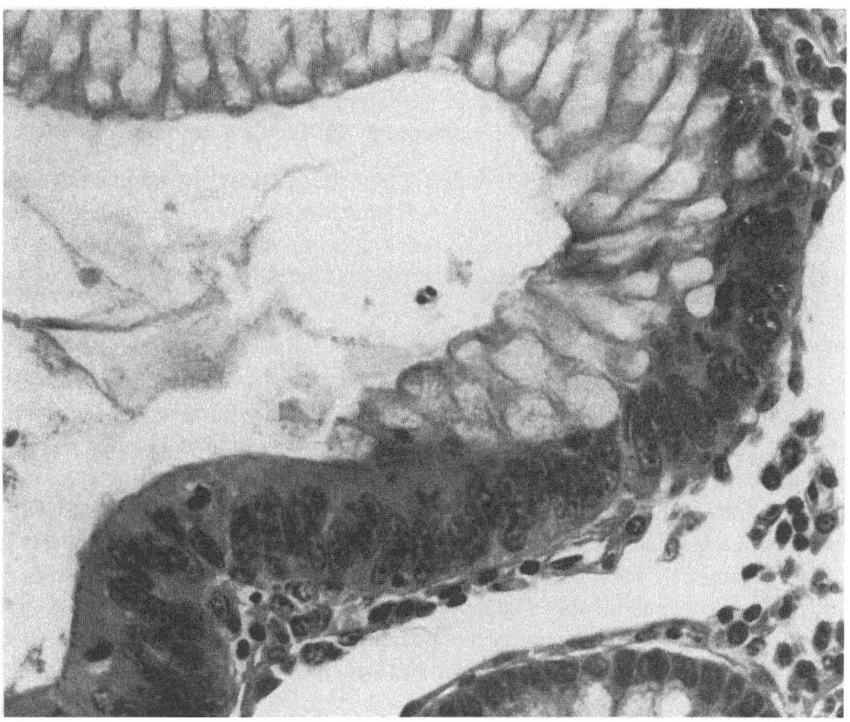

Fig. 19. Junction of adenoma and normal glandular epithelium. Note subtending of adenomatous epithelium below normal epithelium at point of replacement. X 400

Both Paneth cells and enterochromaffin cells may be present in a random manner in all types of adenoma (and carcinoma), in contrast to their presence only in the crypt bases of polyps of other types (*Morson* and *Dawson*, 1972a).

Chromosomal studies on adenomas are scanty. *Messinetti* et al. (1968) reported normal chromosome sets in adenomas except in the presence of "carcinomatous transformation."

Other workers (*Enterline* and *Arvan*, 1967; and *Mark* et al., 1973) have found pseudodiploid sets or the addition of extra chromosomes in the C & D groups to be common in adenomas without atypia. All agree that marked chromosomal abnormalities are present in adenomas containing areas of invasive or non-invasive carcinoma.

It has been well shown that normal colonic and rectal epithelium is composed of a highly dynamic cell population with cells dividing in the base of the crypts, maturing as they are pushed to the surface, and being shed at the surface. The whole process only occupies several days. Ultrastructural studies (*Kaye* et al., 1973) have shown that the epithelium of normal large bowel and of metaplastic polyps is less differentiated in the base of the crypts and steadily differentiates as the cell is pushed towards the surface of the gland. Adenomatous epithelium in contrast does not appear to differentiate beyond an intermediate stage. Studies with tritiated thymidine (*Bottomley* and *Cooper*, 1973; *Cole* and *McKalen*, 1963; *Lipkin*, 1974, and *Wiebecke* et al., 1974) have shown that the normal suppression of DNA synthesis and therefore cell replication in the mid portion of the crypt does not occur in adenomas. Cell replication in adenoma is a random phenomenon occurring at any level including the surface. A change in cell membrane properties of adenomas (*Lipkin*, 1974) may enable cells to persist longer and this, plus the failure of control of replication, leads to the development of a mass, i.e. adenoma.

All of these lines of evidence strongly indicate that adenomas in their numerous variants are indeed true neoplasms and differ sharply from other polyps of inflammatory, hamartomatous, or metaplastic nature. Serial section studies on small adenomas by *Lane* and *Lev* (1963) have shown that these neoplasms arise in the deep, germinative portion of a crypt or crypts.

The histology varies from the tubular often branched pattern of the typical tubular adenoma to the papillary pattern of the villous adenoma. The gross appearance also is variable from the smooth but lobulated structure of the common adenoma to the shaggy appearance of the typical villous form. Whether or not a given adenoma is pedunculated or sessile is not strictly size related. Any type of adenoma may be pedunculated, though the villous adenomas are characteristically sessile and spreading. It is generally considered that pedunculation occurs in a mechanical way by the adenoma being "caught" by peristolic action, the stalk being formed by the loose mucosa and submucosa adjacent to the adenoma. In any event, the stalk of a pedunculated adenoma is composed of normal mucosal and submucosal elements. Because of their vascularity and possibly because of hemorrhage secondary to trauma, adenomas are usually considerably darker than the normal mucosa surrounding them.

6. Terminology

In the past it was usual to sharply separate adenomatous polyps and villous (papillary) adenomas. In recent years it has become generally accepted that intermediate forms not only occur, but are common (*Fund* and *Goldman*, 1970). This is a size related phenomenon (*Enterline*, 1975) (Bar graph). Various terms have been used for these bridging forms. In this chapter I shall adhere to the recommendation of the World Health Organization Committee for classification of intestinal tumors (WHO, 1976). Commonly used synonyms are indicated in parenthesis. These terms are as follows:

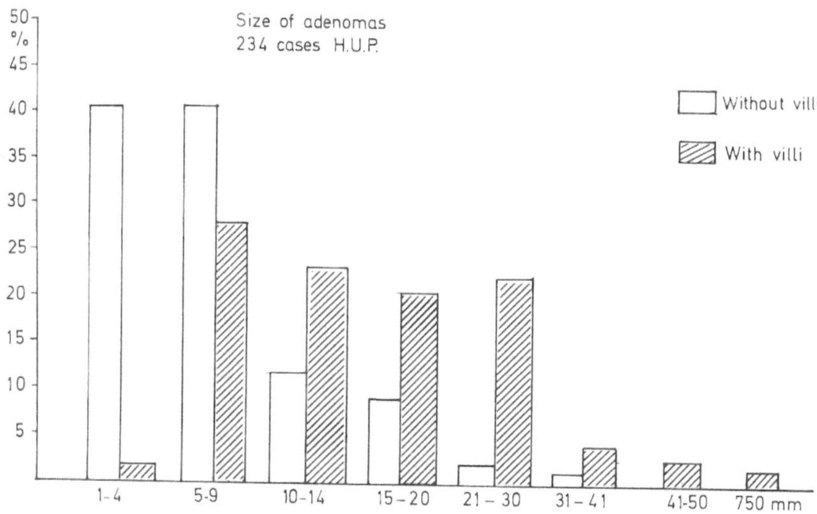

Bar Graph: Size distribution of 234 consecutive adenomas diagnosed at the Hospital of the University of Pennsylvania

1. Tubular adenoma (glandular adenoma, adenoma). "An adenoma composed predominantly of branching tubules embedded in or surrounded by lamina propria" (Fig. 20).

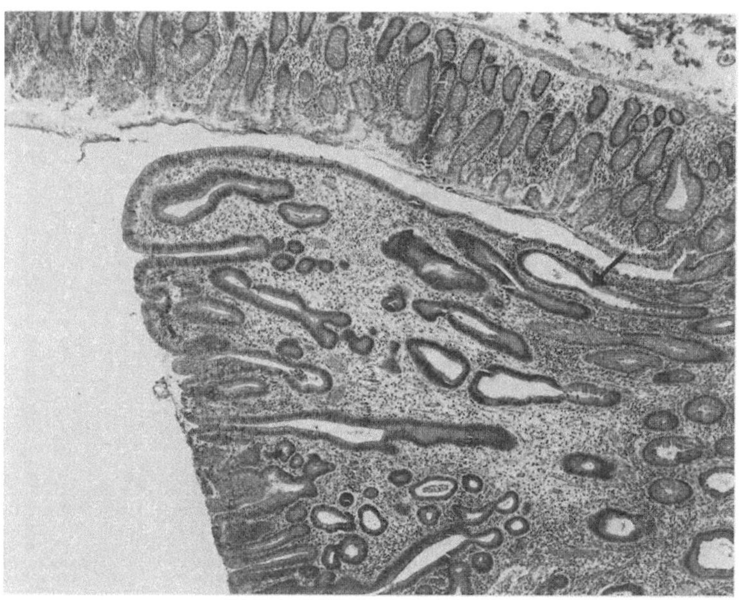

Fig. 20. Tubular adenoma. Edge of sessile tubular adnoma. Note junction with normal glands (arrow), lack of papillary fronds and tendency to branching of tubules. X 40

2. Villous adenoma (papillary adenoma). "An adenoma composed of pointed or blunt finger-like processes of lamina propria covered by epithelium which reaches down to muscularis mucosa" (Fig. 21).

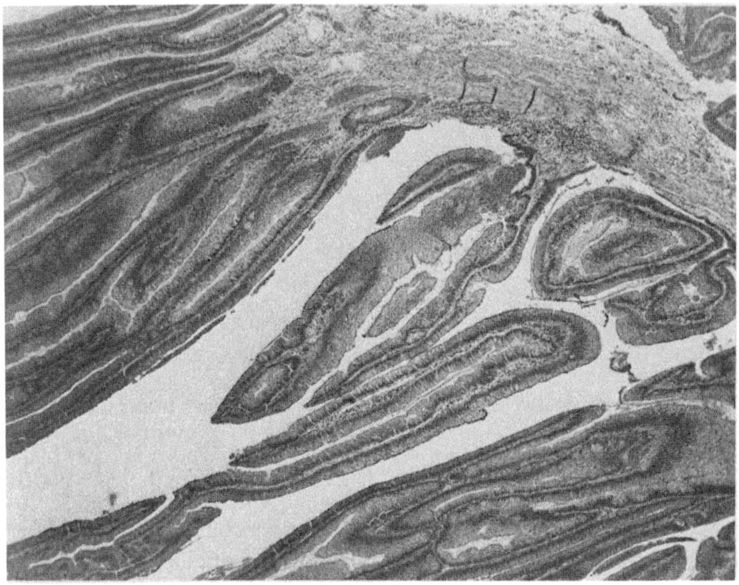

Fig. 21. Villous adenoma. Note long fronds. Invasive carcinoma was present elsewhere in this tumor. X 40

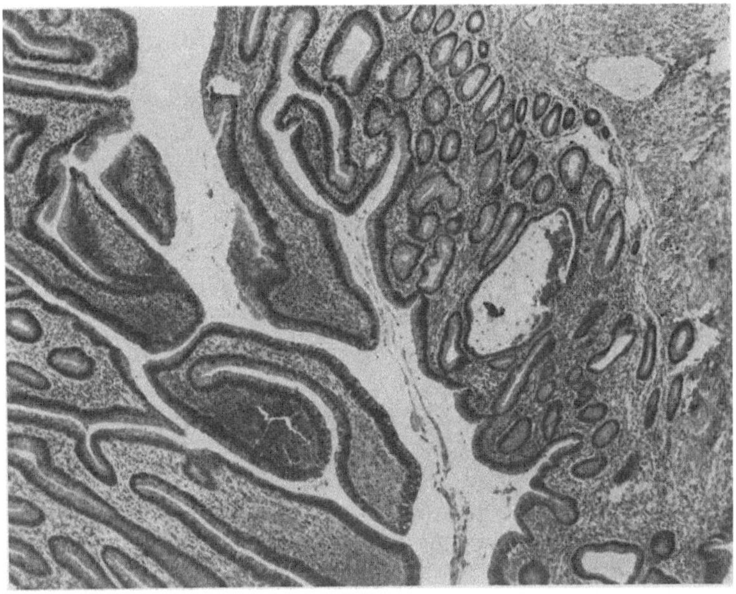

Fig. 22. Tubulo-villous adenoma. Tubular portion to right of photograph with portions of villous elements on left. X 40

3. Tubulo-villous adenoma (mixed adenoma, villoglandular adenoma). "An adenoma which may have both tubular and villous patterns or a pattern which seems intermediate between tubular and villous" (Fig. 22).

The significance of these variations will be discussed below. Adenomas of any type may uncommonly occur elsewhere than the colon, but these will not be considered here.

4. Adenomatosis (adenomatous polyposis coli, familial adenomatous polyposis, multiple polyposis). "A condition in which numerous adenomas are present in the large intestine."

These may be of any of the three types listed. A dividing line between true adenomatous polyposis and multiple adenoma as stated by *Morson* (1972) and recommended by WHO (1976) is that the presence of over 100 adenomas in a colon should be considered adenomatosis. The distinction is of importance since adenomatosis and its variant forms, such as Gardner's syndrome, is inherited as a Mendelian dominant of varying penetrance. This is not true of adenoma, whether single or multiple, although genetic factors may be implicated in a less obvious way. The term "Gardner's Syndrome" is widely recognized and acceptable. However, rather than proliferate epinymics to indicate the association of adenomatous polyposis with extra colonic lesions of various sorts, it seems best to use the term "adenomatous polyposis" and add to it the appropriate lesion indicated, such as with fribromatosis (*Simpson* et al., 1964), with thyroid carcinoma (*Smith* and *Kern*, 1973), with glioma (*Turcot* et al., 1968), with sarcoma (*Fraumeni* et al., 1968), and so forth. I have defined the terms listed below as follows:

a) Atypia

An adenoma of any type, whether or not in adenomatosis, may contain foci in which nuclei are more irregular and less polarized than in the usual adenoma. If the growth pattern of the tubules or villi is not markedly distorted I refer to this as atypia (Fig. 23).

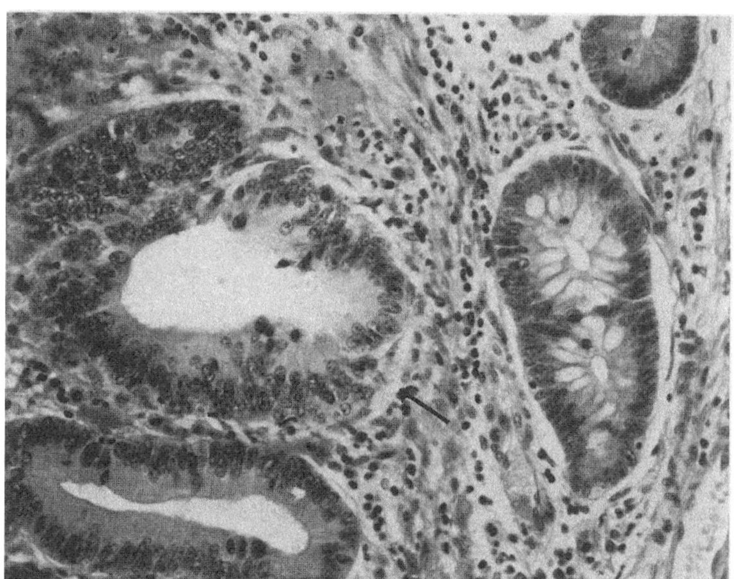

Fig. 23. Atypia in adenoma. Arrow points to gland with moderate atypia showing loss of polarity and size variation in nuclei. Adenomatous gland beneath it shows a minimal atypia. Contrast to normal gland to right as to nuclear size and normal goblet cells. X 250

b) Carcinoma In Situ

An adenoma containing a focus or foci of cells as described under atypia, and in addition obvious distortion of the growth pattern (i.e. irregular budding, cribiform areas), but which lack a desmoplastic reaction or otherwise fail to show evidence of invasion (Fig. 24).

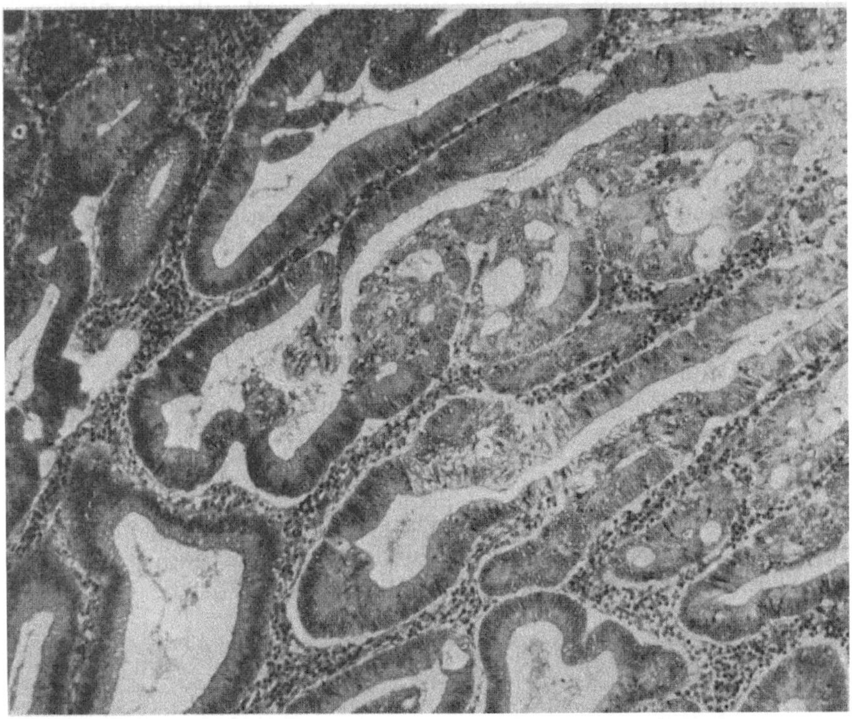

Fig. 24. Carcinoma in situ in adenoma. Note cribiform pattern of gland and loss of nuclear polarity. In situ area appears paler here, but may be more hyperchromatic than surrounding adenoma in other areas. X 200

c) Intramucosal Carcinoma

A focus or foci of cells in an adenoma which show both irregularities of cytology and histology as defined above under atypia and in situ carcinoma, and in addition show clear evidence of invasion as denoted by a desmoplastic reaction and/or by the presence of single cells or clusters of cells obviously not confined within a tubule or villous structure, such invasion not extending beyond the muscularis mucosa (Fig. 25).

d) Invasive Carcinoma

An area in an adenoma as defined above under intramucosal carcinoma, but with clear evidence of extension beyond the limits of the muscularis mucosa (Figs. 26 and 27).

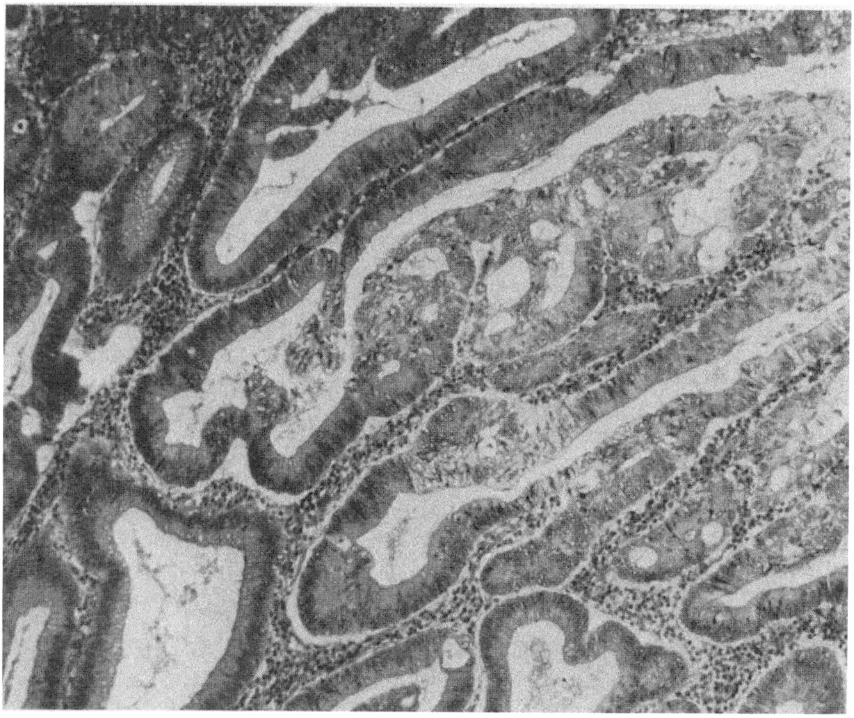

Fig. 25. Intramucosal carcinoma in adenoma. Note areas of adenocarcinoma enmeshed in bundles of smooth muscle from muscularis mucosae. X 150

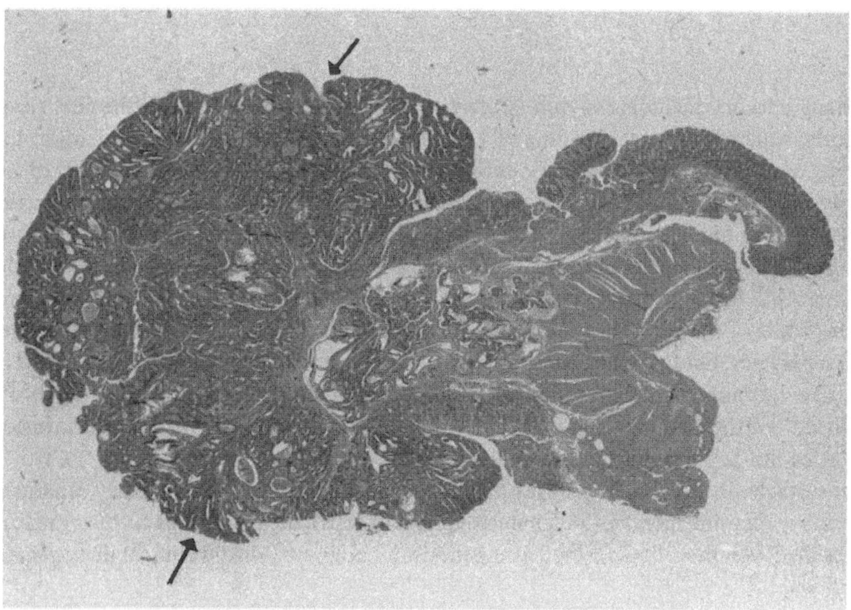

Fig. 26. Invasive carcinoma in adenoma. Adenoma-carcinoma junction approximately indicated by arrows. Note short thick pedicle with tumor invasion to muscularis. X 4

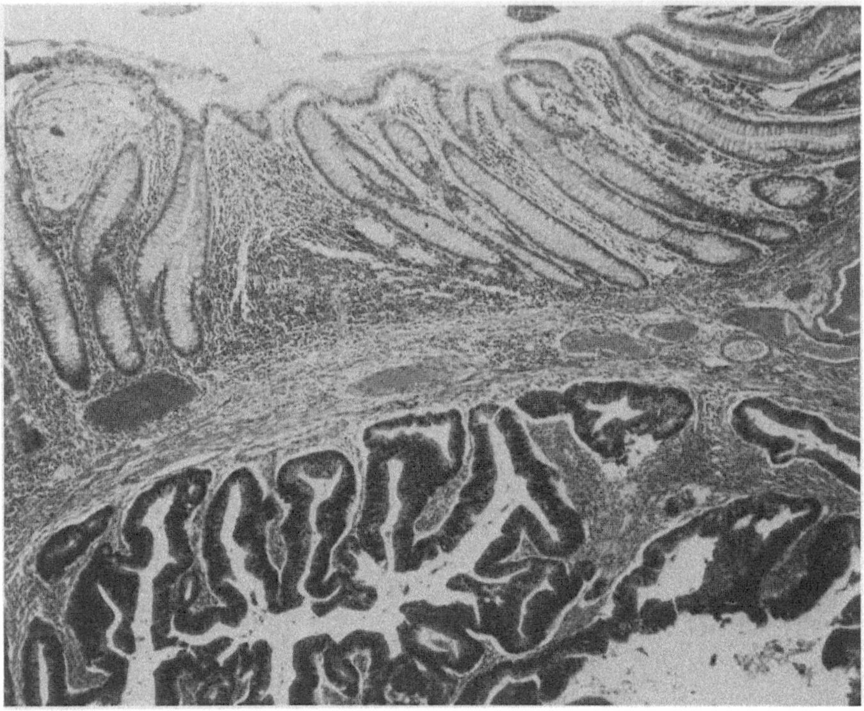

Fig. 27. Invasive carcinoma in adenoma. Well differentiated adenocarcinoma in stalk of adenoma. Stalk mucosa of normal glands. Adenoma not in field. X 65

Many authors, including myself (*Enterline* et al., 1962), have lumped the first three categories under the general heading of "Atypia" or "Dysplasia." I see no objection to this as long as the term used are clearly defined. The justification given is that, short of invasion beyond the muscularis mucosa, the diagnosis of carcinoma is too subjective. On the other hand, it is no more subjective than similar judgments elsewhere, such as in dysplasia and carcinoma in situ of the cervix. There are infinite gradations from one category to the next. There will be some variation of opinion as to where a certain case fits. I would agree that the limits of the muscularis mucosa is the critical one from some standpoints as we will discuss later. On the other hand, the muscularis mucosa in an adenoma, at least if pedunculated, is not a sharply defined structure but sprayed out and often fills much of the "head" of the adenoma. Thus fairly sizable foci of carcinoma with obvious invasion may yet be not beyond this mesh of smooth muscle. To call these "atypia" or "in situ" seems unsuitable. It is highly important that those writing on the subject clearly separate their cases so that independent judgments can be made by their reader as to the conclusions reached, whether it be on the pathogenesis of carcinoma or the clinical management of polyps.

Gross findings, site and incidence of adenomas of various types will be discussed below together with a discussion on the pathogenesis of adenocarcinoma of the colon.

XI. Basic Histogenesis of Colonic Adenocarcinoma

The frequency of colonic adenocarcinoma varies widely geographically (*Burkitt*, 1971). The incidence of carcinoma in the colon of immigrants to high incidence sites, such as Europe and North America, tends to approach that of the adopted country (*Stemmerman*, 1970). This strongly suggests environmental rather than genetic factors as being of major importance. Experimental work has shown that known carcinogenic substances are bound to glucuronide in the liver and that certain colonic bacteria are capable of splitting such substances thus activating these carcinogens within the colon. This provides a potential for tumor growth within the exposed mucosal field (*Hill*, 1974). To what degree such potential carcinogens are endogenous and exogenous is not clear though diet is certainly strongly implicated (*Burkitt*, 1971). This information suggests an attractive hypothesis, i.e. that western highly refined low roughage diets produce either more carcinogens or carcinogens acting over a longer period of time on the colon. Activations of such carcinogens by colonic bacteria would be expected to produce their maximum effect on the left side of the colon as water is absorbed from the fecal stream, which of course fits well with the known site of predilection of large bowel carcinoma. The response to such carcinogenic stimuli, presumably is modified to an unknown degree by genetic factors, as in adenomatosis.

Of more immediate concern to the clinician is whether adenocarcinoma, however produced on a basic level, develops de novo from previously normal mucosa, or only or predominantly within preexisting adenomas. This point is of great practical importance in management aspects of the patient with adenoma.

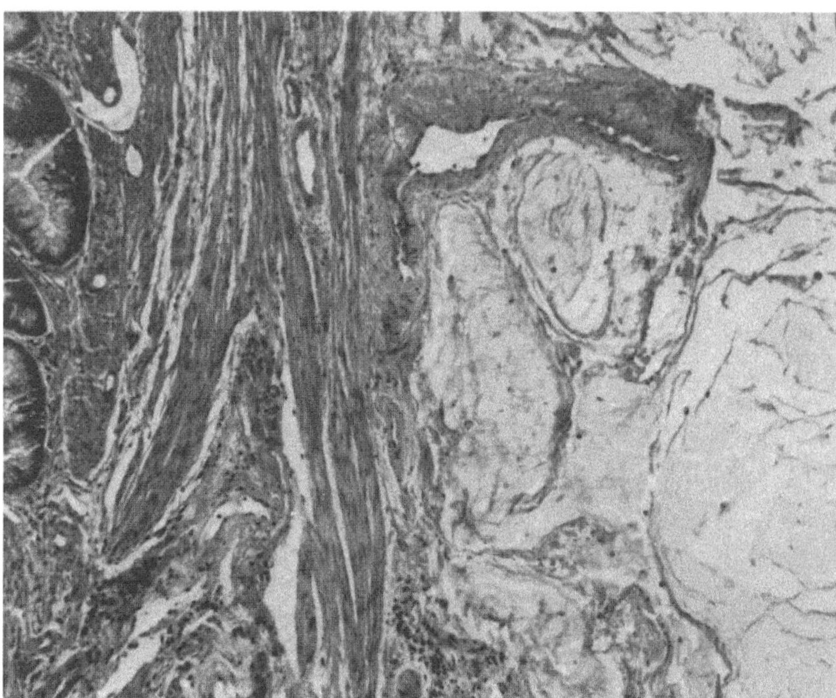

Fig. 28. Pseudoinvasion in adenoma. Pools of mucin in submucosa of adenoma. X 100

1. Pseudo Invasion

Before considering the question of carcinoma arising in adenoma it is necessary to be aware of various histologic patterns mimicking carcinoma.

Castleman and *Krickstein* (1962) emphasized that many adenomas reported as containing invasive carcinoma were in reality merely examples of adenomatous epithelium in which the plane of section cut through the irregular glandular base, thus presenting as islands of epithelium apparently within the stroma. More recently it has been shown that true isolated patches of glandular, but benign, epithelium may exist in the submucosa of adenomas (*Fechner*, 1973; *Muto* et al., 1973; *Greene*, 1974). The terms "misplacement" and "pseudo invasion" have been used for this phenomenon. This is not a rare occurrence and has been found by *Greene* (1974) in 6% of patients with adenoma and in 38% of adenomas associated with carcinomas. Pools of mucin without apparent epithelium in the submucosa of adenomas may also appear in a particular plane of section (Figs. 28 and 29). Pathologists must be altert to this phenomenon if error is to be avoided. The differential diagnosis is usually not difficult. Three points are most helpful in this differentiation:

(1) The cytology is identical to adenomatous or rarely to normal epithelium. The cell clusters of colloid carcinoma and the nuclear atypia of carcinoma are not seen (Fig. 30).

(2) There is usually deposition of hemosiderin in the vicinity indicating old hemorrhage, either secondary to trauma or to vasoocclusive phenomena.

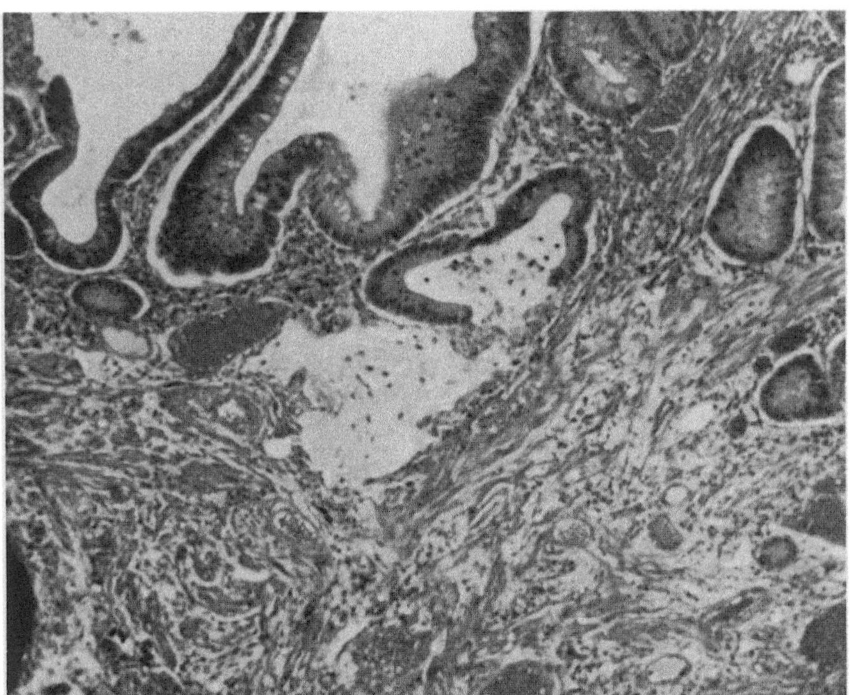

Fig. 29. Pseudoinvasion in adenoma. One mechanism by which mucin may be extravasated into stroma. Note ruptured adenomatous gland with outpouring of mucin. X 100

(3) There is usually no desmoplastic reaction as would be expected in an invasive carcinoma.

Pseudo invasion in adenomas is more common in larger adenomas and in the sigmoid (*Greene*, 1974). It is assumed that pseudo invasion is due to displacement of epithelium through a defective muscularis mucosa with subsequent regeneration and continued secretion. Rupture of glands with release of mucin is another possible mechanism (Fig. 29).

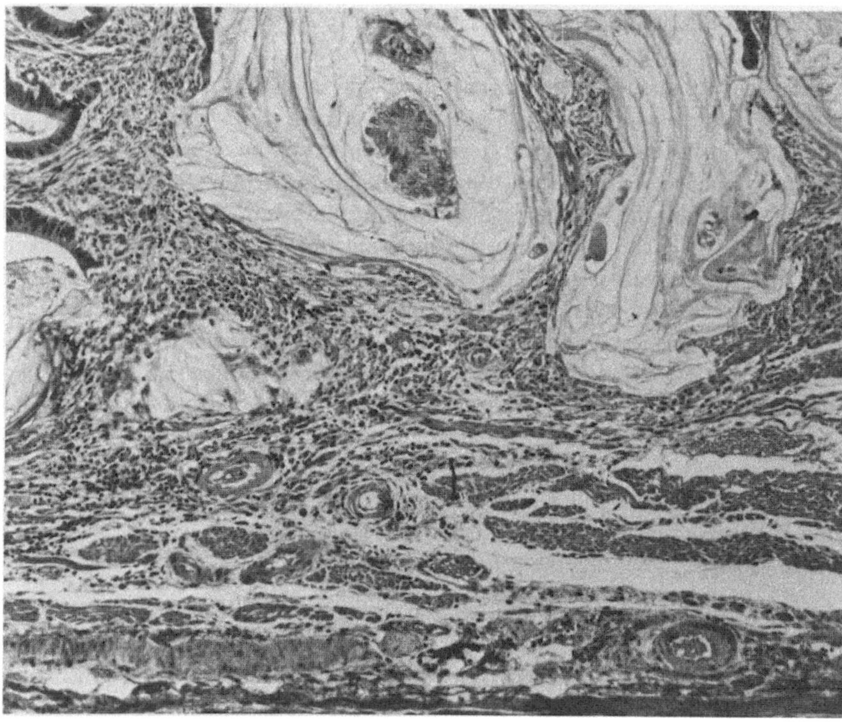

Fig. 30. True invasion. Invasive mucinous adenocarcinoma in adenoma. Note mucin pools with cell clusters. Adenoma not in field. X 65

2. Villous Adenoma

This will be discussed separately since these tumors in their classical form have never been part of the controversy of the adenoma-carcinoma sequence.

While there is no doubt that intergrades are common, the fully villous adenoma is a fairly distinctive entity. While occasionally pedunculated, the classic lesion is usually sessile and often quite large. In *Bacon*'s series (*Bacon* et al., 1971), 35% of his cases of villous adenomas involved the entire circumference of the bowel. The lesions are usually soft and shaggy and easily missed by rectal examination. Firm areas nearly always indicate coexisting invasive carcinoma (*Quan* and *Castro*, 1971). The average age of patients with these tumors is slightly higher, 62 years, than for other types (*Enterline* et al., 1962). About two-thirds of these tumors present in the rectum and only about 10% are proximal to the sigmoid

(*Olson* and *Davis*, 1969). About 85% of the patients are symptomatic (*Quan* and *Castro*, 1971), usually presenting with bleeding or diarrhea. Of interest is the fact that some of these tumors apparently act as selective excreters of potassium. This may produce hypokalemia leading to sudden collapse, confusion and coma precipitated by heat or by fluid or salt restriction (*Babior*, 1966).

3. Development of Carcinoma in Villous Adenoma

Even those who have considered adenomas in general to be of no importance in cancer pathogenesis (*Castelman* and *Krickstein*, 1962; *Spratt* and *Ackerman* (1962) have admitted that carcinoma occurs frequently in villous adenomas. The reported incidence of carcinoma varies widely (*Nicoloff* et al., 1969) depending in part on selection. Some authors have only reported on those tumors which by clinical inspection or biopsy were considered initially benign. The incidence of invasive cancer must be at least 25% and more likely closer to 50% of total villous adenomas. In addition, at least half of the villous adenomas without invasive carcinoma will be found to have varying degrees of dysplasia. Such invasive carcinomas as do arise are fully capable of metastasis (*Enterline*, 1962). Prognosis should be judged as one would judge any colonic carcinoma of like size, depth of penetration and degree of differentiation. There is a direct relationship of size of the villous adenoma and incidence of invasive carcinoma, though invasive carcinoma has been reported in villous adenomas of less than 2 cm (*Quan* and *Castro*, 1971). Biopsy has been notoriously unreliable as a means of ruling out the presence of carcinoma, because the desmoplastic reaction of invasive cancer tends to "stitch" such areas into place allowing the loose submucosa to prolapse presenting the benign portion for biopsy.

A reasonable treatment approach appears to be local excision of the entire adenoma, careful study of the excised tissue for the presence of invasive carcinoma, and a follow-up more radical procedure if thus proven necessary. *Quan* and *Castro* (1971) report a 12% local recurrence rate and a 71% five year survival in a group of 125 villous adenomas with carcinoma. This includes, however, cases with carcinoma in situ.

In our original study, 17 of 81 villous adenomas were associated with other tumors of the colon, of which 16 were carcinoma and three of these 16 had more than one carcinoma (*Enterline*, 1962). The Memorial Hospital study (*Quan* and *Castro*, 1971) reports 16% of their cases to be associated with other cancers of the colon and 49% to be associated with other adenomas. It is clear that the management of a villous adenoma demands careful study of the entire large bowel and careful followup studies in addition to the therapy for the villous adenoma itself.

4. The Relationship of Adenoma to Adenocarcinoma

The question of the importance of adenomas in the pathogenesis of carcinoma may be sought at two levels. At one level is such information as age and site comparisons of adenoma and carcinoma, and evidence on whether or not the association of carcinoma and adenoma is more than random. Such lines of evidence can be expected to establish or disprove whether there is some link between adenoma and carcinoma. It can do no more, however, than establish a "fellow traveller" status for adenoma. At another level are reports on such questions as in what background minute carcinomas are found, i.e. in normal mucosa or adenoma; chromosomal and histochemical observations in adenomas and carcinomas; and finally, whether surgical prophylactic excision of adenomas has any influence on the incidence of subsequent carcinoma. These will be discussed in order.

5. Age of Patients with Adenoma and Carcinoma

If adenomas precede and give rise to carcinomas, one would expect that they would occur in a younger age group. In our own study (*Enterline*, 1962) we would find no such difference, the average age of adenoma being 59 years and of carcinoma, 60. This was also true of *Grinell* and *Lane*'s (1958) study, whose series of adenomas averaged 62 and of carcinomas, 58. These authors, however, point out the difficulties in determining age of onset of adenomas from ordinary surgical experience, and suggest that figures from cancer detection clinics, where asymptomatic patients of all ages are examined, are probably much closer to the true age. These figures show average ages of 50.2 for adenoma and 57.6 for carcinoma – a seven year differential. *Morson* (1974b) estimates an eight year differential between the peak ages of adenoma and of carcinoma. He also states that the average of the appearance of adenomas in familial adenomatous polyposis is 15 years earlier than the average of carcinomas in such patients. It would appear that there is a significant time lapse between the appearance of adenoma and carcinoma quite sufficient to postulate the latter arising from the former.

6. Site of Adenomas and Carcinomas

The location of adenoma and carcinoma within the large intestine has been extensively reported. Although the sites of predilection of carcinoma are clear enough (*Falterman* et al., 1974), there are problems both of incidence and location in the reporting of adenomas. Authors subdivide the division between colon and rectum in differing fashion and many reports fail to distinguish between metaplastic and adenomatous polyps. In many series not all polyps found were examined microscopically. Thus *Blatt* (1961) reports that over 50% of polyps less than 3 mm in his series were of the metaplastic type. Series based on surgical material accentuate rectal and sigmoid lesions because of cases diagnosed during routine sigmoidoproctoscopic examinations. Autopsy figures are presumably more accurate and show less of a sigmoid-rectal predominance. I have listed some selected reports on sites of adenoma in Table 2 and have used *Falterman* et al.'s (1974) huge series of carcinomas for contrast. Those reporting extremely high incidence figures of adenoma, *Chapman* (1963), also report a relatively more uniform distribution of polyps in the large intestine. Many of these may be metaplastic. *Ekelund*'s studies (1974) and those of *Ekelund* and *Lindstrom* (1974) are in some respects unique and very valuable. They are dealing with a stable and relatively isolated population in which nearly all patients are seen at one hospital and in which the autopsy rate is 99%. *Ekelund* and *Lindstrom* (1974) conclude from both their autopsy and surgical material that "the subsite frequency distribution of solitary polyps is similar to that for solitary carcinomas. When solitary and multiple polyps were taken together – the distribution of benign polyps was relatively more even than that of carcinoma." There is a general, but not exact, concordance of site of adenoma and carcinoma. Compared with carcinoma there is some excess of adenomas in the right colon and some deficit of adenomas in the sigmoid and rectal region.

Table 2.

	Caecum Ascending Colon	Transverse Colon	Descending Colon	Sigmoid and Rectum
Adenoma				
Helwig (1947) 1437 autopsies	22%	15%	11%	48%
Edwards and *Jackman* (1957) 802 autopsies	35%	12%	13%	48%
Blatt (1961) 446 autopsies	37%	25%	11%	27%
Ekelund (1974a) 3041 autopsies	24%	19%	11%	45%
Ekelund (1974a) 456 surgical	26%	12%	10%	52%
Grinnell and *Lane* (1958) 1640 surgical	6%	9%	5%	79%
Carcinoma				
Falterman et al. (1974) 2313 cases	18%	9%	7%	65%

Spratt and coworkers (1958) had also concluded that distribution of adenomas and carcinomas are not homogeneous and therefore, in their opinion, not related. They have shown that given patients with both adenomas and carcinomas, the adenomas tend to be more distal in the caecum and ascending colon and more proximal in the rectum and sigmoid. They argue that if indeed adenomas are the source of carcinoma, the distribution of adenomas in such cases should be randomly distributed in relation to the carcinomas. This view can only be considered valid if it is assumed that all adenomas have the same propensity for carcinoma regardless of site. *Ekelund* (1974) has studied this question in a slightly different fashion and has shown that segment for segment, in patients with both adenomas and carcinomas, the adenomas were most frequently found in the same segment as the carcinoma.

7. Incidence of Adenoma and Coexistence with Carcinoma

Incidence reports of adenomas from clinical studies have varied between 5.3% and 11.6% (*Blatt*, 1961), and in autopsy studies from *Helwig*'s (1947) 9.5% to *Chapman*'s (1963) 51%.

There is no mention of metaplastic polyps in this latter series. *Ekelund*'s (1974) autopsy figure was 12.5%. In the same series he found that 5.9% of the cases harbored one or more carcinomas. *Helwig* (1947) reported 40 carcinomas in 1460 consecutive autopsies (2.7%), of which 25 were large, frank carcinomas (1.7%). These figures are typical for European and North American populations. There are marked geographical variations. For instance, in the Bantu of South Africa, both adenomas and carcinomas are extremely rare (*Bremner* and *Ackerman*, 1970).

Adenomas and carcinomas are very uncommon below 30, and all reports show a direct relationship of adenoma incidence with age reaching 25% to 40% of the population above 70 (*Blatt*, 1961; *Edwards* and *Jackman*, 1957). Similarly, carcinoma shows a rapidly increasing incidence after the age of 40 (*Falterman* et al., 1974).

Most series report a slight, but definite male predominance for adenoma. The same slight male predominance seems to be also present for carcinoma (*Berg* and *Howell*, 1974), despite some reports to the contrary (*Falterman* et al., 1974).

Morson and *Dawson* (1972) state that about one-third of all resected colons with carcinomas will have one or more adenomas in addition to the carcinoma. Other estimates are somewhat less than this figure. It has been reported that cancer is from three to five times more frequent in patients with adenomas than in those without (*Goldgraber* and *Kirsner*, 1957; *Rider* et al., 1959). Thus *Rider* et al. (1959), reporting on 1932 patients, showed that of those without adenoma the incidence of carcinomas was 2.1%, with one adenoma the figure was 11.6%, and was 21% in those with multiple adenomas. *Grinell* and *Lane* (1958) have pointed out that patients with carcinoma have twice the frequency of multiple adenomas than those without carcinoma. *Bussey* and coworkers (1967) state that patients with partial resections of colon for carcinoma who have coexisting adenomas, have twice the expected (3.4%) incidence of metachronous independent carcinomas elsewhere in the colon. *Ekelund* (1974) reported that of 115 patients with polyps, new polyps developed in 24 and carcinoma developed in three during an average followup of 102 months. In a control group of 115 patients, in which adenomas were not found, only eight patients developed adenomas and none developed carcinoma in a similar period of time.

From all of these lines of evidence one can conclude that (1) adenomas and carcinomas are frequently associated in the same colon; (2) that this association is not random, the adenomas tending to be most frequently found near the carcinoma; (3) patients with adenoma are at an increased risk of developing carcinoma.

It seems clear that whatever basic carcinogenic factors are operative in the production of adenoma are also operative for carcinoma. It neither proves nor disproves the origin of carcinoma from adenoma as opposed to origin in "normal" mucosa.

More direct lines of investigation are concerned with chromosomal, histochemical and histologic studies of individual adenomas of various types.

Chromosomal studies of adenomas are scanty, as previously mentioned, and are reviewed by *Mark* and coworkers (*Mark* et al., 1973). Abnormalities of the C and D group are common in adenomas and adenomas showing areas of "atypia" or carcinoma in situ show abnormalities approaching the marked aneuploidy and abnormal individual chromosomes seen in colonic carcinoma (*Enterline* and *Arvan*, 1967).

Studies of enzyme systems of adenoma with atypia again show many similarities to those of adenocarcinoma (*Czernobilsky* and *Tsou*, 1968).

There is no question that areas in adenomas show variations in cytology in the direction of loss of polarity, cellular pleomorphism, loss of normal tubular configuration, and at times, clear cut invasive carcinoma. In reading various reports it is difficult to compare figures. There is no good agreement on degrees of atpyia. Some divide their case by "degree of differentiation," some lump atypia, in situ and intramucosal carcinoma with invasive carcinoma. This accounts for much disparity of figures, but nonetheless much valuable information can be gleaned. It is clear that the occurrence of dysplasia and carcinoma is not a random event and certainly that not all adenomas become malignant. Factors of age, site, size and proximity to a large carcinoma and type of polyp play a role.

In deciding where in the spectrum of atypia, in situ and invasive carcinoma a given case fits, it is important that the adenoma be step sectioned before deciding on the extent of such change if present. I have seen adenomas which, in some sections showed minor atypia, in other intramucosal carcinoma, and in still others, invasive carcinoma extending almost to be the base of the stalk.

XII. Relation of Age to Atypia and Carcinoma in Adenoma

There are conflicting reports as to whether there is a higher incidence of atypia and carcinoma in adenomas from older patients (*Sato*, 1974; *Silverberg*, 1970; *Potet* and *Soullard*, 1971). Of course, most adenomas containing focal carcinomas are in older patients since the incidence of adenomas in general rises with age. Carcinoma within adenoma is exceedingly rare below 30 and very uncommon below 40.

XIII. Relation of Site to Atypia and Carcinoma in Adenoma

Ekelund (1974) states that the average "grade of differentiation" of adenomas is lower (i.e. more dysplastic) the closer an adenoma is to the anus. *Silverberg* (1970), who lumped noninvasive and invasive carcinomas together, found 24% of his sigmoid adenomas to contain areas of "malignancy" in contrast to 7.5% of adenomas from the rectum. Our studies (*Enterline*, 1962) reported that 7.6% of rectal adenomas contained carcinomas as contrasted to 12% of those from the sigmoid. In *Grinnell* and *Lane*'s (1958) large series 2.3% of adenomas proximal to the sigmoid contain invasive carcinoma, 3% of those in the sigmoid did so and 2.8% of those in the rectum, a relative uniform incidence throughout. All but eight of his 47 adenomas containing invasive carcinoma, however, were in the rectum or sigmoid. All series show a similar preponderance in surgical material of rectal and sigmoid lesions. In most series the percentage of adenomas with dysplasia or carcinoma is somewhat lower in the rectum as compared to the sigmoid.

It is clear that the majority of adenomas encountered surgically that contain areas of dysplasia or carcinoma are in the sigmoid and rectum. In part this is because these are the most common sites for adenomas, but also probably because of a somewhat increased percent of atypia and carcinoma in adenomas from these sites.

XIV. Relation of Size of Adenoma to Atypia and Carcinoma

Whether one measures atypia, carcinoma in situ, or invasive carcinoma, there is a clear direct relationship to the size of the adenoma in question. Such changes are uncommon in adenomas less than 5 mm and quite common in large adenomas. In our surgical material, (*Enterline*, 1962) atypia was seen in 3% of those under 1 cm and in 25% of those over 2 cm. *Culp*'s (1967) figures for adenomas under 5 mm were 6%, for those over 1 cm, 24%. Many authors have reported that the average size of adenomas containing areas of carcinoma is at least double that of adenomas lacking such change (*Enterline* et al., 1962; *Grinnell* and *Lane*, 1958; *Silverberg*, 1970). *Grinnell* and *Lane* (1958) have shown this to be true of invasive carcinoma which was present in less than 1% of those under 1 cm and in 16% of those over 2.5 cm. *Morson*'s (1974a) figures were 1.3% of those less than 1 cm, 9.5% of those from 1 to 2 cm, and 46% of those over 2 cm. Other figures for invasive carcinomas are comparable. Villous adenoma shows a less striking relationship of the presence of carcinoma to size, perhaps because very small villous adenomas are seldom reported as such.

For these reasons it is thought to be safe to follow rather than exterpate polypoid lesions under 1 cm if their removal presents a hazard to the patient. The advent of the flexible colonoscope has permitted removal of polyps high in the colon without laporoscopy.

XV. Pedunculated vs Sessile

In our experience (*Enterline*, 1974), 46 of 61 adenomas with areas of invasive carcinomas were in pedunculated adenomas. Thus, though the presence of a stalk provides a safety margin as we will discuss, it does not guarantee a benign adenoma.

XVI. "Satellite" Adenomas in Patients with Carcinoma

Several authors (*Ekelund* and *Lindstrom*, 1974; *Silverberg*, 1970; *Potet* and *Soullard*, 1971), have reported that dysplasia and carcinoma are distinctly more common in adenomas from patients with associated frank carcinoma and in adenomas close to such carcinomas. This supports the theory that whatever carcinogenic stimuli for carcinoma adenoma exist tend to be maximally expressed in the same subsite of the colon.

Putting this another way the patient discovered to have an adenoma with a focus of carcinoma is at high risk, perhaps as high as 20%, of having independent metachronous or synchronous carcinoma (*Enterline*, 1975).

XVII. Relation of Carcinoma to Type of Adenoma

The high incidence of invasive carcinoma in villous adenoma is recognized by all observers. In the past these have been considered quite distinct from other adenomas. Now, however, the presence of intermediate types – in part villous, in part tubular – is generally accepted. Focal villous change is reported to be present in as high as 35% of adenomas, and such changes appear to be size related (*Fung* and *Goldman*, 1970; *Enterline*, 1974). *Fung* and *Goldman* (1970) found such focal villous elements in 6% of adenomas from colons not containing villous adenomas or carcinoma, in 19% of adenomas from colons with coexisting carcinoma, and in 65% of adenomas which contained a focus of adenocarcinoma. Similarly *Kurzon* et al. (1974) found carcinoma in only 1% of adenomas lacking villous areas, in 18% of mixed lesions and in 48% of the pure villous adenomas. The latter author suggests that the papillary pattern heralds an increase in malignant potential. My own experience (*Enterline*, 1974) leads me to agree that invasive carcinoma as well as atypia and in situ carcinoma is much less common in the pure adenoma than in the mixed form. However, I found that only 1.2% of adenomas lacking any villous characteristic were larger than 2 cm and 80% were less than 1 cm, while in the mixed type 28% were larger than 2 cm (Table 3). Size for size, however, the incidence of in situ carcinoma was comparable (Table 4). Thus, in the 5 to 9 mm group, 7% of the tubular adenomas and 4.6% of the mixed forms contained in situ carcinoma. While in the 10 to 14 mm range figures were 21% and 22% respectively. I would suggest that the increased malignant potential observed is more a function of size. Obviously, however, villous pattern and size seem tied together.

Table 3. Incidence of in situ and invasive carcinoma in tubular adenomas and tubulo-villous adenomas in series from Hospital of the Universit of Pennsylvania (modified from Annals of Clinical and Laboratory Science volume 4, number 3, 1974)

		In situ Ca.		Invasive Ca.	
	Total	No.	%	No.	%
Tubular adenoma	174	12	7	1	.6
Tubulo-villous adenoma	80	15	18.7	3	3.75
Total	254	27	10.6	4	1.5

Table 4. Incidence of in situ carcinoma in tubular and tubulo-villous adenomas by size. Series from Hospital of the University of Pennsylvania (modified from Annals of Clinical Laboratory Science volume 4, number 3, 1974)

	Tubular Adenoma			Tubulo-villous Adenoma		
Size mm	Total No.	No. in situ Ca.	% in situ Ca.	Total No.	No. in situ Ca.	% in situ Ca.
1- 4	70	0	0	1	0	0
5- 9	69	5	7.2	22	1	4.6
10-14	19	4	21	18	4	22
15-20	14	2	14.3	16	4	25
21-30	1	0	0	17	4	23

XVIII. Significance of Carcinoma in Adenomas

Spratt and *Ackerman* in their 1958 report (*Spratt* and *Ackerman*, 1958), found that 43 of 434 polyps contained areas of micro carcinoma of which only one invaded the stalk. At that time they stated "although the type of carcinoma which is excluded from the stalk has the histologic appearance of carcinoma, it does not behave biologically as cancer." Neither they, nor later *Castleman* and *Krickstein* (1962) have seen metastases from such a lesion. My own experience has been similar in that I have not yet seen metastases from carcinoma confined to the "head" of a stalked adenoma. The latter authors reviewed 60 examples which had been diagnosed as carcinoma in adenoma at their hospital and rejected all but one case. Most were considered to be either examples of atypia or of pure polypoid carcinoma with the remainder being examples of villous adenomas with or without carcinoma. They were in agreement that, though carcinomas and adenomas were linked in some fashion, the adenomas could not be an important predecessor of clinically aggressive carcinoma. However, well documented examples of metastases from carcinoma in adenomas including those with pedicles are now in the literature (*Fenoglio* and *Lane*, 1974; *Strauss* and *Pascal*, 1975). In addition *Strauss* and *Pascal* (1975) have demonstrated a tumor associated antigen in intramucosal as well as invasive portions of such a carcinoma and in its lymph node metastases. Despite this, metastasis from such carcinomas is rare, a fact which has important surgical connotations.

To my knowledge it has not been proven that metastases in such situations occur without extension at least into the muscularis mucosa, whether or not the adenoma is pedunculated. An explanation for this has been offered in the recent demonstration (*Fenoglio* and *Lane*, 1973), that effective lymphatics do not exist superficial to the muscularis mucosa.

That metastases should occur at all is extremely surprising. We are considering here minute carcinomas often measured in millimeters, and of limited degrees of invasion. To conclude that these tiny cancers are therefore biologically not malignant would seem fallacious since their natural history has been abruptly interrupted by the act of excision of their host adenoma. Metastases from polypoid carcinomas in which no adenomatous remnants can be discovered are also only seen in cases in which at least the submucosa of the colon has been invaded.

Though percentages may differ, and allowing for variation in interpretation, there is no question that tiny neoplasms identical with adenocarcinoma occur in tubular and mixed adenomas with some frequency. One can develop a series of cases showing every stage from tiny foci of dysplasia through carcinoma in situ to truly invasive carcinomas. These, in turn, show variation from minimal submucosal invasion to involvement of much of the stalk of the polyp with replacement of all but a small fragment of the original adenomatous epithelium.

In general, extensive stalk invasion appears to correlate with shortening and thickening of the pedicle due to the accompanying fibrosis (Fig. 26). The presence of a long, thin pedicle nearly always means that if carcinoma is present it has not invaded the stalk to any marked degree. With continued invasion plus surface ulceration, all adenomatous remnants, and indeed the stalk if present, could be expected to disappear, leaving an ulcerated plaque of carcinoma bordered by non-adenomatous mucosal epithelium. Those who favor an adenomatous origin for carcinoma point out that many so-called "independent" small carcinomas reported may well have such an origin. Sessile villous adenomas, often involving large areas of mucosa, would logically be expected to retain adenomatous elements despite rather advanced invasive carcinoma, and indeed this is a common experience. In contrast, one would expect the tubular adenoma and mixed forms, especially those on pedicles, to rarely persist in the presence of advanced cancer.

Spratt et al. (1958) failed to find adenomatous remnants in a series of 323 carcinomas. *Castleman* and *Krickstein* (1962) concurred. *Enterline* et al. (1974) reported one percent of a series of some 600 adenocarcinomas to show evidence of marginal adenomatous tissue. At that time we were very careful to exclude cases in which adenomatous tissue showed any foci of villous pattern, and were investigating only large clinical cancers. *Morson* (1974a) reported that the incidence of such remnants was a function of the extent of the carcinoma, being present in 56% of small Dukes A carcinomas, in 18% of those with invasion of the muscularis propria, and 7.6% of Duke C carcinomas. *Fenoglio* et al. (1973) state that their experience agrees with that of *Morson*. An interpretative problem exists since there is some tendency for adenocarcinoma of the colon to be better differentiated peripherally and rarely one may see highly differentiated foci of adenocarcinomas deep within the muscularis propria (Fig. 6). Nevertheless, it seems clear that tissue histologically identical to adenoma may persist at times in even well advanced carcinomas.

XIX. Evidence for Minute Carcinomas Independent of Adenomas

The most convincing evidence of the development of carcinoma independent of adenoma would be the demonstration of minute areas of carcinoma in situ similar to those found so commonly in adenomas. I'm not aware of any such reports. Next most convincing would be very small, though invasive, carcinomas without ulceration, to eliminate the chance that these were merely the ulcerated base of what had formerly been an adenoma. Some cases of minute allegedly independent carcinomas have been published, though reports of carcinoma of 5 mm or less unassociated with adenoma are very rare. Of 20 cases of small cancers reported by *Spratt* and *Ackerman* (1962), only two were in this range, and one of these showed distinct ulceration. *Weingarten* and *Turell* (1952) reported a 2 mm lesion of the rectum which years later was excised (at the time measuring 2.5 mm) which was diagnosed as adenocarcinoma. The photograph is of too poor quality to judge whether adenomatous epithelium is at its edge. The surface is ulcerated. *Turell* (1959) states that he has observed two carcinomas of 2 mm and 3 mm in diameter. No photographs accompany the report. One of these two may be from the earlier report (*Weingarten* and *Turell*, 1952). I have seen only one carcinoma, not in an adenoma, in this size range. It measured 5 mm, was heavily ulcerated, and could well have represented the ulcerated base of a sloughed-off larger lesion.

Though admittedly a tiny carcinoma in an adenoma is easier to detect than an equally tiny carcinoma in a background of normal mucosa, it seems inconceivable, considering the number of proctoscopic and sigmoidoscopic examinations performed, that numerous examples of tiny independent carcinomas less than 5 mm would not be encountered and reported if indeed this is the usual mode of origin of rectal and sigmoidal adenocarcinoma.

Certainly many tiny metaplastic polyps of this size range are removed and diagnosed. A special case might be made for carcinoma arising in ulcerative colitis. Precancerous changes consistent with a diagnosis of carcinoma in situ can be found in that condition. Even here, however, villous changes have been described (*Morson* and *Pang*, 1967).

XX. Results of Prophylactic Removal of Adenomas

Finally, if indeed adenomas give rise to colonic carcinoma, prophylactic removal of all adenomas found in a population should have the effect of markedly reducing the incidence of clinical carcinoma subsequently observed in that population. This assumption is complicated in that it has been shown that the presence of adenoma defines a population at higher risk of colonic cancer than true of the general population. Two good studies are available. *Prager* and coworkers (1974) reported a population of 4400 patients of which 305 had adenomas discovered and removed by proctosigmoidscopy. They achieved a 93% follow-up. Twelve of the 305 were later discovered to have carcinoma within 15 years. This was twice the expected number of cancers. However, all carcinomas discovered were beyond reach of the sigmoidoscope. *Gilbertsen* (1974) recently reported on an ongoing study of 25 years duration. The study population consisted of 18,000 patients of age 45 or older at entrance to the study. All benign polyps encountered at annual proctoscopies were removed. The number of rectal cancers expected was between 75 and 80. The number encountered was 11. All of these were localized and only one of the 12 had extended to the muscularis propria. None had lymph node metastases. The most advanced cancer had been followed for a two and one-half year period before the patient would permit its removal. These two studies indicate that indeed the development of cancer, at least in an accessible site, is markedly reduced by the routine and systematic removal of adenomas.

1. Summary of the Adenoma-Carcinoma Sequence

It has been shown that:

1. Carcinoma and adenoma of the colon and rectum are linked in incidence in high and low risk geographic areas.
2. That patients with adenomas are at an increased risk of carcinoma.
3. That there is a rough, if not exact, subsite relationship between the distribution of adenomas and carcinomas within the large bowel.
4. That carcinoma does develop within adenomas and such change is a function of size (? duration) and type of adenoma.
5. That a series of adenomas can be collected showing all changes from focal atypia to full-blown clinical carcinoma.
6. That truly minute carcinoma rarely, if ever, are discovered independent of adenoma.
7. That systematic removal of adenomas does result in a sharply lowered incidence of later cancer in the segments of large bowel so managed.

It has been customary to preface articles on this subject with such statements as "the question of the relationship of adenoma to carcinoma of the colon has been the subject of much controversy." Indeed this is true. As a result of this "controversy" a great deal of information has accumulated in the past 15 years. In my opinion, this information has, beyond reasonable doubt, established that most if not all colonic carcinoma begins within a nexus of adenoma. While it would be both hazardous and unnecessary to claim such origin for every colonic carcinoma, the development of carcinoma in some other fashion must be the uncommon exception. Certainly only a small percentage of adenomas undergo this sequence. The sequence itself must be a slow process, but clinical prophylaxis of colonic cancer must be directed at the adenoma.

2. Practical Application of Current Knowledge of the Adenoma-Carcinoma Sequence

The clinician is faced with a polypoid lesion of the colon or rectum, however discovered. The gross appearance of polyps is not sufficiently distinctive to permit diagnosis short of excision and histologic examination. A possible exception is the common metaplastic (hyperplastic) polyp which the experienced clinician can learn to recognize and ignore. Pedunculated polyps give rise to metastases so rarely whether the polyp is an adenoma with carcinoma or a polypoid carcinoma; that if the base of the stalk is free of carcinoma, local excision plus followup is adequate therapy. Frozen sections transverse to the base of such lesions are helpful and are preferred to frozen section sampling of the "head." Large sessile lesions are best treated by colonic segmental resection since the incidence of cancer in those over 2.5 cm is at least 25%. A frozen section cannot be relied upon on such lesions to eliminate the possibility of carcinoma. Similar lesions and villous adenomas in the rectum are best treated by initial local resection with later therapy planned after thorough histologic examination and not by frozen section. The presence of one proven adenoma of the colon or rectum places the patient in a higher risk category for the development of carcinoma. This risk is increased in those with multiple adenomas and also is very high in those with villous adenomas or with adenoma of whatever type containing in situ or invasive carcinoma. Such patients demand very careful and long term followup with examination of the entire colon by whatever means at intervals best not exceeding one year. Patients with adenomatous polyposis of course require colectomy. Those in which a rectal stump is permitted to exist require additional close attention and frequent examination.

XXI. Summary

I have attempted to show the diversity of types of lesions which may present as polyps of the colon or rectum, their identifying characteristics and their relation, if any, to carcinoma. Of these the colonic adenoma and its variants have been shown to be significantly associated with carcinoma. Of adenomatous polyps the large polyps, of the mixed and villous forms, are at the highest risk of developing carcinoma within them. There is good and compelling evidence to indicate that most carcinomas of the colon develop within adenoma.

References

Ajdukiewicz, A.B., Youngs, G.R., Bouchier, I.A.D.: Nodular lymphoid hyperplasia with hypogammaglobulinaemia. Gut 13, 589-595 (1972).

Alexander, R.H., Beckwith, J.B., Morgan, A., Bill, A.H.: Juvenile polyps of the colon and their relationship to allergy. Amer. J. Surg. 120, 222-225 (1970).

Allen, M.S., jr.: Hamartomatous inverted polyps of the rectum. Cancer 19, 257-265 (1966).

Arthur, J.F.: Structure and significance of metaplastic nodules in rectal mucosa. J. Clin. Path. 21, 735-743 (1968).

Babior, B.M.: Villous adenoma of the colon. Study of a patient with severe fluid and electrolyte disturbances. Amer. J. Med. 41, 615-621 (1966).

Bacon, H.E., Eisenberg, S.W.: Papillary adenoma or villous tumor of the rectum and colon. Ann. Surg. 174, 1002-1008 (1971).

Bartholomew, L.G., Moore, C.E., Dahlin, D.C., Waugh, J.M.: Intestinal polyposis associated with mucocutaneous pigmentation. Surg. Gynec. Obstet. 115, 1-11 (1962).

Behringer, G.E.: Polypoid lesions of the colon. Which should be removed? Surg. Clin. North Amer. 54, 699-712 (1974).

Berardi, R.S.: Carcinoid tumors of the colon (exclusive of the rectum): Review of the literature. Dis. Colon Rectum 15, 383-391 (1972).

Berg, J.W., Howell, M.A.: The geographic pathology of bowel cancer. Cancer 34, 807-814 (1974).

Blatt, L.J.: Polyps of the colon and rectum. Incidence and distribution. Dis. Colon Rectum 4, 277-282 (1961).

Bottomley, J.P., Cooper, E.H.: Cell proliferation in colonic mucosa and carcinoma of the colon. Proc. Roy. Soc. Med. 66, 1183-1184 (1973).

Bremner, C.G.,Ackerman, L.V.: Polyps and carcinoma of the large bowel in the South African Bantu. Cancer 26, 991-999 (1970).

Brown, N.K., Smith, M.P.: Neoplastic diathesis of patients with carcinoid. Cancer 32, 216-222 (1973).

Buckwalter, J.A., jr., Kent, T.H.: Ectopic submucosal glands in the colon. Arch. Path. 93, 562-564 (1972).

Burkitt, D.P.: Epidemiology of cancer of the colon and rectum. Cancer 28, 3-13 (1971).

Bussey, H.J.R., Wallace, M.H., Morson, B.C.: Metachronous carcinoma of the large intestine and intestinal polyps. Proc. Roy. Soc. Med. 60, 208-210 (1967).

Capitanio, M.A., Kirkpatrick, J.A.: Lymphoid hyperplasia of the colon in children. Roentgen observations. Radiology 94, 323-327 (1970).

Castleman, B., Krickstein, H.I.: Do adenomatous polyps of the colon become malignant? New Eng. J. Med. 267, 469-475 (1962).

Chapman, I.: Adenomatous polyp of large intestine: Incidence and distribution. Ann. Surg. 157, 223-226 (1963).

Cole, J.W., McKalen, A.: Studies on the morphogenesis of adenomatous polyps in the human colon. Cancer 16, 998-1002 (1963).

Crocker, D.W., Veith, F.J.: Focal primary mucosal hyperplasia of the colon. The case for its importance in the pathogenesis of cancer. Ann. Surg. 160, 215-225 (1964).

Cronkhite, L.W., jr., Canada, W.J.: Generalized gastrointestinal polyposis: An unusual syndrome of polyposis, pigmentation, alopecia, and onychotrophia. New Eng. J. Med. 252, 1011-1015 (1955).

Culp, C.E.: New studies of the colonic polyp and cancer. Surg. Clin. North Amer. 47, 955-960 (1967).

Czernobilsky, B., Tsou, K.-C.: Adenocarcinoma, adenomas and polyps of the colon. Histochemical study. Cancer 21, 165-177 (1968).
Danis, R.K.: Lymphoid hyperplasia of the ileum – always benign disease? Amer. J. Dis. Child. 127, 656-658 (1974).
Dawson, I.M.P., Pryse-Davies, J.: The development of carcinoma of the large intestine in ulcerative colitis. Brit. J. Surg. 47, 113-128 (1959).
Donnelly, W.H., Sieber, W.K., Yunis, E.J.: Polypoid ganglioneurofibromatosis of large bowel. Arch. Path. 87, 537-541 (1969).
Dozois, R.R., Judd, E.S., Dahlin, D.C., Bartholomew, L.G.: The Peutz-Jeghers Syndrome – Is there a predisposition to the development of intestinal malignancy? Arch. Surg. 98, 509-516 (1969).
Edwards, C.C., Jackman, R.J.: Unsuspected and subclinical lesions of the large intestine found at autopsy. Surg. Gynec. Obstet. 105, 754-758 (1957).
Ekelund, G.: On colorectal polyps and carcinoma with special reference to their interrelationship. Lund: Studentlitteratur 1974, pp. 1-80.
Ekelund, G., Lindstrom, C.: Histopathological analysis of benign polyps in patients with carcinoma of the colon and rectum. Gut 15, 654-663 (1974).
Enterline, H.T., Arvan, D.A.: Chromosome constitution of adenomas and adenocarcinoma of the colon. Cancer 20, 1746-1759 (1967).
Enterline, H.T., Evans, G.W., Mervado-Lugo, R., Miller, L., Fitts, W.T., jr.: Malignant pottential of adenomas of colon and rectum. J.A.M.A. 179, 322-330 (1962).
Enterline, H.T.: Pathology of colonic polyps as it relates to surgical management. Ann. Clin. Lab. Sci. 4, 145-150 (1974).
Enterline, H.T.: Management of polypoid lesions. J.A.M.A. 231, 967-968 (1975).
Falterman, K.W., Hill, C.B., Markey, J.C., Fox, J.W., Cohn, I., jr.: Cancer of the colon, rectum and anus: A review of 2313 cases. Cancer 34, 951-959 (1974).
Fechner, R.E.: Adenomatous polyps with submucosal cysts. Amer. J. Clin. Path. 59, 498-502 (1973).
Fenoglio, C.M., Kaye, G.I., Lane, N.: Distribution of human colonic lymphatics in normal, hyperplastic, and adenomatous tissue. Its relationship to metastasis from small carcinomas in pedunculated adenomas, with two case reports. Gastroenterology 64, 51-66 (1973).
Fenoglio, C.M., Lane, N.: The anatomical precursor of colorectal carcinoma. Cancer 34, 819-823 (1974).
Filipe, M.I.: Value of histochemical reaction for mucosubstances in the diagnosis of certain pathological conditions of the colon and rectum. Gut 10, 577-586 (1969).
Fraumeni, J.F., jr., Vogel, C.L., Easton, J.M.: Sarcomas and multiple polyposis in a kindred. A genetic variety of hereditary polyposis? Arch. Int. Med. 121, 57-61 (1968).
Fung, C.H.K., Goldman, H.: The incidence and significance of villous change in adenomatous polyps. Amer. J. Clin. Path. 53, 21-25 (1970).
Gannon, P.G., Dahlin, D.C., Bartholomew, L.G., Beahrs, O.H.: Polypoid glandular tumor of the small intestine. Surg. Gynec. Obstet. 114, 666-672 (1962).
Gilbertsen, V.A.: Proctosigmoidoscopy and polypectomy in reducing the incidence of rectal cancer. Cancer 34, 936-939 (1974).
Goldgraber, M.B., Kirsner, J.B.: Polyps and carcinoma of the colon. Arch. Int. Med. 100, 669-677 (1957).
Greene, F.L.: Epithelial misplacement in adenomatous polyps of the colon and rectum. Cancer 33, 206-217 (1974).
Greenwood, S.M., Huvos, A.G., Erlandson, R.A., Malt, S.H.: Rectal carcinoid and rectal adenocarcinoma: A case report and review of the literature. Dis. Colon Rectum. 17, 644-655 (1974).

Grinnell, R.S., Lane, N.: Benign and malignant adenomatous polyps and papillary adenomas of the colon and rectum. An analysis of 1,856 tumors in 1,335 patients. Surg. Gynec. Obstet. 106, 519-538 (1958).
Gruenberg, J., Mackman, S.: Multiple lymphoid polyps in familial polyposis. Ann. Surg. 175, 552-554 (1972).
Haggitt, R.C., Pitcock, J.A.: Familial polyposis of the colon. Cancer 26, 1232-1238 (1970).
Hayashi, T., Yatani, R., Apostol, J., Stemmermann, G.N.: Pathogenesis of hyperplastic polyps of the colon: A hpothesis based on ultrastructure and in vitro cell kinetics. Gastroenterology 66, 347-356 (1974).
Helwig, E.B.: The evolution of adenoma of the large intestine and their relation to carcinoma. Surg. Gynec. Obstet. 84, 36-49 (1947).
Helwig, E.B., Hansen, J.: Lymphoid polyps (benign lymphoma) and malignant lymphoma of rectum and anus. Surg. Gynec. Obstet. 92, 233-243 (1951).
Hill, M.J.: Bacteria and the etiology of colonic cancer. Cancer 34, 815-818 (1974).
Holgersen, L.O., Miller, R.E., Zintel, H.A.: Juvenile polyps of the colon. Surgery 69, 288-293 (1971).
Horrilleno, E.G., Eckert, C., Ackerman, L.V.: Polyps of rectum and colon in children. Cancer 10, 1210-1220 (1957).
Jeghers, H., McKusick, V.A., Katz, K.H.: Generalized intestinal polyposis and melanin spots of the oral mucosa, lips and digits: A syndrome of diagnostic significance. New Eng. J. Med. 241, 933-1005, 1031-1036 (1949).
Kaschula, R.O.C.: Mixed juvenile, adenomatous and intermediate polyposis coli. Dis. Colon Rectum 14, 368-374 (1971).
Kaye, G.I., Fenoglio, C.M., Pascal, R.R., Lane, N.: Comparative electron microscopic features of normal, hyperplastic, and adenomatous human colonic epithelium. Variations in cellular structure relative to the process of epithelial differentiation. Gastroenterology 64, 926-945 (1973).
Kurzon, R.M., Ortega, R., Rywlin, A.M.: The significance of papillary features in polyps of the large intestine. Amer. J. Clin. Path. 62, 447-454 (1974).
Lane, N., Lev, R.: Observations on the origin of adenomatous epithelium of the colon. Serial section of minute polyps in familial polyposis. Cancer 16, 751-764 (1963).
Lane, N., Kaplan, H., Pascal, R.R.: Minute adenomatous and hyperplastic polyps of the colon: Divergent patterns of epithelial growth with specific associated mesenchymal changes. Contrasting roles in the pathogenesis of carcinoma. Gastroenterology 60, 537-551 (1971).
Lipkin, M.: Proliferative changes in the colon. Amer. J. dig. Dis. 19, 1029-1032 (1974).
Long, G.C., Dockerty, M.B., Waugh, J.M.: Lipoma of the colon. Surg. Clin. N. Amer. 29, 1233-1243 (1949).
Lukash, W.W., Morgan, R.I., Sennett, C.O., Nielson, O.F.: Gastrointestinal neoplasms in von Recklinghausen's disease. Arch. Surg. 92, 905-908 (1966).
Mark, J., Mitelman, F., Dencker, H., Norryd, C., Tranberg, K.-G.: The specificity of the chromosomal abnormalities in human colonic polyps. A cytogenetic study of multiple polyps in a case of Gardner's syndrome. Acta path. microbiol. scand. Section A, 81, 85-90 (1973).
McColl, I., Bussey, H.J.R., Veale, A.M.O., Morson, B.C.: Juvenile polyposis coli. Proc. Roy. Soc. Med. 57, 896-897 (1964).
Messinetti, S., Zelli, G.P., Marcellino, L.R., Alcini, E.: Benign and malignant epithelial tumors of the gastrointestinal tract. Chromosome analysis in study and diagnosis. Cancer 21, 1000-1010 (1968).
Morson, B.C.: Some peculiarities in the histology of intestinal polyps. Dis. Colon Rectum 5, 337-344 (1962).

Morson, B.C.: The polyp-cancer sequence in the large bowel. Proc. Roy. Soc. Med. 67, 451-457 (1974a).

Morson, B.C.: Evolution of cancer of the colon and rectum. Cancer 34, 845-849 (1974b).

Morson, B.C., Dawson, I.M.P.: Inflammatory Disorders. In: Gastrointestinal Pathology. Oxford–London–Edinburgh–Melbourne: Blackwell Scientific Publications, 1972a, pp. 471-474.

Morson, B.C., Dawson, I.M.P.: Benign epithelial neoplasms. In: Gastrointestinal Pathology. Oxford–London–Edinburgh–Melbourne: Blackwell Scientific Publications, 1972b, p. 529.

Morson, B.C., Pang, L.: Rectal biopsy as an acid to cancer control in ulcerative colitis. Gut 8, 423-434 (1967).

Muto, T., Bussey, H.J.R., Morson, B.C.: Psuedo-carcninomatous invasion in adenomatous polyps of the colon and rectum. J. Clin. Pathol. 26, 25-31 (1973).

Nicoloff, D.M., Ellis, C.M., Humphrey, E.W.: Management of villous adenomas of the colon and rectum. Arch. Surg. 97, 254-260 (1968).

Olson, R.O., Davis, W.C.: Villous adenomas of the colon, benign or malignant? Arch. Surg. 98, 487-492 (1969).

Orimo, H., Fujita, T., Yoshikawa, M., Takemoto, T., Matsuo, Y., Nakao, K.: Gastrointestinal polyposis with protein-losing enteropathy, abnormal skin pigmentation, and loss of hair and nails (Cronkhite-Canada syndrome). Amer. J. Med. 47, 445-449 (1969).

Peutz, J.L.A.: On a very remarkable case of familial polyposis of the mucous membrane of the intestinal tract and the nasopharynx accompanied by peculiar pigmentation of the skin and mucous membranes. (DUT) Nederl. Maandschr. v. Geneesk. 10, 134-146 (1921).

Ponka, J.L., Walke, L.: Carcinoid tumors of the rectum. Dis. Colon Rectum 14, 46-56 (1971).

Potet, F., Soullard, J.: Polyps of the rectum and colon. Gut 12, 468-482 (1971).

Prager, E.D., Swinton, N.W., Young, J.L., Veidenheimer, M.C., Corman, M.L.: Follow-up study of patients with benign mucosal polyps discovered by proctosigmoidoscopy. Dis. Colon Rectum 17, 322-324 (1974).

Quan, S.H.Q., Castro, E.B.: Papillary adenomas (villous tumors): A review of 215 cases. Dis. Colon Rectum 14, 267-280 (1971).

Report of the Meeting of Investigators of the IRC for the Histological Classification of Intestinal Tumors. Nov. 1973. World Health Organization (to be published). Probably in 1976.

Rider, J.A., Kirsner, J.B., Moeller, H.C., Palmer, W.L.: Polyps of colon and rectum. J.A.M.A. 170, 633-638 (1959).

Robinson, M.J., Pardon, S., Rywlin, A.M.: Enterocolitis lymphofollicularis. Morphologic, pathologic, and serum immunoglobulin patterns. Arch. Path. 96, 311-315 (1973).

Roth, S.I., Helwig, E.B.: Juvenile polyps of the colon and rectum. Cancer 16, 468-479 (1963).

Sachatello, C.R.: Polypoid diseases of the gastrointestinal tract. J. Kentucky Med. Ass. 70, 540-544 (1972).

Sato, E.: Adenomatous polyps of large intestine in autopsy and surgical material. GANN 65, 295-306 (1974).

Scully, R.E.: Sex cord tumor with annular tubules, a distinctive ovarian tumor of the Peutz-Jeghers syndrome. Cancer 25, 1107-1121 (1970).

Shermeta, D.W., Morgan, W.W., Eggleston, J., White, J.J., Haller, J.A.: Juvenile retention polyps. J. Ped. Surg. 4, 211-215 (1969).

Shull, L.N., jr., Fitts, C.T.: Lymphoid polyposis associated with familial polyposis and Gardner's syndrome. Ann. Surg. 180, 319-322 (1974).
Silverberg, S.G.: Focally malignant adenomatous polyps of the colon and rectum. Surg. Gynec. Obstet. 131, 103-114 (1970).
Simpson, R.D., Harrison, E.G., jr., Mayo, C.W.: Mesenteric fibromatosis in familial polyposis: A variant of Gardner's syndrome. Cancer 17, 526-534 (1964).
Smith, W.G., Kern, B.B.: The nature of the mutation in familial multiple polyposis; papillary carcinoma of the thyroid, brain tumors and familial multiple polyposis. Dis. Colon Rectum 16, 264-271 (1973).
Spratt, J.S., jr., Ackerman, L.V.: Pathologic significance of polyps of the rectum and colon. Dis. Colon Rectum 3, 330-335 (1960).
Spratt, J.S., jr., Ackerman, L.V.: Small primary adenocarcinomas of the colon and rectum. J.A.M.A. 179, 337-346 (1962).
Spratt, J.S., jr., Ackerman, L.V., Moyer, C.A.: Relationship of polyps of colon to colonic cancer. Ann. Surg. 148, 682-696 (1958).
Stemmerman, G.N.: Patterns of disease among Japanese living in Hawaii. Arch. Environ. Health 20, 266-273 (1970).
Stemper, T.J., Kent, T.H., Summers, R.W.: Juvenile polyposis and gastrointestinal carcinoma – a study of a kindred. Ann. Int. Med. 83, 639-646 (1975).
Strauss, R.A., Pascal, R.R.: Invasive and metastasizing carcinoma in a small adenomatous polyp of the colon: Report of a case with demonstration of a tumor associated antigen. Human Path. 6, 256-259 (1975).
Swain, V.A.J., Young, W.F., Pringle, E.M.: Hypertrophy of the appendices epiploicae and lipomatous polyposis of the colon. Gut 10, 587-589 (1969).
Turcot, J., Despres, J.P., St. Pierre, F.: Malignant tumors of the central nervous system associated with familial polyposis of the colon. Dis. Colon Rectum 2, 465-468 (1959).
Turell, R.: Adenoma and cancer of rectum and colon. Surg. Clin. North Amer. 39, 1291-1308 (1959).
Utsunomiya, J., Gocho, H., Miyanaga, T., Hamaguchi, E., Kashimure, A., Aoki, N.,Komatsu, I.: Peutz-Jeghers syndrome: Its natural course and management. The Johns Hopkins Med. J. 136, 71-82 (1975).
Veale, A.M.O.: Juvenile polyposis coli. J. Med. Gen. 3, 5-16 (1966).
Virchow, R.: Die krankhaften Geschwulste. Vol. 1, Berlin 1863, p. 243.
Wayte, D.M.,Helwig, E.B.: Colitis cystica profunda. Amer. J. Clin. Path. 48, 159-169 (1967).
Wattenberg, L.W.: A histochemical study of succinic dehydrogenase and cytosome oxidase in proliferative lesions of the large intestine. Cancer Res. 19, 1118-1123 (1959).
Weingarten, M., Turell, R.: Carcinomatous mucosal excrescence of the rectum. J.A.M.A. 149, 1467-1468 (1952).
Weisburger, J.H.: Colon carcinogens: Their metabolism and mode of action. Cancer 28, 60-69 (1971).
Wiebecke, B., Brandts, A., Eder, M.: Epithelial proliferation and morphogenesis of hyperplastic adenomatous and villous polyps of the human colon. Virch. Arch. Path. Anat. and Hist. 364, 35-49 (1974).
Williams, J.P., Knudsen, A.: Peutz-Jeghers syndrome with metastasizing duodenal carcinoma. Gut 6, 179-184 (1965).

Mucin Histochemistry of the Colon

M.I. FILIPE and A.C. BRANFOOT

I. Introduction

"Of all branches of technology capable of conferring on histopathology an increase in objectivity, histochemistry must take first place" (*Pearse*, 1975). Pathologists often face diagnostic problems which are difficult or impossible to solve by routine histological methods, but which may be resolved by histochemical techniques for the detection in cells and tissues of a variety of enzyme activities, specific substances and reactive groups.

Enzyme histochemistry has been applied to benign and malignant tumours of the large bowel in an attempt to assess their malignant potential and prognosis, but the results have not encouraged the use of such methods in diagnosis (*Wattenberg*, 1959; *Willighagen* and *Planteydt*, 1959; *Czernobilsky* and *Tsou*, 1968; *Filipe*, 1971a; *McGinty* et al., 1973; *Marsden* and *Dawson*, 1974). Likewise, changes described by *Monis* and *Mendeloff* (1965) as characteristic of ulcerative colitis have not been confirmed (*Melnyk* et al., 1967; *Filipe*, 1971a), and up to now enzyme histochemistry has failed to help diagnostically.

However, advances in the chemical identification of mucosubstances and a better knowledge of how to stain them have transformed this field of research, now providing a promising instrument for diagnosis, as well as giving insights into the synthesis and secretion of mucus. Further advances in the biological role of these compounds will depend on close collaboration between histochemistry, biochemistry and immunology.

The study of mucins in the normal colonic mucosa and their variations in neoplasia and inflammatory states appears rewarding. The first results have aroused great expectations and these will be discussed as follows:

a) Detection of early malignancy in the general population;

b) Identification of the origin of metastatic adenocarcinoma;

c) Classification of polyps and assessment of their malignant potential;

d) Prediction of malignant change in patients at risk with inflammatory bowel disease;

e) Differential diagnosis of ulcerative colitis and Crohn's disease.

It should be noted at once that histochemical demonstration of mucosubstances offers advantages over many other branches of technology in the simplicity of handling and preparation of material, technical assistance and laboratory facilities required, for these are little more than those routinely employed.

II. Classification of Mucosubstances

Mucosubstances is the general term proposed by *Spicer* et al. (1965) to include all the carbohydrate-containing compounds which can be detected in cells and tissues by histochemical methods. The word *mucin* is reserved for epithelial mucosubstances, whilst *mucopolysaccharide* should be used only for those present in connective tissue.

Although well aware of the differences between histochemical methods applied to tissue sections and chemical reactions taking place in vitro, we think it advisable, whenever possible, to correlate histochemical results with those of biochemical analysis. Bearing this in mind, we may say that mucosubstances visualized histochemically in colonic epithelium (mucins), correspond with glycoproteins of biochemical nomenclature (*Jeanloz*, 1960, 1963).

Glycoproteins, as defined by *Gottschalk* (1966), are conjugated proteins which have as prosthetic groups one or more heterosaccharides with a relatively low number of sugar residues, that lack a serial repeating unit and are bound covalently to the polypeptide chain. In glycoproteins many of the short carbohydrate units have a terminal sialic acid group. Only a few types of sugar occur, the most common being D-mannose, D-galactose, L-fucose, N-acetyl D-galactosamine, and the N- and O-acetyl and N-glycolyl derivatives of neuraminic acid. Ester sulphates can also be found in glycoproteins, and sometimes both sialic acid and ester sulphate are present in the same molecule. Uronic acid is not found. The carbohydrate moiety is linked to the polypeptide chain by an O-glycosidic bond between the aminoacids serine or threonine and N-acetyl-D-galactosamine (*Gottschalk,* 1966; *Spiro*, 1969a, b, 1973).

Glycoproteins are the major components of epithelial mucous secretions.

Mucosubstances, in general, can be classified by their histochemical properties into two main groups:

1. **Neutral mucosubstances:** These contain sugar units with a neutral charge, such as D-galactose, D-mannose, L-fucose, and the N-acetyl derivatives of hexosamines. They are readily detected by the PAS technique.

2. **Acid mucosubstances:** These contain acidic groups which have a strong negative charge and include uronic acid, phosphates, sialic acids and sulphate groups. They are usually identified by their affinity for basic and metachromatic dyes. They can be further subdi-

Table 1. Histochemical Methods to Visualize Epithelial Mucins

Method	Interpretation
Light Microscopy	
Fixation in 10% neutral formol-calcium; paraffin sections	
Periodic acid-Schiff (PAS)	Magenta: All MS containing hexoses and deoxyhexoses with vic-glycol groups; glycogen, neutral MS, some non-sulphated acid MS.
Alcian blue pH 2.5 (AB 2.5)	Basophilia: weakly sulphated MS, carboxyl groups of sialomucins.
Alcian blue pH 1.0 (AB 1.0)	Basophilia: sulphated MS.
High iron-diamine (HID)	Brown-black: sulphated MS. Sialomucins unstained.
High iron-diamine-Alcian blue pH 2.5 (HID-AB)	Brown-black: sulphated MS. Basophilia: Non-sulphated acid MS (sialomucins)
Methylation-HCL, followed by saponification	Complex mechanism. Possible effects: a) Esterification of carboxyl groups: eliminates basophilia of sialomucins. Carboxyl groups regain basophilia after saponification. b) Carboxyl groups form lactones. c) Hydrolysis of sulphate esters. d) De-O-acylation; de-N-acylation. e) Cleavage of ketosidic bonds between terminal sialic acids and the glycoprotein.
Neuraminidase digestion	Hydrolysis of sialic acids, some sialomucins lose basophilia. O-acetyl derivatives are resistant.
Electron Microscopy	
Fixation in glutaraldehyde. Resin embedding.	
Periodic acid-Chromic acid-silver methenamine (PA-CrA-Silver)	As PAS.

vided, according to the absence or presence of one or other acid groups, by varying the pH or the salt concentration of the staining solutions, and by the use of iron-diamine techniques. The specificity of the methods to identify the various acidic groups can be increased by selective enzymatic digestion (e.g. Vibrio cholerae sialidase) and blocking techniques (e.g. methylation). They may also contain vic-glycol groups and so give a PAS reaction.

The histochemical methods used for the detection of mucosubstances depend on the chemical groups present in the carbohydrate moiety, and those more commonly used at light and electron microscopic levels are shown in Table 1.

III. Histochemical Properties of Colonic Mucins

Histochemical techniques reveal neutral, acid sulphated, and acid non-sulphated mucosubstances in normal colonic epithelium (*Filipe*, 1969; *Gad*, 1969; *Filipe*, 1971b; *Mäkelä* et al., 1971) (Table 2).

Table. 2. Distribution of epithelial mucins in the large intestine: normal and ***transitional*** mucosa

	MUCOSA	PAS	AB 2.5	AB 1.0	AB-$MgCl_2$	HID	HID-AB.	Type of Mucin
A	1 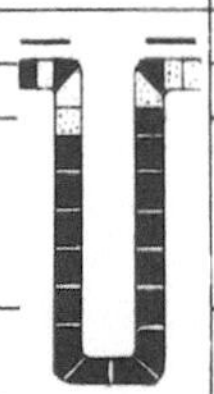	+	+	+	0.4M +	+	Brown	Sulphomucin
	2	+	+	0	0.2M +	0	Basophilia	Sialomucin
	3	+	+	+	0.4M + 0.2M +	+	Brown	Sulphomucin
	4	+	+	+	0.4M + 0.2M +	+	Brown	Sulphomucin
B	1 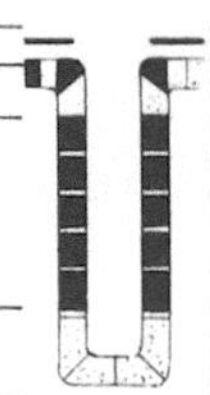	+	+	+	0.4M +	+	Brown	Sulphomucin
	2	+	+	0	0.2M +	0	Basophilia	Sialomucin
	3	+	+	+	0.4M + 0.2M +	+	Brown	Sulphomucin
	4	+	+	0	0.2M +	0	Basophilia	Sialomucin
C	1 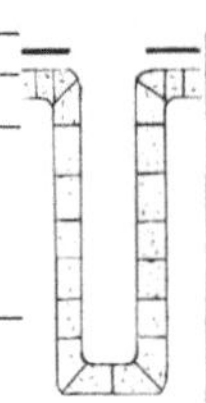	+	+	+	0.4M +	+	Brown	Sulphomucin
	2	+	+	0	0.2M +	0	Basophilia	Sialomucin
	3	+	+	0	0.2M +	0	Basophilia	Sialomucin
	4	+	+	0	0.2M +	0	Basophilia	Sialomucin

Key: A = normal mucosa (left colon); B = normal mucosa (right colon); C = "transitional" mucosa.
1 = cell coat; 2= surface and upper crypt; 3= middle crypt; 4= lower crypt.

Goblet Cell Mucin (GCM): The secretory product of the goblet cell is complex and displays both neutral and acid groups. *Neutral mucins* are all periodate-reactive, giving a positive PAS reaction which is not modified by prior diastase digestion. They contain hexoses, such as glucose, galactose and mannose, and the methyl pentose, fucose, which all have vic-glycol groups readily oxidized by periodic acid to form dialdehydes. These aldehydes will then react with Schiff's reagent to form a substituted red dye. Neutral mucins are not a significant constituent of the GCM, but there may be other substances in the secretory product, such as derivatives of sialic acids, which will also give a positive PAS reaction (*Montreuil* and *Biserte*, 1959; *Esterley* and *Spicer*, 1968; *Pearse*, 1968). Many other substances like polysaccharides (e.g. glycogen), certain carbohydrate-protein complexes, and glycolipids can all react similarly with periodic acid and combine with Schiff reagent (*Pearse*, 1968), but in paraffin-embedded material, after diastase digestion and with controlled oxidation by periodic acid for only 10 min, the PAS reaction demonstrates vic-glycols which are present only in *neutral* and *some acid mucosubstances (sialomucins).*

Sulphomucins and sialomucins: These are the main carbohydrateprotein complex in GCM. They both react with cationic dyes, the most common of which is Alcian blue: the negatively-charged ionized groups in the acid mucins react with the positively-charged dye, most probably through the formation of salt linkages. The separation of the two main acid radicals in the acid mucins (i.e. the carboxyl groups of the sialomucins and the sulphates) can be attempted in various ways.

Alcian blue solutions can be used at different pHs. Both sulphomucins and sialomucins show basophilia with Alcian blue at pH 2.5 (*Mowry* and *Morard*, 1957), but when the pH is lowered to 1.0 basophilia persists only in those goblet cells containing strongly sulphated mucin (*Lev* and *Spicer*, 1964).

By adding various concentrations of $MgCl_2$ to the Alcian blue solution at pH 5.8, it is possible, according to the *"critical electrolyte concentration"* (CEC) concept of *Scott* and *Dorling* (1965), to differentiate carboxyl groups which cause basophilia at low electrolyte concentration, from sulphate groups which have higher CECs. CGM shows intense basophilia at 0.2M concentration of $MgCl_2$, indicating the presence of acid mucosubstances, but at a higher molarity (0.4M $MgCl_2$) basophilia disappears or decreases in goblet cells containing sialomucins, whilst it persists, though weakly, in those where sulphated groups predominate.

The distinction between sulphomucins and sialomucins can be successfully achieved in colonic epithelium by diamine methods. The high iron-diamine (HID) method specifically stains sulphomucins brown-black, but leaves sialomucins unstained (*Spicer*, 1965; *Gad* and *Sylven*, 1969; *Sorvari* and *Arvilommi*, 1973). When followed by Alcian blue at pH 2.5, the sulphated groups in the GCM react with the diamines to give a brown-black colour, whilst the sialomucins react with Alcian blue and are coloured blue. It is not infrequent to find both types of acid mucin in the same cell. The method is essentially based on the reaction taking place between the two isomers, *m* and *p* of diamines and periodate-engendered aldehyde groups. The reaction is accelerated by adding ferric chloride as oxidant. Ferric chloride also lowers the pH of the solution (*Sorvari*, 1972) and thus prevents the ionization of carboxyl groups which could react with the positively-charged diamine complex. Ferric ions may also have a greater affinity than diamines for nucleic acids, and thus render the technique more specific. The high iron-diamine method followed by Alcian blue at pH 2.5 (HID-AB) is routinely and successfully applied to colonic biopsies in our laboratory to reveal sulphomucins and sialomucins simultaneously.

Further characterization of the carboxyl and sulphated radicals in the GCM is obtained by methylation and sialidase digestion. Strong methylation with methanol-HCl (*Spicer* and *Lillie*, 1959) results in a complete absence of colour reaction with HID-AB. Mild methylation fails in most cases to remove the basophilia attributed to carboxyl groups. Methylation using thionyl chloride solution (*Stoward*, 1967, 1968) reduces the staining of sulphomucins by HID, thus making the affinity of carboxyl groups for Alcian blue more apparent in the HID-AB sequence. The mechanism of methylation is complex and the results are difficult to interpret. Formerly these solutions were thought to esterify the carboxyl groups in acid mucosubstances and proteins and to remove sulphate hemi-ester groups. More recent work, however, suggests that carboxyl groups undergo transformation to lactones rather than become esterified (*Sorvari* and *Stoward*, 1970a, b). Also reactions such as de-O-acylation, de-N-acylation and the cleavage of the ketosidic bonds linking terminal sialic acid residues to glycoproteins may take place (*Reid* et al., 1974). The treatment of sections by KOH in methanol (saponification) restores the basophilia due to carboxyl groups removed by previous methylation. But it may also produce an increase in PAS reactivity (KOH-PAS effect), possibly owing to the greater number of 1-2 glycol groups and/or α-amino alcohols available (*Culling* et al., 1971). Recent work suggests that the presence of O-acylated sialic acids in GCM may be responsible for the KOH-PAS effect (*Reid* et al., 1973; *Culling* et al., 1974). An increase in basophilia with Alcian blue at pH 1.0 and HID staining after saponification also occurs in GCM, a change attributed to unmasking of sulphate or other highly acidic groups.

The staining properties of GCM are variably affected by treatment of the sections with Vibrio cholerae neuraminidase (*Sorvari* and *Lauren*, 1973), some being resistant, whilst other goblet cells show a decreased affinity for Alcian blue at pH 2.5 after incubation with the enzyme. The presence of neuraminidase-resistant sialomucins has been described throughout the gastrointestinal tract (*Lev* and *Spicer*, 1965; *Filipe*, 1971b; *Mäkelä* et al., 1971; *Culling* et al., 1974). Biochemical estimation of the sialomucins in our material from human colon reveals that 50-60% are resistant to enzymatic hydrolysis (*Filipe* and *Cooke*, 1974; *Rogers* et al., in preparation). These are most probably O-acetyl derivatives, which have been found to be resistant to neuraminidase hydrolysis (*Andrews* et al., 1967; *Ravetto*, 1968; *Drzeniek*, 1973; *Sorvari* and *Lauren*, 1973; *Culling* et al., 1974).

Cell Coat: Histochemical techniques at light and electronmicroscopic levels reveal the presence of a carbohydrate-rich layer covering the free surface of the epithelial cells (*Ito*, 1965a; *Rambourg* and *Leblond*, 1967). It is tightly bound to the plasma membrane and must be considered an integral part of it (*Winzler*, 1970; *Rambourg*, 1971). In colonic epithelium it stains like sulphated acid mucins: a strong basophilia with Alcian blue at pH 2.5 and pH 1.0, and a brown-black colour with the HID technique. A positive reaction with PAS not modified by prior diastase digestion is attributable to both fucose and sialic acid residues. The glycoprotein nature of the cell coat is clearly revealed at EM level by an intense silver deposit by PA-CrA-silver methenamine (*Rambourg* and *Leblond*, 1967; *Rambourg*, 1973) or by *Thiéry*'s (1972) periodic acid-thiocarbohydrazide-silver technique, and with Hale's colloidal iron stain (*Ito*, 1965a). The presence of sulphate groups has been confirmed by uptake studies with $^{35}SO_4$ (*Ito* and *Revel*, 1964; *Ito*, 1965b).

The glycoprotein composition of the cell coat is thus not unlike that of goblet cell mucus (*Forstner*, 1970; *Lukie* and *Forstner*, 1972), but there is strong evidence that the surface coat carbohydrate is synthesized in absorptive rather than in goblet cells (*Ito* and *Revel*, 1964; *Ito*, 1965a, b; *Neutra* and *Leblond*, 1966a, b; *Rambourg* and *Leblond*, 1967; *Rambourg* et al., 1969; *Bennett* and *Leblond*, 1970).

IV. Mucin Distribution within the Crypt and its Regional Variations

A variety of epithelial cells is found in the crypt and luminal surface of colonic mucosa, each crypt level being characterized by a cell population which chiefly reflects different degrees of maturation (*Pittman* and *Pittman*, 1966; *Kaye* et al., 1973; *Dawson* and *Filipe*, 1976a).

Histochemical, biochemical and ultrastructural changes take place during this regular process of cell differentiation. Undifferentiated and immature cells, capable of DNA synthesis and proliferation, predominate at the bottom of the crypt (*Lipkin* et al., 1963; *Immondi* et al., 1969; *Deschner*, 1970). As the cells migrate towards the surface, they lose their capacity for DNA synthesis and mitotic activity, to develop ultrastructural features of mature goblet and absorptive cells in the middle and upper crypt. In the surface epithelium the cells eventually degenerate, lose their mucin content and die, finally being extruded into the lumen. Parallel with cell differentiation there seems to be a gradient of glycoprotein synthesis, incomplete glycoproteins being found in the surfaces of less mature cells, and in the small intestine there are differences in the glycosyl and galactosyltransferases of the immature crypt and mature villous cells. These findings suggest that there may be similarities between immature mitotically-active intestinal cells and their counterparts in both fetal gut and neoplasms (*Weiser*, 1973a, b; *Isselbacher*, 1974).

The mucins of the goblet cells have also been shown to vary with their level in the crypt (Table 2). In the left colon, sulphomucins predominate in the lower half of the crypt. In the upper crypt one may see the same pattern as in the lower half, but more often both sulphomucins and sialomucins are present. In the surface epithelium both types of acid mucin can be found, either separately in single cells or together in variable proportions in the same cell. Neutral mucins may also be found: in moderate amounts in the upper crypt and surface epithelium, and less in the lower crypt.

The composition and distribution of goblet cell mucins described above has been seen by us in more than 100 left colons and are reported similarly by others (*Gad*, 1969; *Mäkelä* et al., 1971). Together they may be taken as the *normal mucous pattern* of the left colon, including descending and sigmoid portions and rectum. In the right colon, which for our purposes seems to include as far as the splenic flexure, the mucous pattern differs from that of the left half (Table 2). In most of our specimens (though not all) sialomucins are present in the lower third of the crypt, whilst sulphomucins occupy the upper two thirds (*Greco* et al., 1967; *Filipe* and *Branfoot*, 1974; *Lev* and *Orlic*, 1974).

It is tempting to correlate the variations in mucins along the crypt with cell differentiation. Neutral mucins predominate in immature cells but are later replaced by strongly acid ones, and, at a final stage in the biological cycle of the cell, weakly acid mucins become the major component. It is interesting to note that in early fetal life colonic mucus contains sialic acids, and that only in later development do ester sulphates appear as part of the goblet cell mucus (*Lev*, 1968; *Lev* and *Orlic*, 1974).

The presence of one or both types of acid mucin in a single goblet cell can possibly be explained by the formation of two separate polymers, or one polymer with varying proportions of sialic acid and sulphate (*Spicer*, 1965; *Spicer* and *Sun*, 1967). There is evidence that sialic acid-producing cells can also synthesize sulphated material (*Draper* and *Kent*, 1963), and the two radicals can co-exist in various mucus-secreting cells (*Bignardi* et al., 1964; *Lamb* and *Reid*, 1969; *Kent*, 1971). The latter provides a logical hypothesis to explain some of the changes seen in malignancy and is discussed below. The regional variations in mucin distribution between left and right colons may be related to differences in embryology and physiology, but they are as yet poorly understood.

V. The Synthesis and Functions of Intestinal Mucins

Glycoproteins are the main carbohydrate-protein component of the mucus secreted in the intestine. They are essentially carbohydrate and protein moieties linked by a covalent bond. Their synthesis takes four main steps:

1. Synthesis of the protein molecule;
2. Linkage of carbohydrate units to the peptide chain;
3. Assembly of the carbohydrate units;
4. Sulphation.

The protein part is a string of aminoacids assembled in the ribosomes under genetic control (*Spiro*, 1973; *Winzler*, 1970). High resolution autoradiography and cell fraction studies with labeled aminoacids show that protein precursors appear at an early stage in the rough endoplasmic reticulum and only later in the Golgi area (*Revel*, 1970; *Shenkein* and *Uhr*, 1970). It is thought that synthesis of the protein is completed independently before any carbohydrate is attached to its peptide chain (*Spiro* and *Spiro*, 1966; *Spiro*, 1969a, 1973).

The carbohydrate units are linked to the aminoacids serine and threonine in the peptide chain, by N-acetyl glucosamine or N-acetyl galactosamine through an O-glycosidic bond (*Spiro*, 1969a, 1973), though the precise site and mode of attachment of the first sugar remain controversial.

Once synthesized the protein molecule is released from the ribosomes and migrates through the channels of the endoplasmic reticulum to the Golgi apparatus, where specific glycosyltransferases attach one by one to its backbone the sugar residues that go to form its carbohydrate side-chains. The synthesis of the carbohydrate parts needs a series of reactions to convert the neutral sugars, glucose and galactose, into reactive nucleotide-sugar intermediates (*Draper* and *Kent*, 1963; *Peterson* and *Leblond*, 1964; *Neutra* and *Leblond*, 1966a, b; *Warren*, 1966). Activated sugars are then transferred to specific acceptors in the carbohydrate chain. The enzymes responsible for this transfer are glycosyltransferases which are specific for the sugar-nucleotide as well as the acceptors.

In vitro and in vivo experiments using $^{35}SO_4$ show radioactive material in colonic goblet cells of animals (*Lane* et al., 1964; *Young*, 1973) and man (*Filipe*, 1971c), and also in the glycoprotein fractions isolated from intestinal mucins (*Kent* and *Pasternak*, 1958; *Pasternak*, et al., 1958). Sulphation seems to take place in two stages: sulphate is first "activated" and then transferred to receptor molecules by specific sulphotransferases (*Wolfe* and *Vickery*, 1964; *Young*, 1973). That sulphation of glycoproteins occurs in the Golgi apparatus is suggested, *inter alia*, by high resolution autoradiographic studies with $^{35}SO_4$: isotope was detected early in the paranuclear part of the Golgi area, then in the supranuclear zone, and finally in the mucous secretory product. No other organelle showed any radioactivity (*Lane* et al., 1964; *Young*, 1973).

The Golgi apparatus seems to play an important role in the synthesis of glycoproteins. Although chain initiation may start in the endoplasmic reticulum, it is believed that the Golgi membranes are the main site for completion of the carbohydrate-protein complex by attachment of the terminal sugars, such as sialic acid and fucose (*Peterson* and *Leblond*, 1964; *Neutra* and *Leblond*, 1966b; *Bennett* et al., 1974), and sulphate (*Young*, 1973).

The cell coat glycoproteins seem to follow an intracellular pathway of synthesis similar to that of the secretory glycoproteins, but it seems to lie in columnar rather than goblet cells. In light and electron microscopic autoradiographic studies with sugar precursors, labeled material appeared in the Golgi area soon after injection and later migrated to the apical coat of columnar cells (*Peterson* and *Leblond*, 1964; *Ito*, 1965b; *Neutra* and *Leblond*, 1966b; *Bennett*, 1970). How material is conveyed is not yet clear, but transport may involve tubules or vesicles. It can be traced cytochemically at EM level from the formation and maturation faces in the Golgi apparatus into vesicles in both absorptive and *intermediate* cells (*Dawson* and *Filipe*, 1976b). A gradient of glycoprotein concentration towards the apical cytoplasm is well recognized, and some of these vesicles are seen to reach and apparently fuse with the cell membrane (*Rambourg* et al., 1969; *Thiéry*, 1972; *Dawson* and *Filipe*, 1976b).

The intracellular synthesis of glycoprotein is a continuous process, and its rate has been estimated. It was calculated that a fresh droplet was released from the Golgi membranes every 2-4 min in the rat (*Neutra* and *Leblond*, 1966a). The factors controlling synthesis, intracellular transport and secretion are complex and not yet fully understood. The assembly of the protein backbone in the ribosomes is determined genetically, while that of the carbohydrate moiety is postribosomal and not directed by a nucleic acid template. However, it is under indirect genetic control, for this operates through the synthesis of glycosyltransferases. Thus genetic, physiological and environmental factors may all induce changes in the composition and secretion of glycoproteins.

Experiments in vivo and in vitro have shown that changes both in the rate of mucous secretion and in its composition can be induced by local irritants and drugs, either directly or through stimulation of colonic nerves. An excessive discharge of mucous droplets leading to goblet cell exhaustion has been described after direct application of an irritant (*Florey*, 1970). Increased goblet cell mucus production is seen after vagal stimulation or parasympathomimetic drugs. *Smith* and *Butler* (1974) have described the effects of various cholinergic and adrenergic drugs on synthesis and secretion of mucus in the colonic mucosa of mice. With β-adrenergic drugs they found increased synthesis and secretion accompanied by changes in composition. Oversecretion of sialomucins followed long-term cholinergic stimulation.

Yet how the nerves act is not clear. Pieces of colonic mucosa in organ culture have been shown to respond to acetyl-choline by increased secretion of glycoprotein, but without any changes in their rate of synthesis (*MacDermott* et al., 1974). Other drugs, such as aspirin and cortisone, seem to reduce mucin secretion in the colon (*Takeuchi* et al., 1972).

It is important to bear in mind that *non-specific* and physiological stimuli like these may affect the synthesis and secretion of glycoproteins in the colon, and so modify the patterns of secretion that seem to characterize some of its pathological conditions.

The biological functions of intestinal mucins are not fully known and there is much yet to be learned about the roles played by their glycoprotein constituents. Mucins have at least two functions, protective and lubricative, and their general properties have been clearly discussed by *Florey* (1970).

1. **Protection** from abrasion by solid faecal matter may be given by mucin in the surface coat which can seal breaches in the epithelium. *Smith* and *Butler* (1974) have noted a remarkable absence of inflammation where such defects have been sealed by mucin in the mouse.

2. **Lubrication** of the faecal mass may facilitate its movement by peristalsis.

3. **Barrier** functions should be added since mucins may reinforce the cell membranes and tight junctions, e.g. in the maintenance of electrolytic gradients across the mucosal surfaces (*Winzler*, 1970), for, even if they are permeable by ions, they may steepen the gradient by retarding diffusion. Thus, sialic acid on the cell surface seems to transport potassium ions through the plasma membrane, and there is also evidence that it may act as a carrier in the transport of protein out of the cell (*Rambourg*, 1971).

Regional variations in these functions may be expected because, as the faeces pass along the intestine, dehydration makes them firmer and more abrasive, whilst reabsorption of ions multiplies their electrolytic differences. Thus the above functions may be distributed between the two main groups of acid mucins:

a) *Sialomucins* are more viscous and likely to be the primary protective. *Smith* and *Butler* (1974) describe how they form an unbroken coat from the bottom of the crypt to the surface in the mouse, and how efficiently they seal epithelial breaches.

b) *Sulphomucins* are less viscid and likely to have a lubricative effect. *Smith* and *Butler* (1974) note their increase in the distal colon of the mouse, and in the human colon we have noted a difference in the mucous patterns of the regions proximal and distal to the splenic flexure.

Glycoproteins in gel form are impermeable to proteolytic enzymes such as trypsin and may thus protect the mucosa, but it has been shown that in the sol state they may actually stimulate proteolytic digestion. Thus bowel contents switching the colloid mucin from gel to sol state may make the mucosa vulnerable (*Shora* et al., 1975).

4. **Mutual cell recognition** is the basis of morphogenesis, for cells must recognize each other to group themselves as tissues and organs. The sugars of cell coat glycoproteins may play a central part in this interplay and mutual recognition of cells. Normal cells stop growing when they make contact with one another by triggering off reactions leading to inhibition of DNA synthesis (*Emmelot*, 1973), whereas growth without restraint characterizes cancer

cells which may have assumed new characters by changing their surface glycoproteins. The possible roles of sialic acid and glycosyltransferases in the cell membrane and their variations in malignant transformation are discussed below.

5. **Intercellular adhesiveness** differs between normal and malignant cells and can be attributed to the greater sialic acid content of the latter's plasma membranes, for after neuraminidase treatment cell adhesiveness increases and so suggests that the charged residues may be responsible (*Deman* et al., 1974).

6. **Antigenicity** of cell membranes is largely due to their carbohydrate components (*Winzler*, 1970). For instance, the genetic basis of blood group antigens has been shown to rest on the specificity of glycosyltransferases (*Kim* and *Perdomo*, 1972). Changes of antigenic specificity as cells become malignant have been reported, but whether or not there are true *tumour-specific* antigens in plasma membranes of neoplastic cells remains to be established (*Winzler*, 1970). Sialic acid in the cell membrane does not seem to have antigenic properties itself, but it may hide the antigenic sites and shield them from immunocompetent cells (*Currie* and *Bagshawe*, 1968).

7. **Enzymatic activity** may reside in the cell coat, as seen in the small intestine, where enzymes like invertase and maltase may carry out terminal hydrolytic digestion of carbohydrates and proteins as they lie on the surface of the microvillous membrane (*Rambourg*, 1971).

VI. Detection of Early Malignancy in the General Population

In Westernized developed countries cancer of the colon and rectum is one of the commonest forms of malignant disease (*Morson* and *Dawson*, 1972). About half can be cured by surgery but good results depend on early diagnosis. Small established carcinomas can often be detected now by air-contrast barium enema and colonoscopy (*Hawley*, 1974), but quite often the tiny biopsies obtained by endoscopy show *histologically normal mucosa* only. There is thus a need for greater accuracy of detection of early malignant transformation in biopsies, before currently recognized cytological criteria are met. Research in this field will increase the chances of predicting better the future behaviour of the patient, and so lead to better cancer control.

Carcinoma of the large intestine should not be regarded as an isolated, focal lesion in an otherwise normal mucosa; it is the end product of a long interaction between carcinogenic factors, genetic and environmental, and the whole wide field of the mucosa (*Burkitt*, 1971; *Bussey*, 1975; *Hill* et al., 1975). Thus one should expect to find throughout specimens resected for carcinoma a complete spectrum of epithelial changes. It is well established that adenomatous polyps and villous adenomas are premalignant lesions (*Morson*, 1971a, 1974a), and in familial polyposis it is possible to trace all stages of polyp growth from epithelial hyperplasia affecting only part of a single crypt (*Bussey*, 1975). However, before epithelial dysplasia is identifiable in haematoxylin-and-eosin-stained sections, the cells seem to undergo changes that can be revealed by histochemical, biochemical and ultrastructural methods.

A detailed macroscopic, histological and histochemical study of 33 specimens resected for colorectal carcinoma showed abnormal epithelial and glandular features which fell short of accepted criteria of *atypia* (*Filipe* and *Branfoot*, 1974). Strips of mucosa were dissected from the whole resected lengths of bowel and coiled up in *swiss rolls*, while extra blocks were cut from the full thickness of the wall where necessary to include any polyps or other macroscopic lesions. The origin of each piece of tissue was recorded on photocopies of the original photograph (Fig. 1). Fixation in 10% buffered formalin or 10% formol-calcium was followed by routine paraffin embedding. The morphology was assessed on HE-stained sections and histochemical techniques applied to the adjacent serial sections to demonstrate mucosubstances. A complete map of mucin distribution and histological features was made

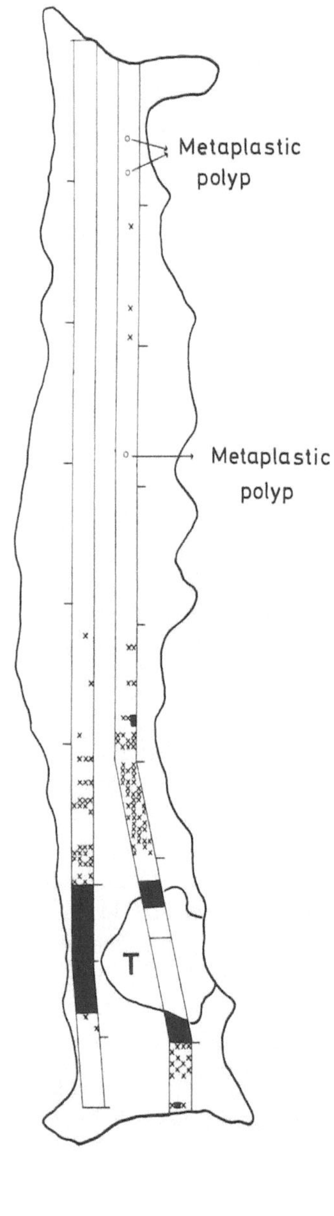

Fig. 1. Diagram of a resected specimen. Tumor area (T) and mucosal strips taken are outlined. Mucin changes: ■ = marked increase in sialomucins; XX = moderate increase in sialomucins; unshaded = normal mucous pattern

by projecting the stained slides onto paper and tracing the mucosal outlines and areas of different mucin content (sulphomucin and sialomucin) (Fig. 2). A rotometer was used to measure the lengths of each mucosal coil and of the zones of differing mucous secretion along it, so that these could be plotted accurately on a chart representing the whole specimen (Fig. 3).

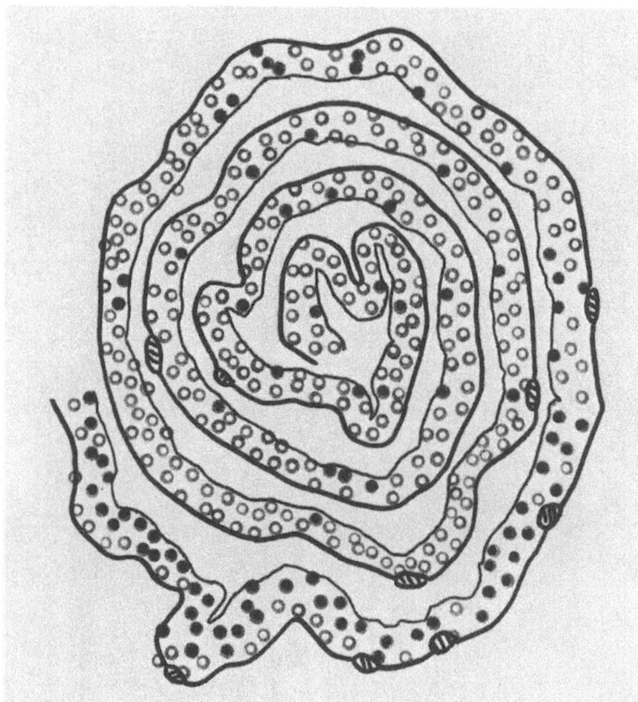

Fig. 2. Tracing of mucosal outlines and mucin distribution of HIB-AB-stained section. Secreting glands indicated as circles, left empty for sulphomucins (○), and blackened for sialomucins (●)

A variety of histological features were seen and these were often accompanied by histochemical changes in the amount and nature of the mucins.

a) *Normal mucosa* in longitudinal section typically has a corrugated surface due to the regular pattern of *anthemia* formed by groups of tubules of varying length (*Filipe* and *Branfoot*, 1974), but the tubules are essentially straight and not usually branched. Electron microscopy can identify at least 8 different types of cell along the crypt (*Kaye* et al., 1973; *Dawson* and *Filipe*, 1976a): undifferentiated, APUD, immature goblet and immature absorptive cells in the lower crypt; mature absorptive and goblet cells and *intermediate* cells in various proportions in the upper crypt. In the surface epithelium, occasional goblet cells, which are often exhausted and empty, are found between mature or senescent absorptive cells.

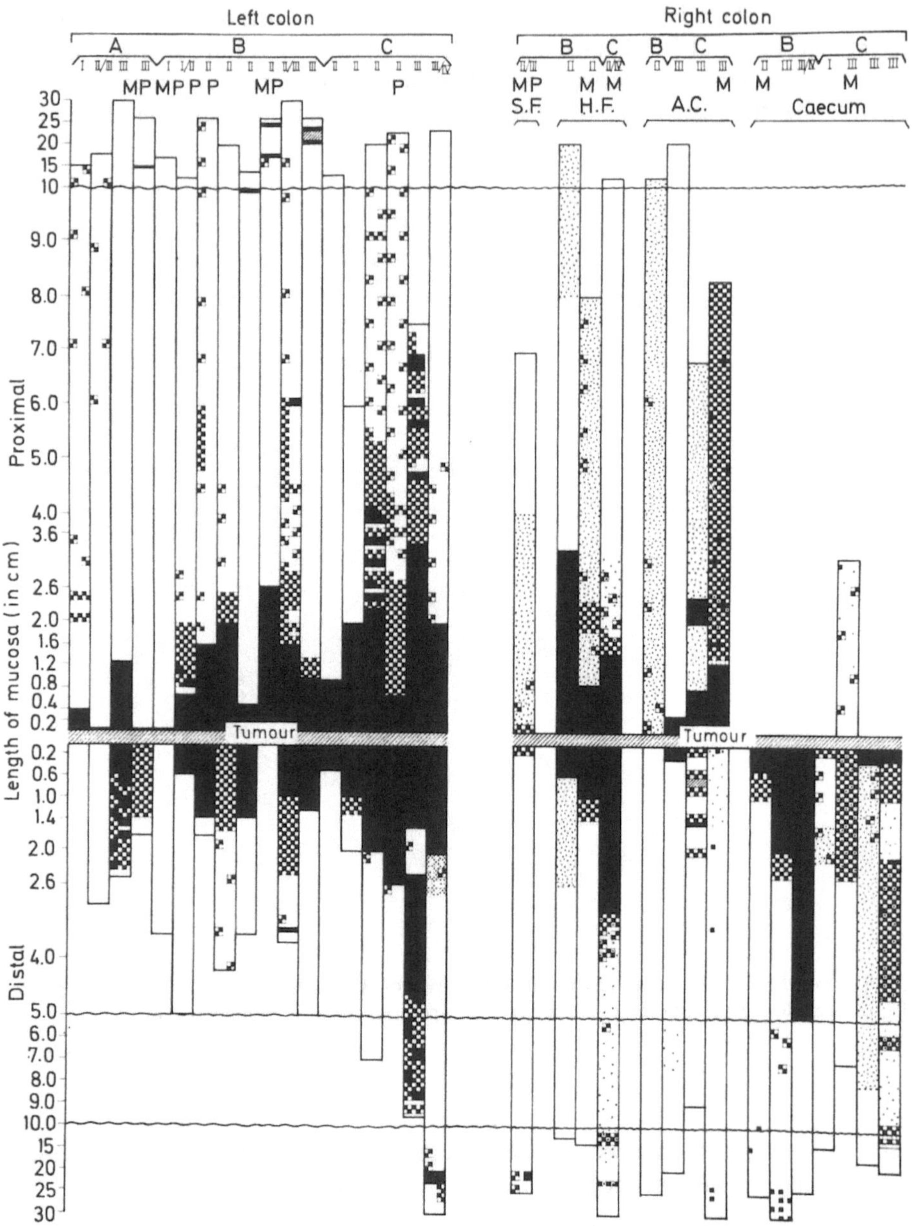

Fig. 3. Patterns of mucous secretion in large bowel bearing carcinoma. ■ = marked increase in sialomucins; ▪ = moderate increase in sialomucins; ▤ = sialomucins present only in the bottom of the crypts (inversion pattern); ▨ = carcinoma; A, B, C = Dukes' Stages; I-IV = Dukes' Grades

Histochemically the goblet cell mucus is predominantly sulphomucin (Fig. 4). Occasionally, however, histologically normal mucosa may show an increase in sialomucins like the *transitional* mucosa described below.

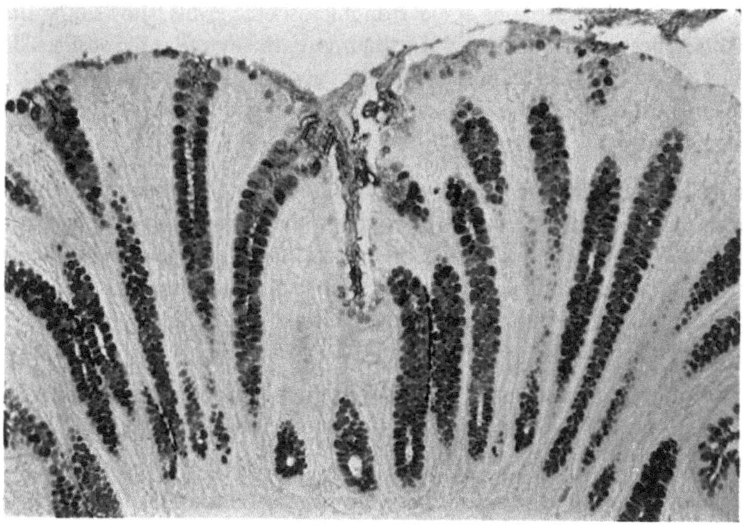

Fig. 4. Normal rectal mucosa showing two anthemia and predominance of sulphomucins (brown) in goblet cells. HID-AB x 45

b) *Transitional mucosa** is usually thicker owing to elongation of the crypts, which are dilated, often branched, and lined by tall goblet cells bulging with mucus. These changes may be minimal or very marked so that all dimensions, both of crypts and cells, are more than double the normal. In the most exaggerated examples the goblet cells may be disrupted, with dislocation of the goblet to a basal position, breach of the basement membrane, and leakage of mucus into the lamina propria. In some crypts full-blown goblet cells are replaced by cells apparently depleted of mucus and having pale eosinophilic ground-glass cytoplasm, a change most commonly seen in the upper half of the crypt. Cytologically the only difference is a tendency for the normally flattened, rather pycnotic nucleus to round up, become more vacuolated and contain more prominent nucleoli. With electron microscopy we have found alterations in the relative proportions of different cell types along the crypt, immature and *intermediate* cells persisting up to higher levels than normal. Mature absorptive cells are fewer and seem to bear an inverse relationship to the high-

* This term may be objectionable but it was first used to describe a zone of transition from frank carcinoma to histochemically normal mucosa, where abnormal secretion was found in the absence of any obvious morphological change.

ly vesiculated *intermediate* cells. On the other hand, goblet cells are increased in number and size and have enlarged and elaborate Golgi zones (*Dawson* and *Filipe*, 1976a).

Histochemically, transitional mucosa shows a consistently abnormal mucous pattern characterized by predominance of sialomucins, along with decrease or absence of sulphated material (Table 2 and Fig. 5). The periodic acid-chromic acid-silver methenamine technique for demonstrating glycoproteins at electron microscopic levels, shows quantitative and qualitative differences from the normal. Furthermore, the cytoplasmic vesicles of both *intermediate* and absorptive cells seem to elaborate a glycoprotein product, and a direct relationship seems to exist between the increased vesiculation and the well developed *fuzzy coat* of this abnormal mucosa (*Dawson* and *Filipe*, 1976b).

In vitro autoradiographic studies with $^{35}SO_4$ show no isotope uptake in the crypt epithelium, though radioactive material may be found in the upper crypt, surface epithelium and cell coat (*Filipe*, 1971c). Biochemical work on mucosal scrapings from the same areas has confirmed that the total hexosamines and sialic acid in transitional mucosa are greater than normal, and accompanied by qualitative changes in sialic acids (*Filipe* and *Cooke*, 1974; *Rogers* et al., in preparation).

These features of *transitional* mucosa were first described in areas adjacent to carcinomas (*Filipe*, 1969, 1971b), but are often seen in patches of mucosa remote from them (*Filipe* and *Branfoot*, 1974).

c) *Foci of epithelial dysplasia in flat mucosa* may be found very close to carcinomas. In these areas mucous secretion appears to be reduced but consists mainly of sialomucins, though some may also be sulphated.

Although not common, frankly dysplastic foci have been found in flat mucosa well away from gross tumours (unpublished observations). In two cases the dysplasia was severe and amounted to carcinoma-in-situ.

d) *Neoplastic* and e) *Metaplastic polyps* are discussed with their histochemical characteristics below.

Changes in composition of goblet cell mucus with increased sialomucins have thus been found in the mucosa of large intestine harbouring carcinoma (Fig. 3). Although they are more marked in so-called *transitional* mucosa next to carcinomas, they may also occur in patches at a distance from the main tumours where the mucosa is either histologically normal or shows features described above as *transitional* or *foci of epithelial dysplasia.* The extent of altered mucosa measured from the edge of the carcinoma ranges from a narrow strip of less than 0.2 cm to a maximum of 5 cm. Isolated patches of markedly abnormal sialomucin secretion are seen in mucosa remote from the tumour in 14 cases.

Our observations suggest that in the left colon there is a direct relation between the extent of mucin changes and the invasiveness of carcinoma (Fig. 3). Also a greater number of isolated patches of increased sialomucins are associated with the more invasive tumours. These relationships are less evident in the right colon. From the distribution of mucin changes it seems that differences exist in the response of the intestinal mucosa to whatever stimuli are disturbing glycoprotein synthesis. The most marked and extensive changes comparable with those in the left colon have been found in the caecum and hepatic flexure, and it is inter-

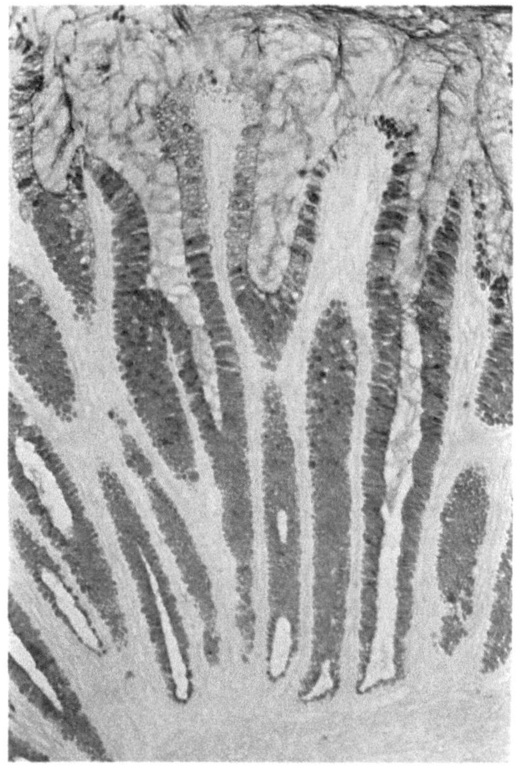

Fig. 5. *Transitional* mucosa. Crypts are longer than in Figure 4 and goblet cells taller, globular and distended with mucus in which sialomucins (blue) predominate. HID-AB x 45

esting to note that the segments of the colon which show more marked mucin changes are those which are more prone to develop carcinoma. Perhaps longer exposure to carcinogens due to slower faecal transit may explain this. In passing it should be noted that we have been unable to relate the intensity and extent of mucin changes to the degree of differentiation or histological pattern of the carcinoma; nor have they any relation to the age or sex of the patients.

The fact that a predominance of sialomucins is seen not only immediately around carcinomas, but also in more remote patches, suggests that these mucin changes reflect a more widespread field of response to unknown stimuli, rather than a local secondary effect of tumour growth. In support of this we have yet to find such changes around secondary tumours ulcerating into the bowel.

Studies in rats in which carcinomas of the large bowel have been induced by weekly subcutaneous injection of 1,2-dimethylhydrazine-2HCl (DMH) provide a suitable animal model for the study of various aspects of carcinogenesis. In our experiments (*Filipe*, 1975) groups of rats, 2 test and 1 control, were sacrificed each week and the whole length of the large intestine was excised and studied by the *swiss roll* technique. In treated rats, histological and histochemical changes were found as early as 4 weeks after the beginning of the experiment. These early changes consist essentially of mild glandular hyperplasia with globular goblet cells distended by mucus. Occasional crypts show mild dysplasia, either with mucin depletion or with changes in mucin composition similar to those described above in human colonic mucosa (Fig. 6). The lesions become more severe after longer periods of treatment: carcinoma-in-situ was found after the 15th injection and frank carcinoma after the 19th. Altered mucin composition, with sialomucins instead of the sulphomucins normally predominant in the left colon of the rat, was consistently found in the glands with mild dysplasia in most of the treated rats after their 5th injection, but never seen in controls (*Filipe*, 1975).

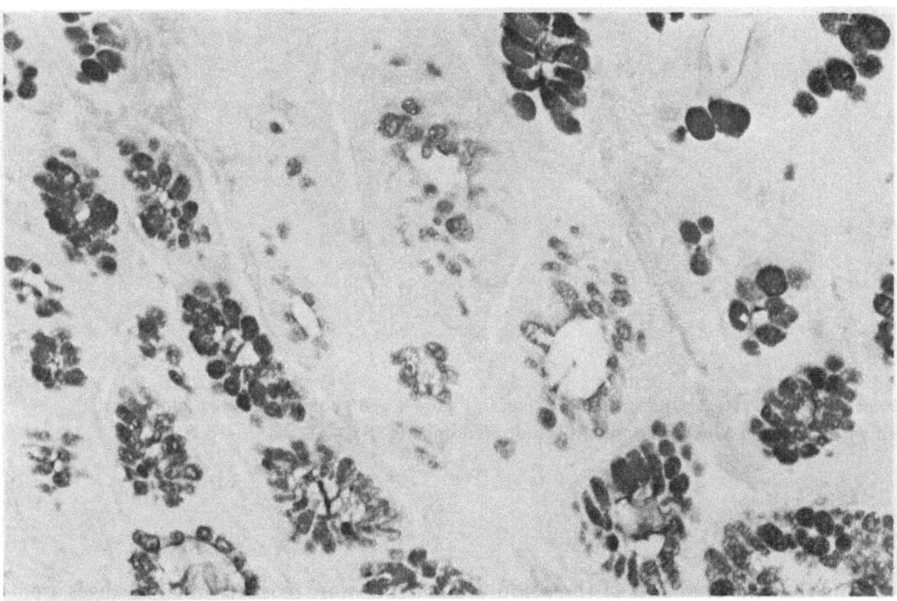

Fig. 6. DMH-treated rat. Sialomucins (grey) in area of dysplasia surrounded by normal glands producing sulphomucins (black). HID-AB x 600

We think at present that modifications in the composition of goblet cell mucin, such as the increase in sialomucins found in the mucosa of colons with carcinoma, may be one feature of early carcinonogenesis. This hypothesis is based on some facts, but is partly speculative, and much has yet to be done to confirm or dismiss our first suspicions.

The fact mentioned above, that changes in glycoproteins were found not only in mucosa next to frank neoplasms but also in isolated patches distant from them, suggests that they are primary rather than secondary to the growth. If they are primary changes, it cannot yet be said whether they are a feature of epithelium irrevocably committed to malignant growth or a nonspecific cellular response to a variety of stimuli. We know that nerve stimulation and certain parenteral drugs may alter the synthesis and secretion of glycoproteins in the intestine. However, one would expect any change they produced to be diffuse, and the focal changes that we have observed seem more likely to be the effect of a local irritant. This may explain some abnormal mucous patterns that we have seen in otherwise unexceptional rectal biopsies from patients with purgative abuse.

The rat model, in which similar mucin changes occur in areas of epithelial dysplasia but never in controls, strongly suggests a relationship between the variations in mucin composition and the process of carcinogenesis.

Whether the raised levels of sialomucins are an expression of cellular immaturity or a direct effect of carcinogens on the mechanism of glycoprotein synthesis we do not know, but we believe there is both morphological and biochemical evidence of cellular immaturity.

Mucin changes are only one expression in the collection of histological, cytological and histochemical features that go to form what we have described as *transitional mucosa.* Taken in isolation such mucin changes may be the result of any of a number of different stimuli. However, we are encouraged to believe that this mucosa does indeed represent early malignant change by a recent report of *Kozuka* (1975). In grading polyps according to their epithelial pseudostratification and branching of glands, he gives under Grade I all the main features that we described in 1974 as typical of *transitional mucosa. Transitional* mucosa may thus be prepolypoid neoplasia in a flat mucosa at a stage not yet sufficiently hyperplastic and irregular to form any macroscopically visible excrescence.

In transitional mucosa the epithelium does not follow the normal course of differentiation, and shows amongst other changes in the goblet cells an increase in sialomucins at the expense of the sulphated. In this and their higher percentage of neuraminidase-sensitive sialic acids they resemble the goblet cells of human fetal colon. This reversion of adult epithelium to an embryonic form receives support from descriptions of tumour cells, which have also been found to have fetal characteristics or produce fetal proteins (*Gold* and *Freedman*, 1965; *Kleist* and *Burtin*, 1969; *Stonehill* and *Bendich*, 1970; *Kleist*, 1971; *Bordes* et al., 1973). The production of embryonic antigens by adult cells undergoing malignant transformation may be due to loss of suppressor genes and a reversion to a more primitive state, a hypothesis supported by alterations in nucleic acid metabolism and proliferative capacity of colonic epithelium adjacent to carcinomas (*Deschner*, 1970; *Deschner* and *Lipkin*, 1970; *Troncale* et al., 1971). Present evidence does not indicate what factors may be responsible for this supposed regression to an embryonic behaviour which alters the normal path of glycoprotein synthesis, but various factors may interfere with this. Protein synthesis is ribosomal and thus genetically determined. Malignant transformation may alter existing regulatory mechanisms and release inactive genes, so that abnormal amounts and forms of protein could be synthesized (*Gurdon*, 1962; *Winzler* and *Bekesi*, 1967). As these proteins pass along the channels of the endoplasmic reticulum there may not always be an opportunity for all the glycosyltransferases to act on the carbohydrate complex, so that variously incomplete or abnormal glycoproteins might be formed. A failure to complete the carbohydrate chains of glycoproteins is likely to be one cause of modification of the cell surface during malignant transformation. Such changes could be brought about by disorders of protein synthesis or of transferase activity as described above (*Kim* et al., 1974).

That carbohydrate metabolism is profoundly altered in malignant cells is supported by cumulative biochemical evidence and sialic acids may play an important role in the behaviour of transformed cells. Their presence in glycoproteins of cell membranes seems to confer certain properties on the membrane which are expressed as cell adhesion (*Deman* et al., 1974), intercellular contact (*Emmelot*, 1973; *Weiss*, 1973), and masking of antigens (*Currie* and *Bagshawe*, 1968; *Rios* and *Simmons*, 1973), and their variations may be related to the differences in behaviour of normal and malignant cells (*Nachbar* et al., 1974). Increased sialic acids and sialyltransferases described in malignant cells may also alter cell contact and the mechanisms controlling cell growth and differentiation (*Emmelot*, 1973).

It has been suggested that tumour cells are coated by neuraminidase-sensitive sialic acids, which may not only hide their antigens from recognition by the host, but also shield them from his immunocompetent cells (*Currie* and *Bagshawe*, 1968; *Rios* and *Simmons*, 1973). If this hypothesis is correct, they may play an important role in immunological reactions to tumour-specific antigens and the control of tumour growth (*Baldwin*, 1970).

From the above and our own experience there is evidence of a relationship between changes in the glycoprotein content of cells and malignant transformation. It thus seemed logical to pursue mucin changes in other cancer fields, such as neoplastic polyps, familial polyposis and inflammatory bowel diseases, and these are discussed below.

VII. Identification of the Origin of Metastatic Adenocarcinoma

The clinical pathologist is often asked to name the probable site of origin of metastatic adenocarcinoma in a lymph node, liver biopsy or omentum, yet he can only guess and long for a specific stain. The amount and histochemical characteristics of the mucin secreted by carcinomas of the large intestine are variable. In most, secretion is scanty or absent; the few goblet cells are either quite empty, or contain only a little mucus as a droplet near the luminal border, or more often as a narrow rim around an otherwise empty theca. In papillary tumours it is common to find *villi* covered by goblet cells, which contain sulphated mucin side by side with others, in which sialomucin predominates. In well differentiated adenocarcinomas one often finds a mixture of neutral and acid nonsulphated mucins in the gland-like lumens. In our experience, mucoid carcinomas, which we define as those in which 50% or more of the cells are floating free in lakes of mucin, are more common in the right colon than the left. Sialomucins generally form the bulk of these tumours but differ from those in the normal goblet cell by their greater susceptibility to sialidase digestion (*Korhonen* et al., 1971). However, the patterns of mucous secretion are so variable from case to case and even in different areas of the same tumour, that we can say that in most adenocarcinomas of the large intestine both types of acid mucin will be found, often swirling together in alternating bands in the larger pools.

From all this it is not surprising that attempts to identify adenocarcinomas of the large intestine have not been successful (*Johnson* and *Helwig*, 1963; *Cook*, 1973). Recently, however, *Culling* et al. (1975) using a technique to discriminate more finely between sialic acid derivatives, claim that it is possible to distinguish carcinomas arising in the lower gastrointestinal tract from all others.

VIII. Classification of Polyps and Assessment of their Malignant Potential

Metaplastic and *neoplastic polyps* are often found in specimens resected for carcinoma. The former are small raised plaques showing no tendency towards neoplasia, whilst adenomatous polyps and villous adenomas are supremely important for their malignant potential (*Morson*, 1974b). The two groups of polyps are quite distinct in their histology and histogenesis (*Lane* et al., 1971; *Kaye* et al., 1973), and these differences are reflected in their liability to undergo malignant change. Metaplastic polyps have no demonstrable malignant potential, whilst that of neoplastic polyps varies with their villosity. Thus, the overall rate of malignant degeneration in adenomatous polyps is about 5%, whilst that of villous adenomas is 40% (*Morson*, 1974a). It is clear therefore that not all polyps will fulfill their malignant potential in a normal lifetime, but why do some evolve, some remain static, and others even regress? Can one predict which polyp will become malignant? These are important questions to answer if successful cancer control is to be achieved.

Experience at St. Mark's Hospital in London gives us a useful prediction of malignancy by computing the size, degree of epithelial dysplasia and tissue architecture of the polyp. Yet a polyp after many years may fail to realize the malignant potential with which it was credited according to these criteria. In an attempt to solve this problem the patterns of mucous secretion have been investigated in isolated polyps (*Filipe*, 1969, 1972) and in familial polyposis (*Filipe* and *Bussey*, in preparation).

The patterns of mucous secretion in metaplastic and neoplastic polyps are quite distinct. In the former, mucins are largely sulphated and thus quite normal and the adjoining mucosa shows no change. The neoplastic adenomatous and villous polyps, on the other hand, present a motley maze of mucous patterns with secretion varying in kind and quantitiy from field to field. In areas of mild dysplasia and no decrease of secretion, a mixture of sulphated and sialomucins is seen. More severe dysplasia and scant secretion makes a pattern like that described in carcinoma, whilst in papillary polyps sulphated mucins predominate in varying amounts. Similar findings are reported by *Mäkelä* et al. (1971) and *Marche* et al. (1972), but we have also found sialomucins predominate in the mucosa around neoplastic polyps, just as they do in *transitional mucosa* around carcinomas. However, no relationship has yet been found between the types of mucin secreted and the degree of differentiation of polyps, as *Goldman* and *Ming* reported in 1968.

In studying our series and trying to compare our findings with those of others, we have felt an urgent need for a comprehensive histological classification of neoplastic polyps. Recently *Kozuka* (1975) has graded them on the basis of epithelial pseudostratification and glandular branching, and describes as Grade I the same enlargement of cells and glandular dimensions, rounding out of nuclei, and branching of glands that we have observed in apparently normal flat mucosa (*Filipe* and *Branfoot*, 1974). This strengthens our argument that transitional mucosa may indeed represent the first morphological sign of malignant change in flat mucosa. So, just as we have been able to relate the mucin changes in flat mucosa around carcinomas to their extent of invasion, we hope that review of our material according to *Kozuka*'s classification may enable us to assess the malignant potential of a polyp, by variations in the mucin secreted by both the polyp itself and the mucosa around it.

The questions asked about isolated polyps apply equally to *familial polyposis.* This rare hereditary disease is another precancerous condition of the colon and rectum. Patients develop numerous adenomatous polyps throughout the large bowel and will, if left untreated, present with carcinoma at an age much earlier than those in the general population (*Morson* and *Bussey*, 1970; *Bussey*, 1975). Such cases offer a unique opportunity to study the histogenesis of cancer through a sequence of increasing grades of dysplasia to adenomatous polyps and invasive carcinoma, and give us material for a study of mucin changes in mucosa showing various *grades of premalignancy.*

No consistent pattern of mucous secretion has yet emerged in the *non-malignant* mucosa between polyps, though there is a tendency towards non-sulphated mucous secretion, a change more apparent in the left colon and rectum than in specimens from the right. This predominance of sialomucins is apparently not related to the degree of dysplasia of the adjacent polyps, but in areas next to proved carcinomas, we have found mucin changes similar to those described in *transitional mucosa* around the common form of large bowel cancer. In the adenomatous polyps, the goblet cell mucins are a mixture of sulphated and non-sulphated, but as in the isolated polyps described above, they show no relation to the degree of cellular atypia. So far we have no strong evidence to suggest that mucin changes in histologically normal mucosa between polyps in familial polyposis will give any indication of their malignant potential (*Filipe* and *Bussey*, in preparation).

IX. Prediction of Malignant Change in Inflammatory Bowel Disease

The description of precancer by *Morson* and *Pang* (1967) held promise of monitoring cases of ulcerative colitis in danger of developing carcinoma, so that quiescent extensive disease might be managed conservatively (*Lennard-Jones* et al., 1974). Furthermore whilst current surgical opinion favours total proctocolectomy as the treatment of choice for intractable colitis, most authorities will agree that there are cases for whom conservation of the rectum and avoidance of ileostomy are desirable. Such patients are especially at risk. There is thus an increasing demand for the recognition and prognosis of precancer, yet its diagnosis and management have in practice proved less certain.

The general features of precancer are agreed and its value has been attested by others (*Yardley* and *Keren*, 1974). However, its patchiness, absence from the rectum when carcinoma is found elsewhere in the bowel (*Evans* and *Pollock*, 1972), danger of overdiagnosis, lack of precise definition, and uncertainty of prognosis remain problematical (*Hulten* et al., 1972; *Keren* and *Yardley*, 1974; *Cook* and *Goligher*, 1975; *Sherlock* and *Kirsner*, 1975). Patchiness may be overcome by multiple biopsies and more accurate sampling by endoscopists with a keener eye for suspicious velvety areas. Absence from the rectum may be circumvented by more extensive biopsies made possible by fibreoptics. But the absence of precise criteria and the dangers of overdiagnosis remain.

The authors are acutely aware of these difficulties for we are concerned with the management of a large number of patients with inflammatory bowel disease who are threatened by malignant change, since total colectomy and ileorectal anastomosis has long been the preferred treatment at the Gordon Hospital (*Aylett*, 1971). Having recognized abnormal mucins in apparently normal mucosa both immediately around and in patches remote from carcinomas of the large intestine in the general population (see above), it was logical to seek this *transitional mucosa* in colitics.

Since 1971 we have been collecting all specimens of inflammatory bowel disease to study prospectively along the whole length of the large intestine how the patterns and extent of mucin changes vary with inflammation, dysplasia and neoplasms. Blocks are first cut from the full thickness of the wall to sample each segment and gross lesion, but later, strips of mucosa are cut from the full length of the specimen. So far we have made only a preliminary survey of 20 cases of carcinoma and 5 of precancer, but we have not completed the mapping of the whole specimens and control cases of total colitis, without malignant changes and matched for age of onset and various durations of disease. Nonetheless, we have already found mucosal changes in long-standing colitis like those we have described above in the general population with cancer.

1. Transitional Mucosa

We have found a predominance of sialomucin secretion in what at first sight seems normal mucosa in ulcerative colitics who have developed carcinoma, just like those in the general population (see above), but seldom so far in those without at least early malignant change. As with cancer in the general population, this *transitional mucosa* can often be suspected in H and E sections (Fig. 7) for dilatation and branching of crypts lined by tall goblet cells

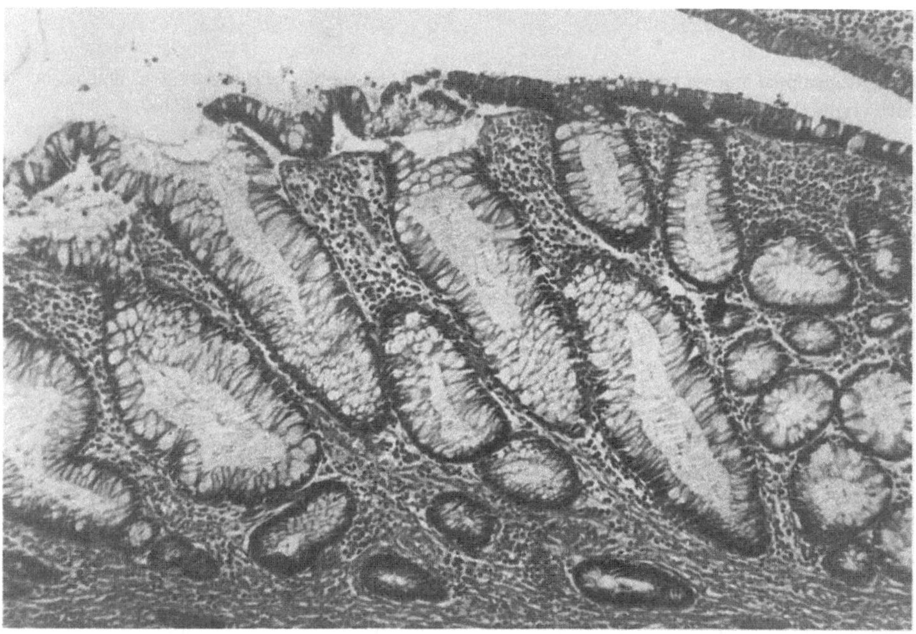

Fig. 7. Transitional mucosa in long-standing colitis. Wide crypts lined by tall goblet cells yet no obvious dysplasia. Histochemically sialomucins predominate. HE x 300

are accompanied by secretion that is largely sialomucins. Likewise, it is found around and mingling with carcinoma and frank precancer (Fig. 8), but also in isolated areas. It thus displays the same patchiness as *Morson* and *Pang*'s precancer (1967), but may be recognized in a small rectal biopsy when the other is absent.

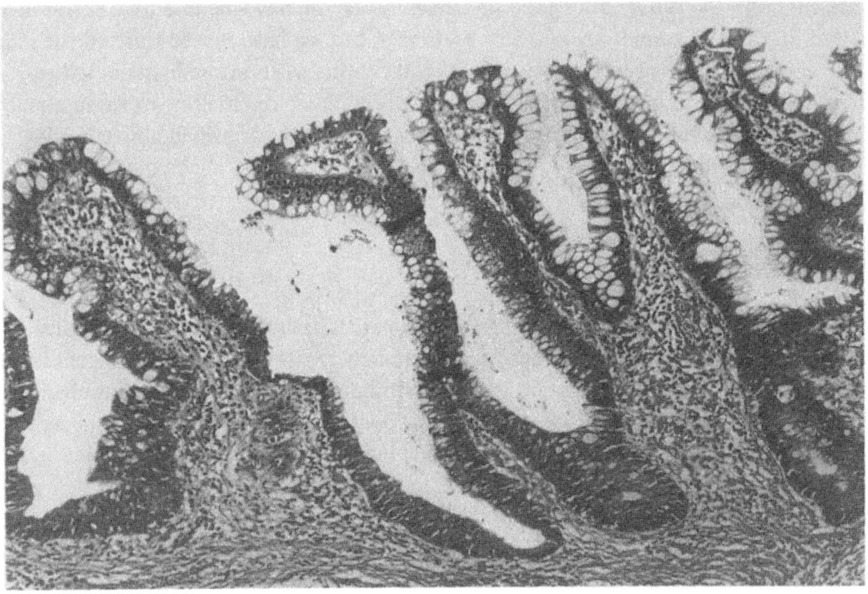

Fig. 8. Transitional mucosa and precancer. Abnormally tall clear goblet cells cover villous mucosa in which crypts show frank dysplasia. Histochemically sialomucins predominate. HE x 300

Morphologically, transitional mucosa in ulcerative colitis tends to differ from that in the general population. Whilst the characteristically enlarged goblet cells and dilated crypts are seen, the mucosa is not usually so thickened by elongation of crypts and seems to share in the atrophic state of *burnt-out* colitis. However, sometimes it is more hyperplastic and presents a villous form (Fig. 8), albeit still stunted, and such an area may merge with the villosity of frank precancer.

2. Villous Mucosa

A villous pattern of mucosa may be seen in at least three conditions:

a) *Normal healing of ulcers* in many kinds of bowel disease and experimental animals may be accompanied by a papillary appearance as the regenerating sheet of epithelium spreads across the ulcer floor, buds downwards into the lamina propria and canalizes to form new tubules. In our own material and published illustrations, these regenerative villi are typically pointed or acuminate (Fig. 9).

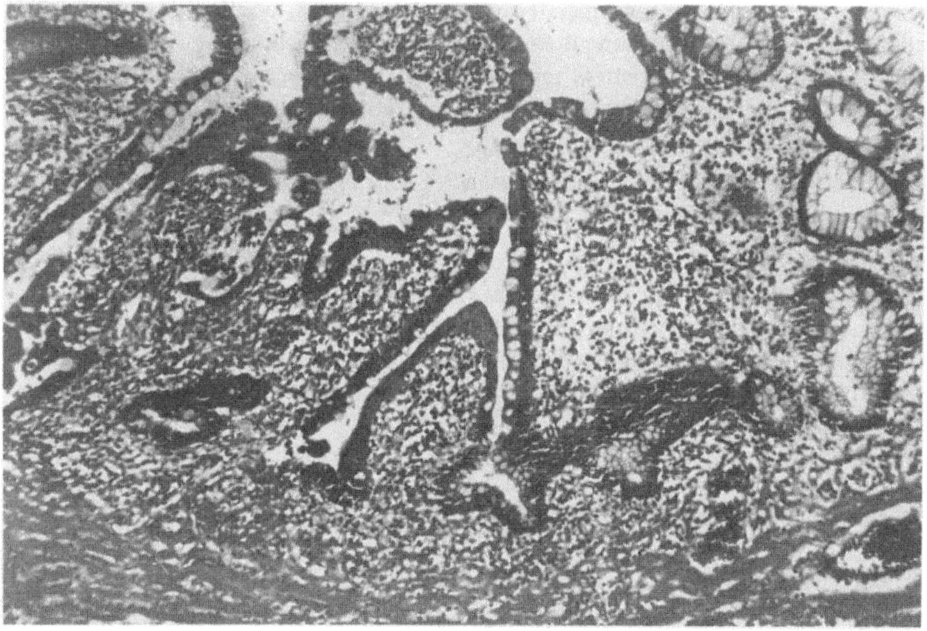

Fig. 9. Acuminate villi characteristic of innocent healing of ulcers. Histochemically normal sulphomucins predominate. HE x 300

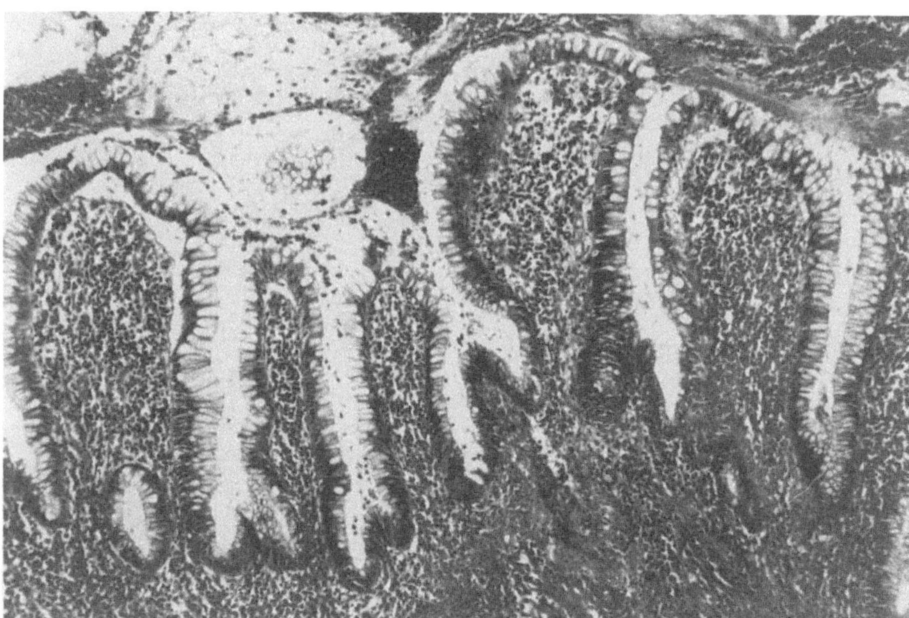

Fig. 10. Villosity of mucosa in long-standing colitis suggests precancer but absence of dysplasia is supported histochemically by a normal mucous pattern. HE x 300

b) *Repair in ulcerative colitis* can generate a uniformly villous surface that is velvety to the naked eye, yet the epithelium shows little or no evidence of dysplasia (Fig. 10). *Morson* (1974c) has noted that this pattern of repair is characteristic of certain patients with long-standing chronic ulcerative colitis and wonders if follow up will show that they are predisposed to malignant change.

c) *Precancer* often takes a villous form and we agree with *Yardley* and *Keren* (1974) that it is an important feature in weighing up the diagnosis.

Recognition that there are these three different forms of villous mucosa is important because overemphasis of villosity can lead in our experience to overdiagnosis of precancer, insufficient weight being given to cytology and inflammation. It is in such difficult cases that we believe histochemistry can make the diagnosis less subjective: in reparative forms the pattern of secretion is normal, but in the precancerous, sialomucins predominate (Fig. 8).

3. Precancer in the Presence of Active Colitis

Most pathologists are reluctant to diagnose precancer in the presence of more than minimal inflammation because regenerating epithelium can appear disturbingly dysplastic, yet so far no strict criteria have been laid down to distinguish such reactive hyperplasia from premalignant dysplasia. We have studied cases of carcinoma, however, with active colitis and have

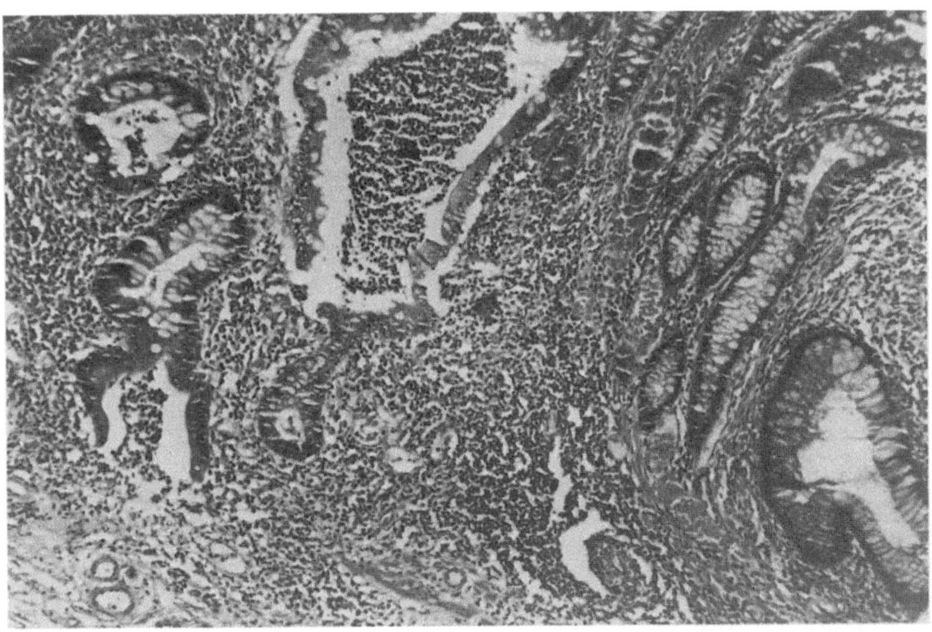

Fig. 11. Active colitis with invasive carcinoma. On the left is a crypt abscess surrounded only by focal transitional change (see text), but on right, dilated branched crypt is lined on its left side by tall basophilic cells characteristic of transitional mucosa and confirmed by histochemistry. HE x 300

found transitional mucosa (Fig. 11). This encourages us to believe that mucin changes may add another dimension in the diagnosis of precancer.

4. Focal Transitional Change

In haematoxylin-and-eosin stained sections the normal tall clear oval goblet cells may be replaced in the upper crypt by cuboidal cells with vacuolated nuclei and a goblet which is spherical, displaced from the nucleus towards the luminal border, and filled with basophilic, coarsely-clumped mucin. Histochemically sialomucins predominate.

A scattering of such cells in crypts largely lined by cubical cells with cytoplasm devoid of mucin and vacuolated nuclei we term *focal transitional change.* It is found in the region of crypt abscesses and we believe it indicates reactive hyperplasia, with the loss of differentiation reflected in the switch to sialomucin. It is quite distinct from the more diffuse change of transitional mucosa, and the two must not be confused, though they may be seen side by side in a case of carcinoma with active colitis.

As for Crohn's disease, we like others (*Keighley* et al., 1975) are finding that some of our carcinomas have arisen in this form of colitis. It is too early to speak of its antecedents, but we have the impression that the difference in mucin patterns of the two conditions is preserved.

Lewis et al. (1971) have sought to increase the value of rectal biopsy in monitoring chronic ulcerative colitis by demonstrating isoenzymes of lactic dehydrogenase characteristic of malignancy. Our results encourage us to hope that mucins will prove another and simpler refinement.

X. The Differential Diagnosis of Ulcerative Colitis and Crohn's Disease

The value of rectal biopsy in the diagnosis of inflammatory bowel disease has been well established, but there remains an obstinate number of cases in which histological appearances are not decisive (*Schachter* and *Kirsner*, 1975), even after applying all currently recognized criteria. This is particularly true of Crohn's disease and ulcerative colitis, for a small fragment of mucosa may show nonspecific chronic inflammatory cell infiltration of the lamina propria with crypt abscesses, but, on the one hand lacking granulomas, histiocytic and patchy infiltrates, or on the other, diffuse neutrophil infiltration, mucus depletion, and shortfall and irregularity of glands, the appearances can only be described as equivocal. The preservation of mucin in the presence of Crohn's disease and its depletion in ulcerative colitis have been emphasized by *Morson* (1971b) but in practice the differences are not always readily apparent in haematoxylin-and-eosin-stained sections, which so often vary in quality. It is here that mucin histochemistry has indeed conferred an increase in objectivity.

Histochemical studies of the enzymes in rectal biopsies of ulcerative colitis and Crohn's disease have revealed few differences (*Filipe*, 1971a) apart from a nonspecific increase in acid phosphatase in ulcerative colitis which may only reflect regeneration (*Dawson*, 1972). *Danovitch* et al. (1972) found parallel increases in other acid hydrolases and some rise in alkaline phosphatases, and derived the former from lysosomes and the latter from some other cells, e.g. neutrophils, but they made no comparative study of other conditions. The results have seemed unrewarding, especially since the methods require fresh tissue and special techniques, but studies of mucins, by contrast have shown much more obvious differences and are readily applicable to routinely processed material.

Hellstrom and *Fischer* (1967) applied mucin stains to surgical specimens and found striking quantitative differences, claiming that mucin depletion was greater in acute than in chronic ulcerative colitis, whilst mucin was preserved in Crohn's disease. *Filipe* and *Dawson* (1970) reported similar sharp discrimination in rectal biopsies, and *Hemet* and *Métayer* (1972) have confirmed this. So long as one ignores areas of severe ulceration and polypoidal hyperplasia (where mucins are respectively absent or increased), the mucins are qualitatively and quantitatively normal even in the presence of inflammation in Crohn's colitis, but in ulcerative colitis they are reduced proportionately with the severity of inflammation. Healing and regeneration in serial biospies are accompanied by restoration of mucin secretion. Preservation of mucins may lead to review of cases of putative ulcerative colitis and alteration of the diagnosis to Crohn's disease. Like *Goligher* (1975) we have found that cases in which the evidence at first seems equivocal often subsequently declare themselves as Crohn's disease.

Differential counting of cells in the epithelium and lamina propria has been recommended by *Korelitz* and *Sommers* (1974) to improve the differential diagnostic criteria. They found that the differences in the number of goblet cells was not statistically significant when the various groups were compared. Cell counts, however, overlook differences in the amount of mucin in individual cells, whose sum may be computed less laboriously by histochemistry at a glance.

Future refinements may stem from recent reports of a rate-limiting enzyme in mucin synthesis, which is increased in the healing phase of ulcerative colitis and also in the apparently normal mucosa of Crohn's disease (*Goodman* et al., 1975). Qualitative differences have also been detected in the carbohydrate components of the mucins (*Teague* et al., 1973; *Fraser* and *Clamp*, 1975). Mannose, which normally forms only a small proportion of colonic mucins and is a product more of serous than goblet cells as in the parotid gland, is increased in ulcerative colitis and may be responsible for a sharp reduction in the mucins' total viscosity.

Acknowledgments: We are grateful for the assistance of all the technical staff and the Department of Medical Photography and also have to thank our secretaries, Miss *J. Carter* and Mrs. *N. Jackson.* This work has been supported by grants from the Westminster Hospital, the Cancer Research Campaign and the Medical Research Council.

References

Andrews, A.T. de B., Herring, G.M., Kent, P.W.: Some studies on the composition of bovine cortical-bone sialoprotein. Biochem. J. 104, 705-715 (1967).

Aylett, S.O.: Ileorectal anastomosis: review 1952-1968. Proc. roy. Soc. Med. 64, 967-971 (1971).

Baldwin, R.W.: Tumour specific antigens associated with chemically induced tumours. Rev. Eur. Etud. Clin. Biol. 15, 593-598 (1970).

Bennett, G.: Migration of glycoproteins from Golgi apparatus to cell coat in the columnar cells of the duodenal epithelium. J. Cell Biol. 45, 668-673 (1970).

Bennett, G., Leblond, C.P.: Formation of cell coat material for the whole surface of columnar cells in the rat small intestine, as visualized by radioautography with L-fucose-^{3}H. J. Cell Biol. 46, 409-416 (1970).

Bennett, G., Leblond, C.P., Haddad, A.: Migration of glycoprotein from the Golgi apparatus to the surface of various cell types as shown by radioautography after labelled fucose injection into rats. J. Cell Biol. 60, 258-284 (1974).

Bignardi, C., Aureli, G., Balduini, C., Castellani, A.A.: Sulfosialopolysaccharide-peptides from dog submaxillary gland. Biophys. Res. Comm. 17, 310-312 (1964).

Bordes, M., Michiels, R., Martin, F.: Detection by immunofluorescence of carcinoembryonic antigen in colonic carcinoma, other malignant or benign tumours, and non-cancerous tissue. Digestion 9, 106-115 (1973).

Burkitt, D.P.: Epidemiology of cancer of the colon and rectum. Cancer 28, 3-13 (1971).

Bussey, H.J.R.: In: Familial Polyposis Coli. Baltimore: Johns Hopkins University Press 1975.

Cook, H.C.: A histochemical characterisation of malignant tumour mucins as a possible aid in the identification of metastatic deposits. Med. Lab. Technol. 30, 217-224 (1973).

Cook, M.C., Goligher, J.C.: Carcinoma and epithelial dysplasia complicating ulcerative colitis. Gastroenterology 68, 1127-1136 (1975).

Culling, C.F.A., Reid, P.E., Burton, J.D., Dunn, W.L.: A histochemical method of differentiating lower gastrointestinal tract mucin from other mucins in primary or metastatic tumours. J. clin. Path. 28, 656-658 (1975).

Culling, C.F.A., Reid, P.E., Clay, M.G., Dunn, W.L.: The histochemical demonstration of O-acylated sialic acid in gastrointestinal mucins: their association with the potassium hydroxide-periodic acid-Schiff effect. J. Histochem. Cytochem. 22, 826-831 (1974).

Culling, C.F.A., Reid, P.E., Dunn, W.L.: The effect of saponification upon certain histochemical reactions of the epithelial mucins of the gastrointestinal tract. J. Histochem. Cytochem. 19, 654-662 (1971).

Currie, G.A., Bagshawe, K.D.: The role of sialic acid in antigenic expression: further studies of the Landschutz ascites tumour. Brit. J. Cancer 22, 843-853 (1968).

Czernobilsky, B., Tsou, K-C.: Adenocarcinoma, adenomas and polyps of the colon. Histochemical study. Cancer (Philad.) 21, 165-177 (1968).

Danovitch, S.H., Gallucci, A., Shora, W.: Colonic mucosal lysosomal enzyme acitivities in ulcerative colitis. Amer. J. dig. Dis. 17, 977-992 (1972).

Dawson, I.M.P.: The histochemistry of Crohn's disease. Clinics in Gastroenterology 1, 309-320 (1972).

Dawson, Penelope A., Filipe, M.I.: An ultrastructural and histochemical study of the mucous membrane adjacent to and remote from carcinoma of the colon. Cancer 37, 2388-2398 (1976a).

Dawson, Penelope A.,Filipe, M.I.: An ultrastructural application of silver methenamine to the study of mucin changes in the colonic mucosa adjacent to and remote from carcinoma. Histochem. J. 8, 143-158 (1976b).

Deman, J.J., Bruyneel, E.A., Mareel, M.M.: A study on the mechanism of intercellular adhesion. Effects of neuraminidase, calcium and trypsin on the aggregation of suspended HeLa cells. J. Cell Biol. 60, 641-652 (1974).

Deschner, E.E.: Autoradiographic studies of synthesis of DNA, RNA, and protein in normal and diseased colonic mucosa. In: Carcinoma of the colon and antecedent epithelium (ed. *W.J. Burdette*), pp. 222-229. Springfield: Charles C Thomas 1970.

Deschner, E.E., Lipkin, M.: Study of human rectal epithelial cells in vitro. III. RNA, protein and DNA synthesis in polyps and adjacent mucosa. J. nat. Cancer Inst. 44, 175-185 (1970).

Draper, P., Kent, P.W.: Biosynthesis of intestinal mucins. Utilization of 1-^{14}C glucose by sheep colonic mucosa in vitro. Biochem. J. 86, 248-254 (1963).

Drzeniek, R.: Substrate specificity of neuraminidases. Review. Histochem. J. 5, 271-290 (1973).

Emmelot, P.: Biochemical properties of normal and neoplastic cells surfaces. A review. Eur. J. Cancer 9, 319-333 (1973).

Esterley, J.R., Spicer, S.S.: Mucin histochemistry of human gall bladder: changes in adenocarcinoma, cystic fibrosis and cholecystitis. J. nat. Cancer Inst. 40, 1-12 (1968).

Evans, D.J., Pollock, D.J.: In-situ and invasive carcinoma of the colon in patients with ulcerative colitis. Gut 13, 566-570 (1972).

Filipe, M.I.: Value of histochemical reactions for mucosubstances in the diagnosis of certain pathological conditions of the colon and rectum. Gut 10, 577-586 (1969).

Filipe, M.I.: Some aspects of the histochemical enzyme distribution in colon and rectum.: Normal and pathological. Acta histochem. Suppl. 9, 333-337 (1971a).

Filipe, M.I.: ^{35}Sulphur uptake in the mucosa adjacent to carcinoma of the large intestine. Histochem. J. 3, 27-35 (1971c).

Filipe, M.I.: The mucous membrane of the normal human large intestine and the changes which occur in it immediately adjacent to proven carcinoma: A histochemical, autoradiographic and chemical study. Ph.D. thesis, London University (1971b).

Filipe, M.I.: The value of a study of the mucosubstances in rectal biopsies from patients with carcinoma of the rectum and lower sigmoid in the diagnosis of premalignant mucosa. J. clin. Path. 25, 123-128 (1972).

Filipe, M.I.: Mucous secretion in rat colonic mucosa during carcinogenesis induced by Dimethylhydrazine. A morphological and histochemical study. Brit. J. Cancer 32, 60-77 (1975).

Filipe, M.I., Branfoot, A.C.: Abnormal patterns of mucous secretion in apparently normal mucosa of large intestine with carcinoma. Cancer 34, 282-290 (1974).

Filipe, M.I., Cooke, K.B.: Changes in the composition of mucin in the mucosa adjacent to carcinoma of the colon as compared with the normal: a biochemical investigation. J. Clin. Path. 27, 315-318 (1974).

Filipe, M.I., Dawson, I.M.P.: The diagnostic value of mucosubstances in rectal biopsies from patients with ulcerative colitis and Crohn's disease. Gut 11, 229-234 (1970).

Florey, H.W.: The secretion of mucus and inflammation of mucous membranes. In: General Pathology (ed. *Lord Florey*) 4th ed., p. 195. London: Publ. Lloyd Luke (Medical Books) Ltd. 1970.

Forstner, G.G.: (1-^{14}C) glucosamine incorporation by subcellular fractions of small intestinal mucosa. Identification by precursor labelling of three functionally distinct glycoprotein classes. J. biol. Chem. 245, 3584-3592 (1970).

Fraser, G.M., Clamp, J.R.: Changes in human colonic mucus in ulcerative colits. Gut 16, 832-833 (Abstract) (1975).

Gad, A.: A histochemical study of human alimentary tract mucosubstances in health and disease. I. Normal and tumours. II. Inflammatory conditions. Brit. J. Cancer 23, 52-68 (1969).

Gad, A., Sylven, B.: On the nature of the high-iron diamine method for sulphomucins. J. histochem. Cytochem. 17, 156-160 (1969).

Gold, P., Freedman, S.O.: Demonstration of tumour-specific antigens in human colonic carcinomata by immunological tolerance and absorption technique. J. exp. Med. 121 439-462 (1965).

Goldman, H., Ming, S.C.: Mucins in normal and neoplastic gastrointestinal epithelium: histochemical distribution. Arch. Path. 85, 580-586 (1968).
Goligher, J.C.: Surgery of the anus, rectum and colon, 3rd ed. London: Baillière Tindall 1975.
Goodman, M.J., Kent, P.W., Truelove, S.C.: Glucosamine synthetase activity in the colonic mucosa in ulcerative colitis and Crohn's disease. Gut 16, 833 (Abstract) (1975).
Gottschalk, A.: Definition of glycoproteins and their delimitization from other carbohydrate-protein complexes. In: Glycoproteins: Their Composition, Structure and Function. London: Elsevier Publ. Co. 1966.
Greco, V., Lauro, G., Fabrini, A., Torsoli, A.: Histochemistry of the colonic epithelial mucins in normal subjects and in patients with ulcerative colitis. A qualitative and histophotometric investigation. Gut 8, 491-496 (1967).
Gurdon, J.B.: Adult frogs derived from the nuclei of simple somatic cells. Develop. Biol. 4, 256-273 (1962).
Hawley, P.R.: Carcinoma in the colon. Brit. J. Hosp. Med. 11, 211-216 (1974).
Hellstrom, H.R., Fischer, E.R.: Estimation of mucosal mucin as an aid in the differentiation of Crohn's disease of the colon and chronic ulcerative colitis. Amer. J. Clin. Path. 48, 259-268 (1967).
Hemet, J., Métayer, J.: Intérêt pratique de l'étude des mucines dans le diagnostic des colites primitives. Ann. Anat. Pathol. 17, 389-392 (1972).
Hill, M.J., Drasar, B.S., Williams, R.E.O., Meade, T.W., Cox, A.G., Simpson, J.E.P., Morson, B.C.: Faecal bile acids and clostridia in patients with cancer of the large bowel. Lancet 1975 I, 535.
Hulten, L., Kerwenter, J., Ahren, C.: Precancer and carcinoma in chronic ulcerative colitis (A histopathological and clinical investigation). Scand. J. Gastroenterol. 7, 663-669 (1972).
Imondi, A.R., Balis, M.E., Lipkin, M.: Changes in enzyme levels accompanying differentiation of intestinal epithelial cells. Exp. cell Res. 58, 323-330 (1969).
Isselbacher, K.J.: The intestinal cell surface: some properties of normal, undifferentiated and malignant cells. Ann. Int. Med. 81, 681-686 (1974).
Ito, S.: The enteric surface coat in cat intestinal microvilli. J. Cell Biol. 27, 475-491 (1965a).
Ito, S.: Radioactive labelling of the surface coat in enteric microvilli. Anat. Rec. 151, 489 (1965b).
Ito, S., Revel, J.P.: Incorporation of radioactive sulfate and glucose in the surface coat of enteric microvilli. J. Cell Biol. 23, 44A-45A (1964)
Jeanloz, R.W.: The nomenclature of mucopolysaccharides. Arthr. and Rheum. 3, 233-237 (1960).
Jeanloz, R.W.: Recent developments in the biochemistry of aminosugars. Advanc. Enzymol. 25, 433-456 (1963).
Johnson, W.C., Helwig, E.B.: Histochemistry of primary and metastatic mucus-secreting tumours. Ann. N.Y. Acad. Sci. 106, 794-803 (1963).
Kaye, G.I., Fenoglio, C.M., Pascal, R.R., Lane, N.: Comparative electron microscopic features of normal, hyperplastic, and adenomatous human colonic epithelium. Variations in cellular structure relative to the process of epithelial differentiation. Gastroenterol. 64, 926-945 (1973).
Keighley, M.R.B., Thompson, H., Alexander-Williams, J.: Multifocal colonic carcinoma and Crohn's disease. Surgery 78, 534-537 (1975).
Kent, P.W.: Biosynthesis of intestinal glycoproteins in animals and man. Gut 12, 417 (Abstract) (1971).
Kent, P.W., Pasternak, C.A.: Biosynthesis of intestinal mucins. 3. Formation of active sulfate by cell-free extracts of sheep colonic mucosa. Biochem. J. 69, 453-458 (1958).

Keren, D.F., Yardley, J.H.: Assessment of precancer in rectal biopsy and colectomy specimens in ulcerative colitis. Lab. Invest. 30, 379 (Abstract) (1974).

Kim, Y.S., Isaacs, R., Perdomo, J.: Alterations of membrane glycopeptides in human colonic adenocarcinoma. Proc. Nat. Acad. Sci. (Wash.) 71, 4869-4873 (1974).

Kim, Y.S., Perdomo, J.: Glycoprotein biosynthesis in small intestine. III. Enzymatic basis for the difference in the antigenicity of mucins. J. clin. Invest. 51, 1135-1145 (1972).

Kleist, S. von: Étude d'un antigène spécifique des tumeurs coliques humaines d'origine embryonnaire. Biol. Med. 60, 237-292 (1971).

Kleist, S. von, Burtin, P.: Isolation of a fetal antigen from human colonic tumours. Cancer Res. 29, 1961-1964 (1969).

Korelitz, B.I., Sommers, S.C.: Differential diagnosis of ulcerative colitis and granulomatous colitis by sigmoidoscopy, rectal biopsy and cell counts of rectal mucosa. Amer. J. Gastroenterol. 61, 460-469 (1974).

Korhonen, L.K., Mäkelä, V., Lilius, G.: Carbohydrate-rich compounds in the colonic mucosa of man. II. Histochemical characteristics of colonic adenocarcinomas. Cancer 27, 128-133 (1971).

Kozuka, S.: Premalignancy of the mucosal polyp in the large intestine. I. Histologic gradation of the polyp on the basis of epithelial pseudostratification and glandular branching. Dis. Colon Rect. 18, 483-493 (1975).

Lamb, D., Reid, L.: Histochemical types of acidic glycoprotein produced by mucous cells of the tracheo-bronchial glands in man. J. Path. 98, 213-229 (1969).

Lane, N., Caro, L., Otero-Vilardebo', L.R., Godman, G.C.: On the site of sulfation in colonic goblet cells. J. Cell Biol. 21, 339-351 (1964).

Lane, N., Kaplan, H., Pascal, R.R.: Minute adenomatous and hyperplastic polyps of the colon: divergent patterns of epithelial growth with specific associated mesenchymal changes. Contrasting roles in the pathogenesis of carcinoma. Gastroenterol. 60, 537-551 (1971).

Lennard-Jones, J.E., Misiewicz, J.J., Parrish, J.A., Ritchie, J.K., Swarbrick, E.T., Williams, C.B.: Prospective study of out-patients with extensive colitis. Lancet 1974 I, 1065-1067.

Lev, R.: A histochemical study of glycogen and mucin in developing human foetal epithelia. Histochem. J. 1, 152-165 (1968).

Lev, R., Orlic, D.: Histochemical and radioautographic studies of normal human fetal colon. Histochemistry 39, 301-311 (1974).

Lev, R., Spicer, S.S.: Specific staining of sulphate groups with Alcian blue at low pH. J. Histochem. Cytochem. 12, 309 (1964).

Lev, R., Spicer, S.S.: A histochemical comparison of human epithelial mucins in normal and hypersecretory states including pancreatic cystic fibrosis. Amer. J. Path. 46, 23-47 (1965).

Lewis, B., Morson, B.C., February, A.W., Hywel Jones, J., Misiewicz, J.J.: Abnormal lactic dehydrogenase isoenzyme patterns in ulcerative colitis with precancerous change. Gut 12, 16-19 (1971).

Lipkin, M., Bell, B., Sherlock, P.: Cell proliferation kinetics in the gastrointestinal tract of man. I. Cell renewal in colon and rectum. J. Clin. Invest. 42, 767-776 (1963).

Lukie, B.E., Forstner, G.G.: Synthesis of intestinal glycoprotein. Incorporation of ($1-^{14}C$) glucosamine in vitro. Biochim. biophys. Acta (Amst.) 261, 353-364 (1972).

MacDermott, R.P., Donaldson, R.M., jr., Trier, J.S.: Glycoprotein synthesis and secretion by mucosal biopsies of rabbit colon and human rectum. J. clin. Invest. 54, 545-554 (1974).

Mäkelä, V., Korhonen, L.K., Lilius, G.: Carbohydrate-rich compounds in the colonic mucosa of man. I. Histochemical characteristics of normal and adenomatous colonic mucosa. Cancer 27, 120-127 (1971).

Marche, C.R., Bocquet, L., Ganter, P.: Caractères histochimiques des mucines épithéliales dans les polypes recto-coliques de l'adulte et de l'enfant. Ann. Anat. path. 17, 393-404 (1972).

Marsden, J.R., Dawson, I.M.P.: An investigation into the enzyme histochemistry of adenocarcinomas of human large intestine and of the transitional epithelium immediately adjacent to them. Gut 15, 783-787 (1974).

McGinty, F., Delides, G., Harrison, D.: The significance of enzyme histochemical patterns in carcinomas of the large intestine in man. Gut 14, 502-505 (1973).

Melnyk, C.S., Braucher, R.W., Kirsner, J.B.: Regeneration of the human colon mucosa. Morphological and histochemical study. Gastroenterol. 52, 985-997 (1967).

Monis, B., Mendeloff, A.I.: Studies in ulcerative colitis: TPN-linked dehydrogenases and nonspecific esterases in rectal biopsy specimens. Gastroenterol. 48, 173-184 (1965).

Montreuil, J., Biserte, G.: Acide sialique et spécificité de la réaction a l'acide periodique-fuchsine de Schiff appliquée à l'électrophorèse sur papier. Exemple particulier de l'orosomucoïdes. Bull. Soc. chim. Biol. 41, 959-973 (1959).

Morson, B.C.: Precancerous conditions of the large bowel. Proc. roy. Soc. Med. 64, 959-962 (1971a).

Morson, B.C.: Pathology of ulcerative colitis. Proc. roy. Soc. Med. 64, 976 (1971b).

Morson, B.C.: The polyp-cancer sequence in the large bowel. Proc. roy. Soc. Med. 67, 451-457 (1974a).

Morson, B.C.: Evolution of cancer of the colon and rectum. Cancer 34, 845-849 (1974b).

Morson, B.C.: The technique and interpretation of rectal biopsies in inflammatory bowel disease. In: Pathology Annual (ed. *S.C. Sommers*), Appleton-Century-Crofts, pp. 209-230 (1974c).

Morson, B.C., Bussey, H.J.R.: Predisposing causes of intestinal cancer. In: Current Problems of Surgery. Chicago: Year Book Med. Publ. Inc. 1970.

Morson, B.C., Dawson, I.M.P.: In: Gastrointestinal Pathology. Oxford: Blackwell Scientific Publ. 539 (1972).

Morson, B.C., Pang, L.S.C.: Rectal biopsy as an aid to cancer control in ulcerative colitis. Gut 8, 423-434 (1967).

Mowry, R.W., Morard, J.C.: The distribution of acid mucopolysaccharides in normal kidneys, as shown by the Alcian blue-Feulgen (AB-F) and Alcian blue-periodic acid-Schiff (AB-PAS) stains. Amer. J. Path. 33, 620-621 (1957).

Nachbar, M.S., Oppenheim, J.D., Aull, F.: Cell surface contributions to the malignant process. Review. Amer. J. Med. Sc. 268, 123-138 (1974).

Neutra, M., Leblond, C.P.: Synthesis of the carbohydrate of mucus in the Golgi complex as shown by electron microscope radioautography of goblet cells from rats injected with glucose-H^3. J. Cell. Biol. 30, 119-136 (1966a).

Neutra, M., Leblond, C.P.: Radioautographic comparison of the uptake of galactose-^3H and glucose ^3H in the Golgi region of various cells secreting glycoproteins or mucopolysaccharides. J. Cell Biol. 30, 137-150 (1966b).

Pasternak, C.A., Kent, P.W., Davies, R.E.: Biosynthesis of intestinal mucins. I. Survey of incorporation of 35S sulphate by isolated gastrointestinal tissues. Biochem. J. 68, 212-217 (1958).

Pearse, A.G.E.: In: Histochemistry – Theoretical and Applied. Vol. 1, 3rd ed. London: Churchill 1968.

Pearse, A.G.E.: The role of histochemistry in increasing objectivity in histopathology. Postgraduate Med. J. 51, 708-710 (1975).

Peterson, M., Leblond, C.P.: Synthesis of complex carbohydrates in the Golgi region, as shown by radioautography, after injection of labeled glucose. J. Cell Biol. 21, 143-148 (1964).

Pittman, F.E., Pittman, J.C.: An electron microscopic study of the epithelium of normal human sigmoid colonic mucosa. Gut 7, 644-661 (1966).

Rambourg, A.: Morphological and histochemical aspects of glycoproteins at the surface of animal cells. Int. Rev. Cytol. 31, 57-114 (1971).

Rambourg, A.: Staining of intracellular glycoproteins. In: Electron Microscopy and Cytochemistry (eds. *E. Wisse, W.Th. Daems, I. Molenaar, P. van Duijn*), pp. 245-253. Amsterdam: North Holland Publ. Co. 1973.

Rambourg, A., Hernandez, W., Leblond, C.P.: Detection of complex carbohydrates in the Golgi apparatus of rat cells. J. Cell Biol. 40, 395-414 (1969).

Rambourg, A., Leblond, C.P.: Electron microscope observations of the carbohydrate-rich cell coat present at the surface of cells in the rat. J. Cell Biol. 32, 27-53 (1967).

Ravetto, C.: A histochemical identification of N-acetyl-O-diacetyl neuraminic acid resistant to neuraminidase. J. Histochem. Cytochem. 16, 663 (1968).

Reid, P.E., Culling, C.F.A., Dunn, W.L.: Saponification-induced increase in the periodic acid-Schiff reaction in the gastrointestinal tract. Mechanism and distribution of the reactive substance. J. Histochem. Cytochem. 21, 473-482 (1973).

Reid, P.E., Culling, C.F.A., Dunn, W.L.: The histochemical interpretation of the complex results of methylation upon gastrointestinal tract mucins with special reference to periodic acid-Schiff reactivity. J. Histochem. Cytochem. 22, 986-991 (1974).

Revel, J.P.: In: Chemistry and Molecular Biology of the Intercellular Matrix. Vol. 3 (ed. *E.A. Balazs*). London: Academic Press 1970.

Rios, A., Simmons, R.L.: Immunospecific regression of various syngeneic mouse tumours in response to neuraminidase-treated tumour cells. J. nat. Cancer Inst. 51, 637-644 (1973).

Schachter, H., Kirsner, J.B.: Definitions of inflammatory bowel disease of unknown etiology. Gastroenterol. 68, 591-600 (1975).

Scott, J.E., Dorling, J.: Differential staining of acid glycosaminoglycans (mucopolysaccharides) by Alcian blue in salt solutions. Histochemie 5, 221-223 (1965).

Shenkein, I., Uhr, J.W.: Immunoglobulin synthesis and secretion. I. Biosynthetic studies of the addition of the carbohydrate moieties. J. Cell Biol. 46, 42-51 (1970).

Sherlock, P., Kirsner, J.B.: Newer techniques for the early detection of gastrointestinal cancer in inflammatory bowel disease. Amer. J. dig. Dis. 20, 649-654 (1975).

Shora, W., Forstner, G.G., Forstner, J.F.: Stimulation of proteolytic digestion by intestinal goblet cell mucus. Gastroenterol. 68, 470-479 (1975).

Smith, B., Butler, M.: The autonomic control of colonic mucin secretion in the mouse. Brit. J. exp. Path. 55, 615-621 (1974).

Sorvari, T.E.: Histochemical observations on the role of ferric chloride in the high-iron diamine technique for localizing sulphated mucosubstances. Histochem. J. 4, 193-204 (1972).

Sorvari, T.E., Arvilommi, H.S.: Some chemical, physical and histochemical properties of three diamine fractions obtained by gel chromatography from the high-iron diamine staining solution used for localizing sulphated mucosaccharides. Histochem. J. 5, 119-130 (1973).

Sorvari, T.E., Lauren, P.A.: The effect of various fixation procedures on the digestability of sialomucins with neuraminidase. Histochem. J. 5, 405-412 (1973).

Sorvari, T.E., Stoward, P.J.: Some investigations of the mechanism of the so-called methylation reactions used in mucosubstance histochemistry. I. Methylation with methyliodide solvents containing either hydrogen chloride or thionyl chloride. Histochemie 24, 106-113 (1970a).

Sorvari, T.E., Stoward, P.J.: Some investigations of the so-called methylation reactions used in mucosubstance histochemistry. II. Histochemical differentiation of lactone and ester groups in methylated mucosaccharides. Histochemie 24, 114-119 (1970b).

Spicer, S.S.: Diamine methods for differentiating mucosubstances histochemically. J. Histochem. Cytochem. 13, 211-234 (1965).
Spicer, S.S., Leppi, T.J., Stoward, P.J.: Suggestions for a histochemical terminology of carbohydrate-rich tissue components. J. Histochem. Cytochem. 13, 599-603 (1965).
Spicer, S.S., Lillie, R.D.: Saponification as a means of selectively reversing the methylation blockade of tissue basophilia. J. Histochem. Cytochem. 7, 123-125 (1959).
Spicer, S.S., Sun, D.C.H.: Gastric pepsin, mucus and clinical secretory studies. II. The role of the mucous barrier in the defense of the stomach vs. peptic ulceration. Carbohydrate histochemistry of gastric epithelial secretions in dog. Ann. N.Y. Acad. Sci. 140, 762-783 (1967).
Spiro, R.G.: Glycoproteins: their biochemistry, biology and role in human disease. I. New Engl. J. Med. 281, 991-1001 (1969a).
Spiro, R.G.: Glycoproteins: their biochemistry, biology and role in human disease. II. New Engl. J. Med. 281, 1043-1056 (1969b).
Spiro, R.G.: Glycoproteins. Adv. Protein Chem. 27, 350-467 (1973).
Spiro, R.G., Spiro, M.J.: Glycoprotein biosynthesis: studies on thyroglobulin. Characterisation of a particulate precursor and radioisotope incorporation by thyroid slices and particle systems. J. biol. Chem. 241, 1271-1282 (1966).
Stonehill, E.H., Bendich, A.: Retrogenetic expression: the reappearance of embryonal antigens in cancer cells. Nature 228, 370-372 (1970).
Stoward, P.J.: The histochemical properties of some periodate-reactive mucosubstances of the pregnant Syrian hamster before and after methylation with methanolic thionyl chloride. J. roy. Micr. Soc. 87, 77-103 (1967).
Stoward, P.J.: The histochemical reactions of methanolic thionyl chloride with the anionic groups and basic protein component of sulphated mucosubstances. J. roy. Micr. Soc. 88, 119-131 (1968).
Takeuchi, T., Ensrud, E.R., Steggerda, F.R.: The effects of large doses of aspirin and cortisone on the goblet cells and the mucosal membranes in the small and large intestine. Amer. J. dig. Dis. 17, 49-53 (1972).
Teague, R.H., Fraser, D., Clamp, J.R.: Changes in monosaccharide content of mucous glycoproteins in ulcerative colitis. Brit. Med. J. 1973 II, 645-646.
Thiéry, J.P.: Ultrastructure, cytochimie et biogenèse des mucines digestives. Ann. Anat. Path. 17, 307-326 (1972).
Troncale, F., Hertz, R., Lipkin, M.: Nucleic acid metabolism in proliferating and differentiating colonic cells of man and in neoplastic lesions of the colon. Cancer Res. 31, 463-467 (1971).
Warren, L.: In: Glycoproteins: Their Composition, Structure and Function (ed. *A. Gottschalk*). London: Elsevier 1966.
Wattenberg, L.W.: A histochemical study of succinic dehydrogenase and cytochrome oxidase in proliferative lesions of the large intestine. Cancer Res. 19, 1118-1123 (1959).
Weiser, M.M.: Intestinal epithelial cell surface membrane glycoprotein synthesis. I. An indicator of cellular differentiation. J. Biol. Chem. 248, 2536-2541 (1973a).
Weiser, M.M.: Intestinal epithelial cell surface membrane glycoprotein synthesis. II. Glycosyltransferases and endogenous acceptors of the undifferentiated cell surface membrane. J. biol. Chem. 248, 2542-2548 (1973b).
Weiss, L.: Neuraminidase, sialic acids, and cell interactions. J. nat. Cancer Inst. 50, 3-19 (1973).
Willighagen, R.G.J., Planteydt, H.T.: Aminopeptidase activity in cancer cells. Nature 183, 263-264 (1959).

Winzler, R.J.: Carbohydrates in cell surfaces. Int. Rev. Cytol. 29, 77-125 (1970).
Winzler, R.J., Bekesi, J.G.: Glycoproteins in relation to cancer. In: Methods in Cancer Research, Vol. 2, pp. 159-202 (ed. *H. Busch*). London: Academic Press 1967.
Wolfe, H.J., Vickery, A.L.: The use of S^{35} labeled sulphate in studies on human normal and neoplastic cartilage tissues. Lab. Invest. 13, 743-751 (1964).
Yardley, J.H., Keren, D.F.: Precancer lesions in ulcerative colitis. Cancer (Philad.) 34, 835-844 (1974).
Young, R.W.: The role of the golgi complex in sulfate metabolism. J. Cell Biol. 57, 175-189 (1973).

The Precarcinomatous Phase of Ulcerative Colitis

R.H. RIDDELL

The first observation of coexistent ulcerative colitis and carcinoma is attributed to *Crohn* and *Rosenburg* who in 1925 described a patient with a 14 year history of ulcerative colitis complicated by carcinoma, and they raised the possibility of an association between these two conditions. In 1927, *Yeomans* reported a further case of colonic cancer in ulcerative colitis but in 1929 *Bargen* presented the first large series with 15 carcinomas in 693 patients, an incidence of 2.1%. These early reports were followed much later by a single paper in 1940 by *Jackman, Bargen* and *Helmholtz* who described the occurrence of carcinoma in 6 of 95 children with ulcerative colitis, an incidence of 6.3%. From 1945 onwards, there were a series of papers which tended to confirm the association between these two diseases and those until 1961 are summarised by *Goldgraber* and *Kirsner*. From this it became clear that there was marked variation in the incidence of colitic carcinomas from different centres with an incidence which varied from 0.6% to 17% in a series of children. However, the acceptance of this association was not without its antagonists. Indeed, as late as 1952, *Felson* and *Wolarsky* concluded that the two diseases were totally independant while in the same year *Otani* and *Snapper* stressed that there are conditions which may be misinterpreted as carcinoma and ulcerative colitis such as the ulceration occasionally seen proximal to a stenosing primary carcinoma, or secondary carcinoma in a patient with ulcerative colitis. In 1964, *Edwards* and *Truelove* concluded that the true incidence of carcinoma in ulcerative colitis lay between 3 and 5%, a figure which has gained wide acceptance. By combining several series, *Mottet* (1971) estimates that 3.1% of colitics will develop carcinoma.

Carcinoma complicating ulcerative colitis accounts for only a very small proportion of large bowel carcinomas and the true figure is probably less than 1%. It has been estimated that there were approximately 100,000 new cases of large bowel cancers in the USA in 1975 (American Cancer Society, 1974), and using this figure only about 1000 will arise as a complication of ulcerative colitis. However, they tend to develop insidiously even when the patient is under active medical care and may not become manifest until advanced. Frequently, tumours are multiple and their detection can be difficult because they may be flat or plaque-like (Figs. 1 and 2) making recognition difficult radiologically or endoscopically. This type of tumour tends to behave aggressively even though well differentiated (Fig. 2). The average age at which these tumours occur is much lower than non-colitic cancers, but a more reliable indication may be the mean age of death which is 46 (*Mottet*, 1971).

This inevitably means that many of these patients have heavy parental and financial responsibilities, while some will be in their twenties or even younger. All of these factors combine to produce a problem for which there is no simple answer and this has resulted in a variety of philosophies of management. The more aggressive of these are based on the identification of a subgroup of colitics in whom virtually all of these carcinoma occur.

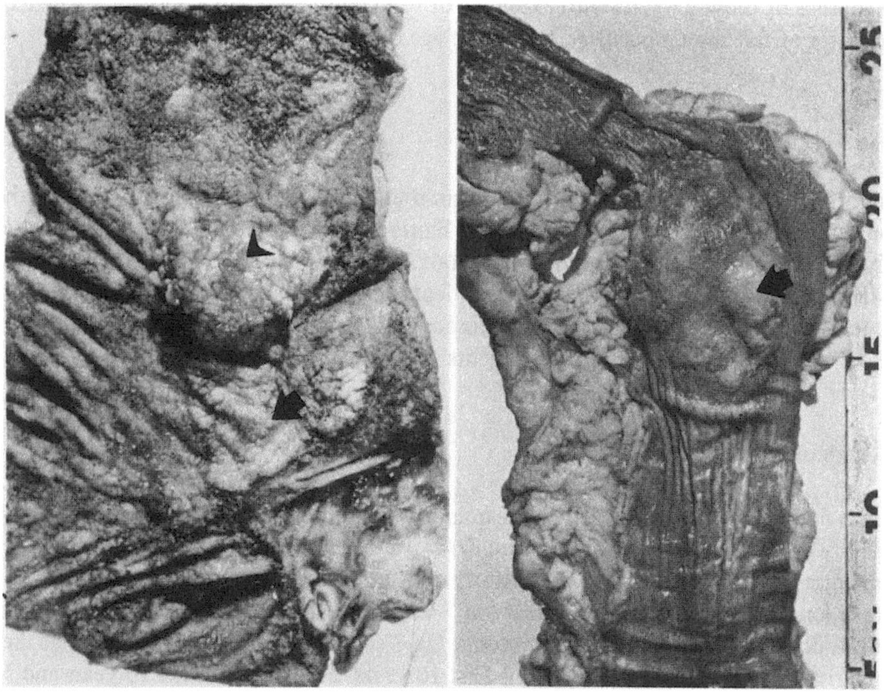

Fig. 1a. Small nodular carcinoma in the ascending colon (arrowhead). The mucosa on either side is rather warty, particularly above. This has a villous appearance microscopically. Note also the plaque of rather nodular tissue immediately beneath the carcinoma (arrowed). The terminal ileum and ileo-caecal valve are bottom right

Fig. 1b. Plaque-like carcinoma at splenic flexure (arrowed). Note that the surrounding mucosa appears more opaque than the mucosa at either end which is markedly atrophic

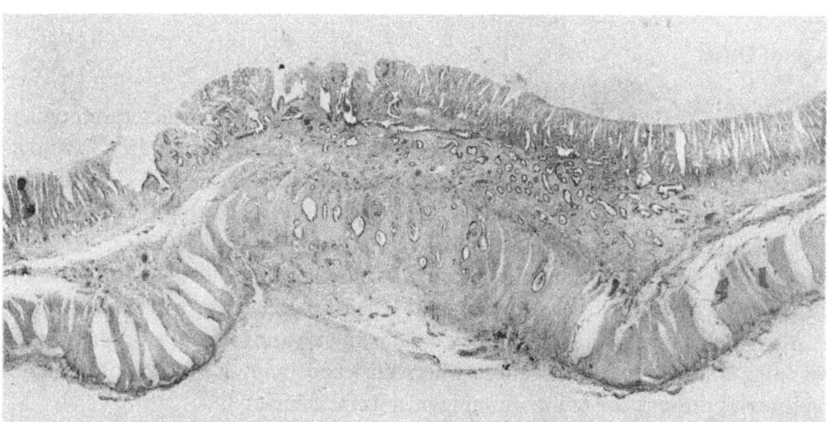

Fig. 2. Low power section through a plaque-like carcinoma. The muscularis propria is almost infiltrated. (H & E x 9)

I. The High Risk Clinical Group

This consists of those patients with extensive or total colitis and a long history, particularly if the onset of the disease occurred before the age of 25.

1. Extent of Disease

Many of the studies of cancer in colitis confirm that extensive or total involvement of the colon is invariably present. Distal colitis (i.e., limited to rectum or left side), is only very rarely associated with carcinoma (*Hinton*, 1966; *Edwards* and *Truelove*, 1964; *MacDougall*, 1964; *de Dombal*, 1966). However, some patients with distal colitis radiologically do in fact have total colitis when examined by colonoscopy with the aid of multiple biopsies (*Dilawari* et al., 1972). This implies that not all patients with pancolitis are recognised clinically.

2. Length of History

There is no doubt that the incidence of carcinoma in colitics correlates well with the length of history as summarized by *Edwards* and *Truelove* in 1964 and by *Goligher* in 1968. Few carcinomas develop before a five year history and the vast majority after a history of 10 years or longer. However, in his summary of 7 series, *Mottet* suggests that 22% of cancers in colitis occur before 10 years of symptoms. On 7 cases only, *Goligher* suggests that the annual risk in total colitis is 0.4% for the first 10 years, 2.0% for the next 10 years and 5.8% for patients with a history of 20-29 years, thus producing a cumulative risk of 41.8% after 25 years. However, *Edwards* and *Truelove* in a much larger series of 624 patients found 22 with carcinoma in whom there was a cumulative risk of 12.6% at 20 years. While the year of age of onset is usually recorded, it is still surprising how often there is "disease since childhood" or a "long history of colitis".

3. Age of Onset

It is noticeable that the percentage of patients with colitis developing carcinoma is markedly elevated when children are included and series only including children have the highest incidence, e.g., *Rosenqvist* et al. 17%, *Devroede* et al. 20% per decade after the first decade. *Edwards* and *Truelove* have summarised the position by suggesting that the younger the patient at the onset of the disease the greater the risk of subsequent cancer. However, many other factors come into this argument, such as the fact that most children developing ulcerative colitis have severe disease that usually reflects extensive or total colitis from an early age. Also, their life expectancy is much greater than, for example, a similar group of patients developing colitis in the sixth decade where life expectancy is much shorter and other common diseases prevent the colitis running its natural course.

4. Other Factors

Other factors that have been suggested as predisposing to cancer are a severe first attack (*Edwards* and *Truelove*, 1964) and the character of the symptomatology. *Edwards* and *Truelove* considered that chronic continuous symptoms predispose to carcinoma while *Svartz* and *Ernberg* (1949) suggested that patients with longstanding quiescent colitis are at greatest risk. *Goligher* has encountered both situations (1968). Personal experience leads me to believe that the patients that do poorly are those who are not under medical supervision and present with symptoms due to their tumour; a large mass or stricture is usually found. Local disease is usually extensive and multiple tumours not infrequent. By contrast those tumours occurring in patients under medical supervision have more often been detected when much smaller and less advanced locally. It must be admitted, however, that patients not under medical supervision usually have either no symptoms or symptoms that they are easily able to manage themselves without resorting to medical advice.

II. Management of the High Risk Clinical Group

The identification of this clinical high risk group has put the clinician in a dilemma. One approach is to submit the whole of this high risk group to proctocolectomy, usually when the disease has been present for 10 years (*Goligher*, 1968; *Rosenqvist*, 1955). However, this wholesale sacrifice of colons has been challenged because apart from the inevitable small mortality, appreciable morbidity, and the effects of permanent ileostomy, only a small proportion of patients even within this high risk group eventually develop carcinoma. It has been estimated that approximately 3.0-3.5 of all colitics develop cancer (*Mottet*, 1975). As about one third of all colitics are total, it follows that in this high risk group about 10% will develop carcinoma. This is in accordance with the 12.5% incidence at 20 years indicated by *Edwards* and *Truelove* although the incidence will probably rise with the length of history. However, this incidence is considered sufficient by some to justify their aggressive management. Others see carcinoma complicating colitis so infrequently that they tend to take no special precautions. Many clinicians tend to follow a middle course and while not advocating proctocolectomy on all their high risk patients, nevertheless become increasingly ready to advise this operation when severe exacerbations of the disease occur which they might otherwise have treated more aggressively by medical methods.

III. The Distribution of Carcinoma in Ulcerative Colitis

It is commonly held that the distribution of colitic cancers varies from that seen in non-colitic cancers in that the former are more commonly seen in the proximal colon. In some studies, this has been marked and *Edwards* and *Truelove* (1964) found only 6 of 27 carcinomas reported in the rectum. Conversely, *Mottet* (1971), by combining several series, suggested that 45% of colitic cancers arise in the rectosigmoid, compared to 60% of non-colitic cancers. This is of some importance as those carcinomas occurring in the rectum are directly accessible by sigmoidoscopy while those proximal require other methods of diagnosis.

1. Site of Carcinomas

The distribution of carcinomas included in this study is shown in Table 1. This was based on 111 colitic carcinomas available for pathologic study from 73 patients at St. Mark's Hospital, London.

Table 1. Comparison of the distribution of multiple and single carcinomas with patients and sex

	Multiple Tumours		Single Tumours			
	Male (9 patients)	Female (9 patients)	Male (21 patients)	Female (34 patients)	Total (73 patients)	% of % of Total
Caecum	3	1	1	1	6	5.4
Ascending Colon	1	0	1	1	3	2.7
Hepatic Flexure	0	4	0	1	5	4.5
Transverse Colon	6	6	0	7	19	17.1
Splenic Flexure	2	4	1	3	10	9.0
Descending Colon	5	2	1	4	12	10.8
Sigmoid Colon	2	6	1	1	10	9.0
Rectum	6	8	16	16	46	41.5
Total	25	31	21	34	111	100.0

In this series rectal cancers accounted for 41.5% of the cancers studied and this is only little short of the figure of 50.0% which is the accepted proportion of carcinomas arising in the rectum in the population at large (*Morson* and *Dawson*, 1972). A significant difference, however, is that in the general population a further 25.0% of carcinomas are expected in the sigmoid area and the remaining 25.0% tend to be fairly equally distributed between the remaining parts of the large intestine (*Morson* and *Dawson*, 1972). In this series it is apparent that the sigmoid colon is the site of only 9.0% of all carcinomas and that as the right side of the colon is approached the incidence gradually decreases. A second peak is encountered in the transverse colon where approximately 1/6 of the carcinomas were found. However, it should be remembered that when compared with the 9.0% found in the vicinity of the splenic flexure and the 10.0% found in the descending colon that this figure is quite in proportion to the relative length of the large intestine. Even accounting for the shortening that occurs in ulcerative colitis it is hard to imagine the length of the transverse colon being less than twice that usually described as being splenic flexure, and yet the splenic flexure alone has approximately 50.0% of carcinomas when compared to the entire transverse colon. This suggests that carcinomas arising in ulcerative colitis do so predominantly on the left side and are more common as the rectum is approached. The right side of the colon accounts for only a small proportion of all carcinomas in ulcerative colitis.

2. Multiple Carcinomas

When the distribution of single and multiple tumours is examined two important factors emerge. In men the vast majority of single tumours occur in the rectum (16 out of 21) while in women 16 out of 34 were in the rectum and there was a much greater tendency for the remainder to be distributed throughout the remaining colon particularly transverse and left side. When multiple tumours are considered, however, the distribution throughout the colon is very similar in both sexes. When compared to the usual distribution of carcinomas in patients not having ulcerative colitis the general trend of rectal carcinomas occurring in males and colonic carcinomas occurring females is maintained.

Table 1 also shows the distribution of the multiple tumours which were present in 18/73 patients (24.7%). The shift to the right is apparent. No combination was seen with undue frequency; the most frequent was that of transverse colon and rectum, but this occurred only in 4 of the 18 patients. In 11/18 the most distal tumour was in the rectum; in a further 3 it was in the sigmoid and in the remainder it was in the descending colon. However, the most distal tumour was not always the most advanced pathologically.

IV. Methods of Cancer Detection in Ulcerative Colitis

1. Conventional Methods

These include barium enema, which is relatively insensitive unless the carcinoma is advanced; sigmoidoscopy, useful because almost half of colitic cancers do so within sigmoidoscopic range (Table 1); colonoscopy, the value of which has yet to be assessed, but should be of greater value than barium enema in the detection of more proximal carcinomas and the evaluation of strictures; and plasma carcino-embryonic antigen activity, which to date has been of little value (*Dilawari* et al., 1974).

V. Epithelial Dysplasia in Ulcerative Colitis

1. The Concept of Dysplasia as a Premalignant Lesion

The concept of a premalignant phase in ulcerative colitis is not new. *Yeomans*, as early as 1927, when describing only the second case of carcinoma developing in ulcerative colitis (the first having been described 2 years before by *Crohn* and *Rosenburg*) raised the possibility that carcinoma might be related to the inflammatory polyps developing in this condition ("pseudo"-polyps is a poor term, for polyps they most assuredly are). This view was expounded by numerous authors subsequently and the entire sequence and previous literature was well described by *Dawson* and *Pryse-Davies* in 1959.

The problem that this raises is in trying to decide whether adenomas arising in ulcerative colitis are true adenomas similar to those seen in non-colitic patients or really represent adenomatous transformation of inflammatory polyps. This is exemplified by *Fenoglio* and *Paschal* (1973) who suggested that adenomatous polyps and intraepithelial anaplasia occurred 7 times more frequently and at a younger age in patients with ulcerative colitis. In contrast, *Swinton* and *Warren* (1939), *Hardy, Brooke* and *Hawkins* (1948) and *Counsell* and *Dukes* (1952) took the view that inflammatory polyps never become neoplastic. The last reference is of interest since I have personally examined pathology reports written by *Cuthbert Dukes* at that time and one of these has reported "extensive premalignant change in ulcerative colitis". This suggests that *Dukes* was certainly familiar with the problem and that this conclusion was based on his considerable experience. An intermediate view was taken by *Warren* and *Sommers* (1949), who stated that "inflammatory polyps .... are considered least likely to undergo malignant change".

In 1967, *Morson* and *Pang* described "precancerous" changes in the mucosa in 23 colectomy specimens resected for carcinoma in ulcerative colitis. These changes were often extensive and involved the mucosa away from the site of the carcinoma as well as in its immediate vicinity. Similar changes were found in a retrospective study of 12 of 134 patients with total colitis undergoing resection – an incidence of 9%. In a retrospective study of 148 rectal biopsies taken from patients with ulcerative colitis, 94 were from patients treated medically and none showed premalignant change while in 16 of 54 biopsies from patients later undergoing colectomy, this "premalignant" change was found (29%), but none of them were accompanied by carcinoma. In a further 9 patients, a report of premalignant change was responsible to some extent for subsequent proctocolectomy and, in 5 of these, a carcinoma was found incidentally in the resection specimen. They point out that these changes may occur in flat or polypoid mucosa and emphasized that irregularity, loss of parallelism, lateral budding of the epithelial crypts and a tendency to adopt a villous configuration was common while the importance of proliferating tubules in the submucosa was stressed. Cytological changes similar to those seen in dysplasia in other sites were described, such as enlarged pleomorphic hyperchromatic nuclei with nuclear stratification and increase in the nuclear-cytoplasmic ratios. They concluded that regular rectal biopsy might be used to demonstrate these changes and to predict which patients were most likely to develop carcinoma even though this may be elsewhere in the colon. *Evans* and *Pollock* (1972), however, investigated the extent of premalignant change as described by *Morson* and *Pang* in 4 patients and found it to be very variable, being absent or restricted in 2, but very extensive in the other 2. Furthermore, in all 4 cases, the rectum was spared in whole or in part and they suggested that rectal biopsy was not a good method for predicting which patients would develop carcinoma. However, *Hulten* et al. (1972), found premalignant change in 22 of 25 patients with ulcerative colitis and carcinoma, and in 12 of these it was in direct continuity with the tumour. They also examined specimens from ulcerative colitis of short duration, ulcerative colitis and lymphoma, and Crohn's disease. While the full picture of premalignant change was not found in these groups, they did find in these specimens nuclear stratification, variation in size and shape of nuclei with hyperchromatism and lateral budding of the tubules, but emphasized that neither loss of nuclear polarity nor true villous growth was observed. Unfortunately, they do not define precisely their criteria for distinguishing between nuclear stratification and loss of polarity.

Myrvold et al. (1974), from the same hospital, described 47 patients subjected to proctocolectomy for ulcerative colitis in whom 3-4 rectal biopsies were taken from different sites prior to operation. Premalignant change was found in 7 of these. In resection specimens of these 7 patients, a carcinoma was found in 5, while in only 1 was it suspected. However, they also described "cellular atypia" in a further 16 patients; while in the resection specimens from this group, 10 had premalignant change, although none had an accompanying carcinoma. Regrettably, there are no illustrations of this change while the text states only that it is not the "full picture of precancerous change". In the other 24 patients in this group with no atypia or precancer on rectal biopsy, 9 had "cellular atypia in the resection specimens, while one had precancer". They also state that although 3-4 biopsies were taken from each patient, precancer was only noted in one or two of these. They concluded that the finding of these changes justified prophylactic proctocolectomy.

Yardley and *Keren* (1974) also attempted to define the "precancer" lesion in patients with ulcerative colitis by examining 41 resected specimens and 412 rectal biopsies taken at the Johns Hopkins Hospital by grading the degree of acute inflammation, the degree of atypia and the degree of villous change. They found "epithelial atypia" in the mucosa adjacent to 7 out of 8 resected for carcinoma and emphasized the importance of villous or polypoid change and mucin depletion. They found similar changes in 3 of the 412 rectal biopsies studied and two of these were found to have invasive carcinoma in the resected colon while the third had diffuse precancerous change throughout his colon in the form of multiple adenomas. However, they also stressed that acute inflammation increased the number of biopsies showing suspicious changes. They also pointed out that some cases of precancer might go undetected if rectal biopsy only was used, and suggested that precancer patients might be more successfully identified using the colonoscope. These reports suggest that an identifiable morphologic precursor to carcinoma in colitis does exist.

To date there are few prospective studies; *Lennard-Jones* (1974) reported 171 patients with extensive colitis who were followed between 1966 and 1973 during which time 14 showed epithelial dysplasia on rectal biopsy. In 7 of these, proctocolectomy was carried out and 3 had carcinoma in the resected specimen, two being small inconspicuous and confined to the bowel wall (Dukes A). The third was larger with slight extension beyond the bowel wall, but no nodal involvement (Dukes B). All were well 2, 6 and 7 years after the resection. In the remaining 7 patients, the dysplasia was inconstant and not severe enough to be regarded as precancerous and they remained under medical care 1-3 years after dysplasia was first noted. During this time, no other carcinoma developed. At first sight, this implies that rectal biopsy is a useful indication of incipient malignancy, but this study is open to the criticism that if a flat plaque-like carcinoma developed in the more proximal colon in one of these patients in the presence of consistently normal rectal biopsies, it could remain undetected until it manifests itself clinically or on barium enema. The fact that this has not happened to date is encouraging.

From these studies, several points are apparent:

First, while frank precancerous change in a rectal biopsy is a useful additional parameter in detecting early carcinoma in colitis, the number of patients already having a carcinoma at the time of operation is high and suggests that it might be more valuable to carry out the operation at an earlier stage in the life history of this process. However, so far only severe dysplasia (precancer) can be diagnosed with confidence, lesser degrees always raising the possibility that an inflammatory or post-inflammatory dysplasia is present. The relationship between inflammatory dysplasia and precancer and methods of distinguishing between them requires clarification.

Second, it appears that there is a significant relationship between rectal precancer and carcinoma. What is not known is the extent of precancer particularly in the rectum because this is the site most accessible to biopsy. If the whole rectum is always affected then a single biopsy would be positive. If the changes are patchy then multiple biopsies would be required. In the event that precancer spares the rectum, then rectal biopsy would be of no value.

VI. Precarcinomatous Change

1. Macroscopic Appearance

a) Flat mucosa: epithelial dysplasia frequently occurs in mucosa showing no distinguishing features from those usually seen in longstanding ulcerative colitis. However, if the mucosa is hyperplastic and of increased thickness the usual atrophic appearance may be absent and underlying vessels difficult to see. Such atypical areas should be biopsied.

b) Villous mucosa: This change is recognizable macroscopically as an indistinct, slightly verrucose appearance because of the villi (Fig. 1b). In the fresh specimen it has a somewhat velvety appearance and the villi vary from just visible on close inspection to readily visible, depending largely on size. Endoscopically this is more difficult to recognize as viewing is necessarily carried out end on rather than by direct vision from above. However, it is occasionally recognized by clinicians as "? villous tumour" from which a biopsy is taken. The recognition of this lesion will clearly be facilitated by a wider knowledge of its existence.

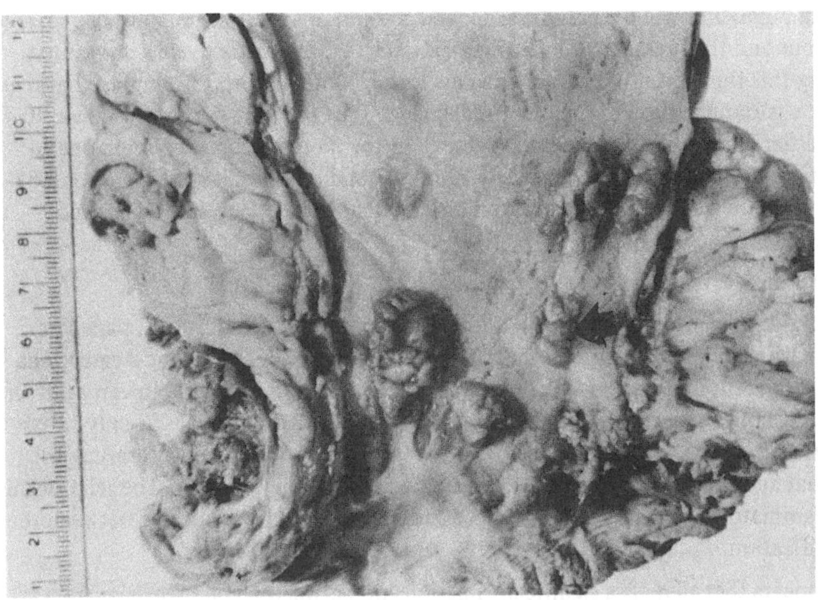

Fig. 3. Discrete polypoid nodules in rectum. One is only just elevated above the surrounding mucosa (arrow). A small carcinomatous plaque was also present (arrowhead). Note also that the intervening mucosa is opaque and appears thickened.

c) **Polypoid mucosa:** This is readily recognized in fresh and fixed specimens as well as endoscopically (Fig. 4). However, there may be difficulty in distinguishing some inflammatory polyps from an adenoma, and this has been shown to be spectrum (*Dawson* and *Pryse-Davies*, 1959). As the incidence of invasive carcinoma in adenomas is closely related to size (*Morson*, 1973), it is clearly advisable to excise endoscopically any polyp in which the head is 1 cm or more in diameter.

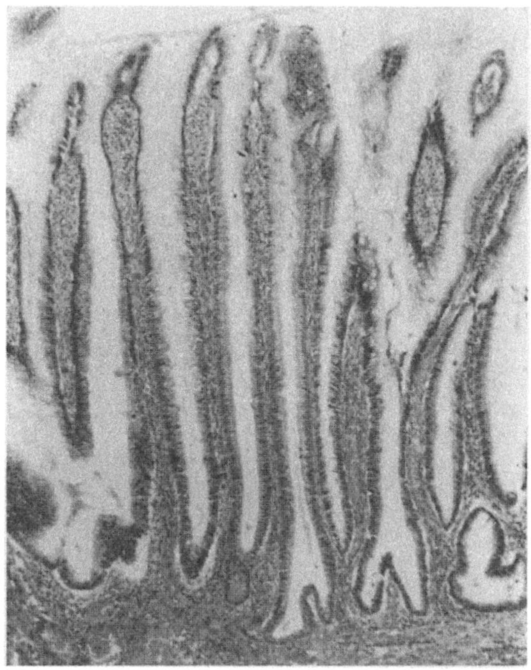

Fig. 4. Adenomatous dysplasia (villous). Tall slender villi are present. (H & E x 75)

2. Microscopic Appearance

A total of 111 carcinomas were subjected to histological examination in an attempt to define any patterns that were present either overlying the carcinoma or at its edge from which there was evidence that the carcinoma was arising. This disclosed 5 basic patterns which appeared to be closely related to the carcinoma and 2 of these were found to relatively common while the other three were comparatively rare.

These are called:	Adenomatous change	Common
	Basal cell change	Common
	In-situ anaplasia	Rare
	Clear cell change	Rare
	Pancellular change	Rare

a) Adenomatous type: This is the classical picture of neoplastic epithelium and occurs in flat, villous and polypoid mucosa (Figs. 1 and 3). When villi are present they vary from rather broad to tall and slender (Fig. 4). Sometimes the villi have small tubules budding into their substance and this produces club-shaped villi (Fig. 5). In most villi the greatest dysplasia is usually seen at the base of the crypts and there is evidence of maturation as the tip of the villus is approached. When club-shaped villi are present the reverse is frequently the case. As the villi decrease in height there is a greater tendency for them to bud, and this may be sufficiently marked as to give rise to a back to back appearance.

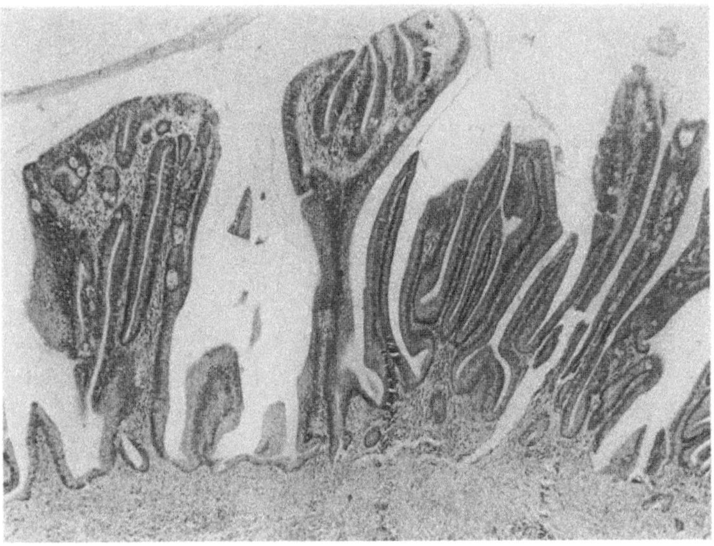

Fig. 5. Adenomatous dysplasia (villous). Well developed slender villi are present but in some of these there are tubules budding into the villus and producing a club-shaped appearance (H & E x 48)

A further feature descernible at low power is the amount of mucus present, and this usually varies inversely with the severity of dysplasia. In areas of severe cytological atypia there is seldom any mucin production and the cytoplasm is eosinophilic. Only an occasional goblet cell, or sometimes a minute amount of mucin in a very regular pattern on the lumenal aspect of the cells, can just be discerned. When dysplasia is less marked there may be moderate amounts of mucin present. Goblet cells can appear normal but sometimes a regular row of goblet cells is present in which the mucus droplet occupies only about half of the cell (Fig. 6). When dysplasia is mild there is frequently a normal or even an excessive amount of mucus (Fig. 7); the cells often appear abnormally large and sometimes the goblet cells lose their polarity. Then the whole cell migrates towards the luminal surface and is poorly oriented so that the nucleus is not on the basal side of the cell. Under these circumstances the cells usually become rounded and take on an appearance resembling signet ring cells (Fig. 12b).

Cytologically cell size is uniform although minor variations are seen, particularly towards the tips of villi. The nuclei show all the characteristic features associated with neoplasia.

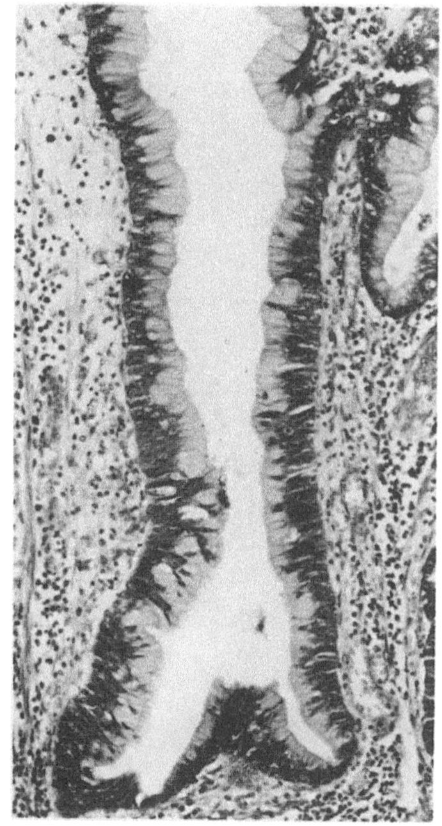

Fig. 6. Adenomatous dysplasia of moderate degree. The nuclei, although hyperchromatic, are largely situated at the base of the cell. The remainder of the cell is mucus (H & E x 120)

These are usually rather uniformly hyperchromatic and elongated and it is difficult to see any nuclear detail. Occasional small nucleoli may be present. Sometimes the nuclei are more vesicular with a heavy hyperchromatic peripheral chromatin rim and one or two prominant nucleoli (Fig. 8).

In the polypoid type of dysplasia there can be difficulty in distinguishing a true adenoma from a dysplastic inflammatory polyp (Fig. 9) and in the late stages it is impossible. While this appears to be semantics it is feasible to treat a solitary adenoma in the absence of dysplasia in the adjacent mucosa by simple polypectomy. However, if the patient has numerous inflammatory polyps several of which show dysplasia, this suggests that a more generalized change is occurring and more radical surgery should be seriously considered. While the adenomatous type of change has been described as occurring in flat, villous and polypoid mucosa, carcinoma arising from a flat mucosa is exceptional and there is usually transformation to a villous or more polypoid form in the immediate vicinity of the carcinoma.

Early adenomatous change is invariably found at the base of the crypts, particularly when these are bifid (Fig. 7). Rarely the luminal surface appears most dysplastic although this is more commonly in the early stages of the "basal cell" type of dysplasia. Figure 7 is probably the earliest lesion that can be considered to have invasive potential, although carcinoma

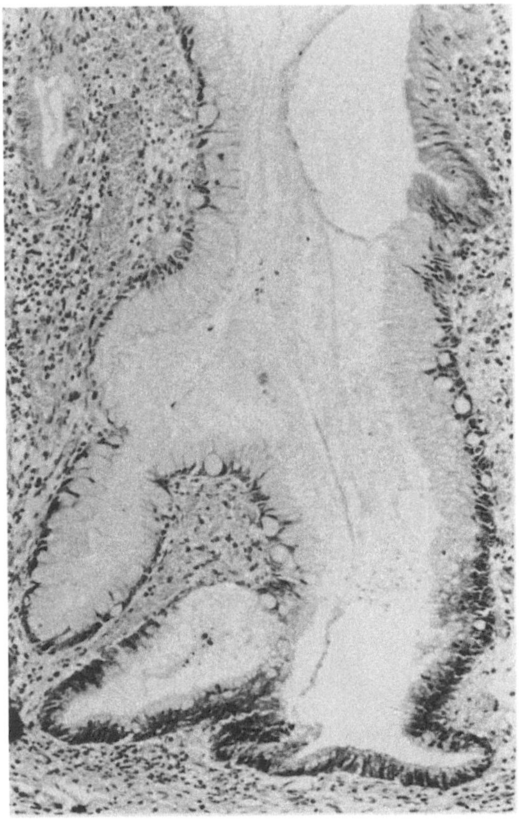

Fig. 7. Mild adenomatous dysplasia. There is marked glandular distortion but the cells are large and in some of the goblet cells the mucus has become trapped and the cell is rounded resembling a signet ring cell. Dysplasia is limited to the base of the crypt. This is one of the earliest phases in which adenomatous dysplasia can be confidently diagnosed (H & E x 120)

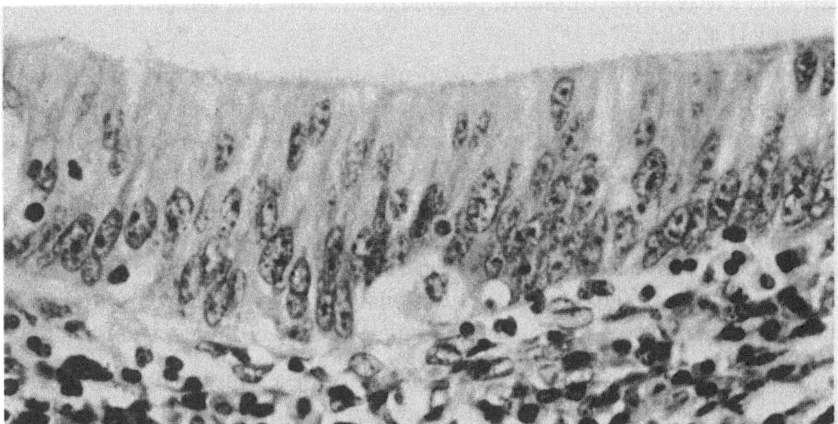

Fig. 8. Mild adenomatous dysplasia with open vesicular nuclei and prominent nucleoli (H & E x 480)

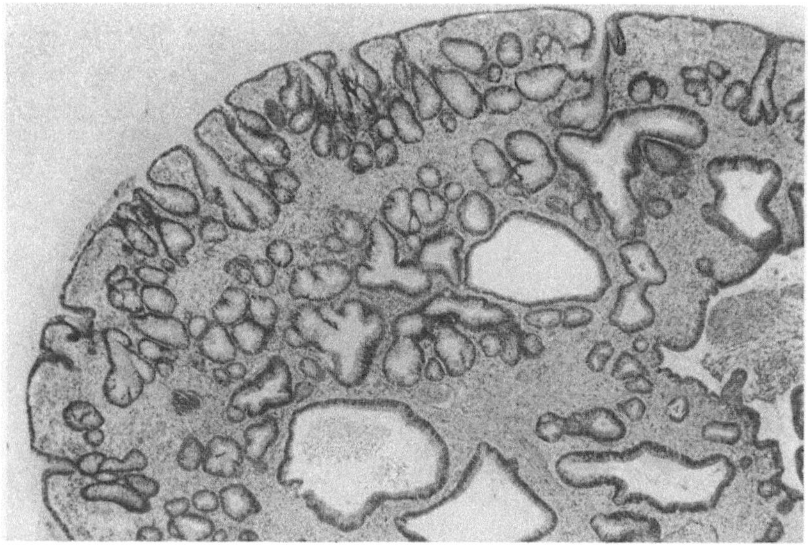

Fig. 9. Adenoma or dysplasia in an inflammatory polyp? The low power appearance here with a poorly organised array of crypts and lamina propria suggest that this may have been an inflammatory polyp. (The similarity of this low power to a juvenile or retention polyp is apparent – H & E x 30)

seldom arises in mucosa showing so little dysplasia. When carcinomas do arise from this type of mucosa they are usually "colloid" cancers, and the epithelium lining the colloid vacuoles similarly shows surprisingly little dysplasia. Furthermore, these tumours may destroy the muscularis propria, an "erosive" process, so that the luminal surface rests directly on the remnants, if any, of the muscularis propria. Biopsies of these lesions may be very difficult to diagnose as carcinoma and this may only become apparent when the resected specimen is examined.

In some biopsies dysplasia is insufficiently severe to classify as early neoplastic and yet is out of proportion to that expected as a response to inflammation even when inflammation present is taken into account. The only logical recourse in these circumstances is to request repeat biopsies.

b) Basal cell proliferation: This is most frequently seen in flat featureless mucosa where it occurs in a relatively pure form, but may be mixed with the adenomatous type of dysplasia. It can arise in mucosa of normal or increased thicknesses. Cell size is often normal or only moderately increased and the characteristic feature is a row of distinct small and intensely hyperchromatic nuclei arranged in a line (Fig. 10). The lack of the typical features of neoplasia including pleomorphism, loss of polarity and nuclear crowding is typical and the appearance is not dissimilar to Beluga caviar arranged in a row (Fig. 11a). Occasional nuclei are slightly vesicular with a dense peripheral chromatin ring, a prominent nucleolus, mild pleomorphism but marked polychromatism (Fig. 11b). The cytoplasm is similarly distinct and is usually markedly eosinophilic to the point of appearing almost oncocytic. Furthermore, an identical appearance is seen throughout the whole length of the tubule, suggesting failure of cellular maturation. Goblet cells are absent. Sometimes evidence of maturation

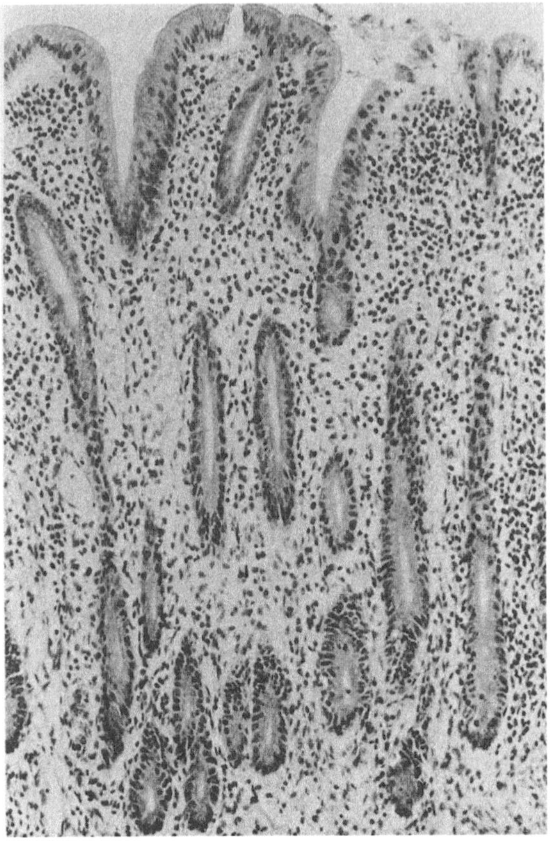

Fig. 10. Basal cell proliferation. The low power appearance may be deceptively unimpressive although occasionally the mucosa is thickened. The major abnormalities are the rather slender crypts, increased mucosal thickness and a total loss of goblet cells. However, even at this magnification mitotic figures can be seen in the mouths of the crypts with no adjacent ulceration (H & E x 120)

is seen as judged by the formation of goblet cells or a small row of mucin droplets close to the luminal border of the cell (Fig. 12a). Mitotic activity is usually readily visible, at times it is intense, and mitotic figures can sometimes be found in the upper third of the crypts. Frequently, argentaffin, other clear cells, and Paneth cells may also be found. Inflammatory changes in the lamina propria are usually mild. The impression then is that the cells at the base of the crypts pass to the surface with very little or no evidence of maturation, and it is for this reason that the term "basal cell" proliferation was chosen.

This is a particularly perplexing lesion as it is difficult to believe from its appearance that it has any neoplastic potential. However, it appears to give rise directly to some of the very poorly differentiated tumours that characterise ulcerative colitis (Fig. 13). The uniform appearance of both nucleus and cytoplasm along the crypt suggest that the cells are failing to mature as they progress towards the surface. When associated with a high mitotic index this might be because the turnover time is insufficient for the cells to mature as in subtotal

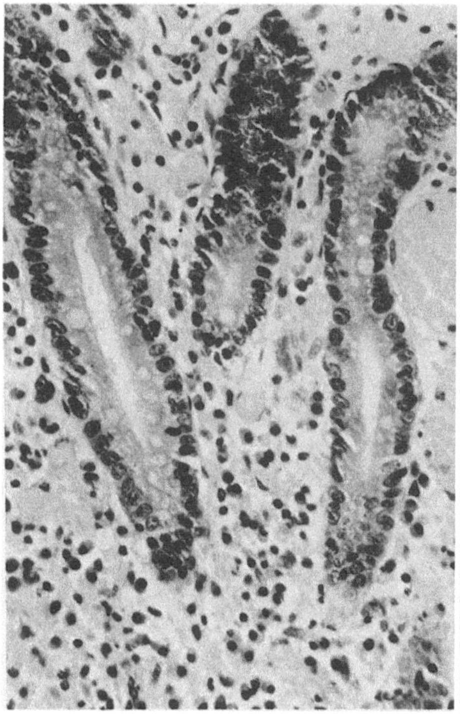

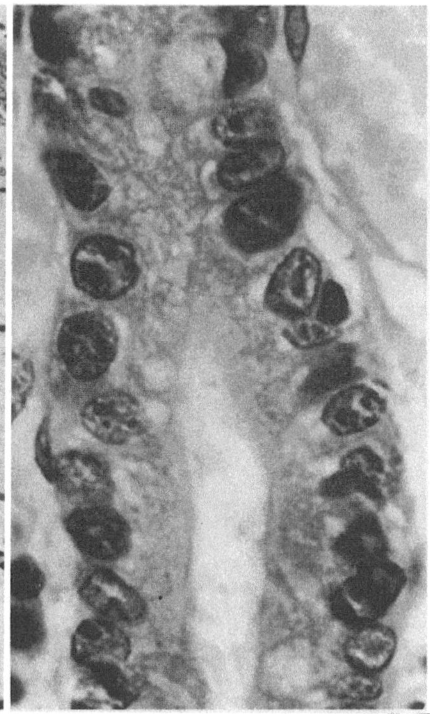

Fig. 11a. Basal cell proliferation. The nuclei are distinct and are polychromatic but have not lost their polarity. This produces the Beluga caviar effect (H & E x 300)

Fig. 11b. Basal cell proliferation. High power view of Figure 11a. Nuclear pleomorphism, occasional prominent nucleoli, and variation in the intensity of staining is apparent. Note the failure of the nuclei either to lose polarity or to overlap (H & E x 1200)

villous atrophy in the jejunum, but when this is not apparent it is possible that the cells just fail to mature. The possibility that these cells are all absorptive cells with primary failure of goblet cell formation has to be considered but the nuclei are not the small rather vesicular normochromatic nuclei with small nucleoli that are typical of these cells. Furthermore, in many instances features of goblet cells can be discerned (Fig. 12). Once the late lesion can be recognized, it becomes much easier to recognise the early stages which in their own way are also characteristic. The most noticeable feature is that only part of the crypt is involved, but because the lesion probably reflects a failure of maturation it is most readily identified in the luminal portions of the crypt where the lack of goblet cells and glassy eosinophilic cytoplasm are seen (Figs. 12 and 13). However, mitoses are not usually present while the characteristic nuclear changes are present but less well developed. Sometimes the changes are rather more obvious in the basal two thirds of the crypts.

c) In-situ anaplasia: This is rare and has only been seen in flat mucosa. When present it is frequently associated with the basal cell type of dysplasia in the adjacent mucosa. It takes one of two forms. In one there is virtually no residual crypt structure but the mucosa consists of a sheet of small undifferentiated cells (Fig. 14) in which signet ring cells can usually

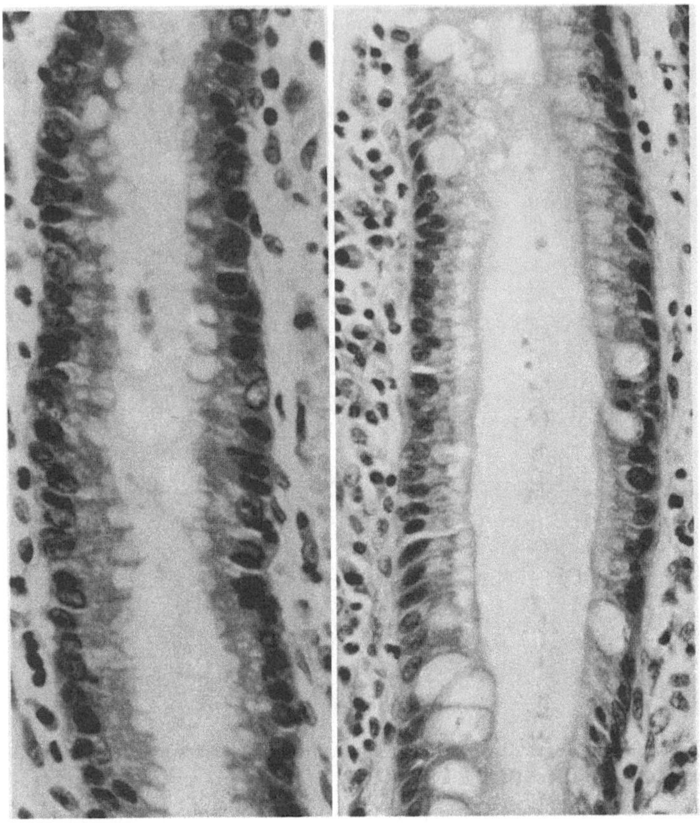

Fig. 12a. Basal cell proliferation. Nuclei remain reasonably distinct and polychromatic but this is less marked than in Figure 11 and mucus droplets are present at the apical border of many of the cells (H & E x 480)

Fig. 12b. Basal cell proliferation – early phase. Many of the cells are distinct and appear to be of one type only, each with an apical mucus droplet. Nuclei are polychromatic and distinct although less so than in Figure 12a. Atypical goblet cells are also present in the crypts (H & E x 300)

be seen and sometimes may predominate. Surprisingly, in spite of the appearance this is often confined by the muscularis mucosae. However, once it becomes invasive vessel permeation is easy to find. In the second variety the crypt structure can still be discerned but the crypts appear to be breaking down. This form is even more uncommon than the first. In all cases examined there was little excess inflammation in the adjoining mucosa.

d) Clear cell type: This a further type of change which at first demands little attention because of its apparently innocuous appearance and occurs as a slightly raised plaque. It is characterized by large clear cells, which stain poorly with either alcian blue (pH 2.5) or by the PAS method. The nuclei are elongated and hyperchromatic and there is some loss of polarity (Fig. 15). Occasional villi may be present (Fig. 16). Carcinomas arising from this mucosa tend to be well differentiated (Fig. 17). Close to the surface the lumen takes

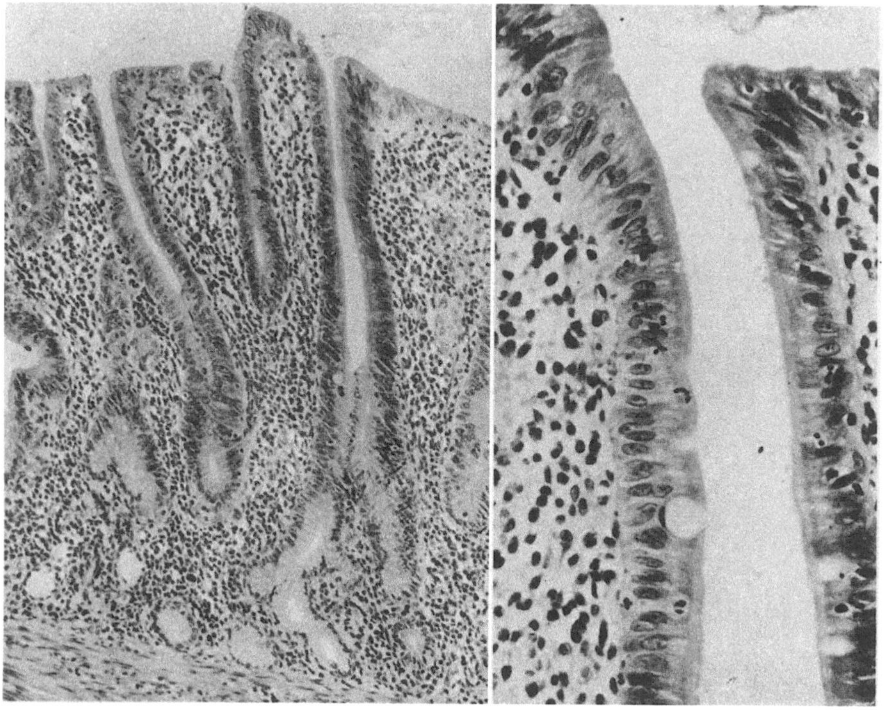

Fig. 13a (left). Basal cell proliferation – early phase. This usually involves the upper half of the crypt where distinct nuclei and no goblet cells are seen. Numerous goblet cells are present in the lower third of the mucosa but these have the appearance of pseudo-pyloric metaplasia rather than normal colonic goblet cells. They stain more intensely with PAS than ordinary goblet cells. Pseudo-pyloric metaplasia can be seen with and without dysplasia in ulcerative colitis (H & E x 120)

Fig. 13b (right). Higher power of Figure 13a showing lack of maturation and enlarged distinct basally situated nuclei. Only minor variations in nuclear staining are present (H & E x 480)

on an irregular arrangement that is reminiscent of the sawtooth appearance seen in metaplastic (hyperplastic) polyps. Paneth and argentaffin cells were not seen and mitotic figures were rare.

e) Pancellular dysplasia: This is seen in flat featureless mucosa and is characterized by dysplasia which is manifest mainly as large hyperchromatic nuclei with loss of polarity, but this affects all cell lines including Paneth, argentaffin and goblet cells. Paneth cells are prominent, found away from their usual position at the base of the crypts and appear to migrate up the crypt. Their nuclei lose their polarity and may be situated on the luminal side of the granules (Fig. 18). Goblet cells tend to be distended with mucus, possibly an indication of an abnormality in the normal release mechanism. When the nucleus loses its polarity and appears as a crescent at the luminal border to the cell the comparison with a signet ring cell seems unavoidable, although it may well be totally inappropriate. Argentaffin cells also appear far more numerous and may entirely surround the crypt giving an appearance resembling an in-situ argentaffinoma (Fig. 19). Any of these types of cell may predominate,

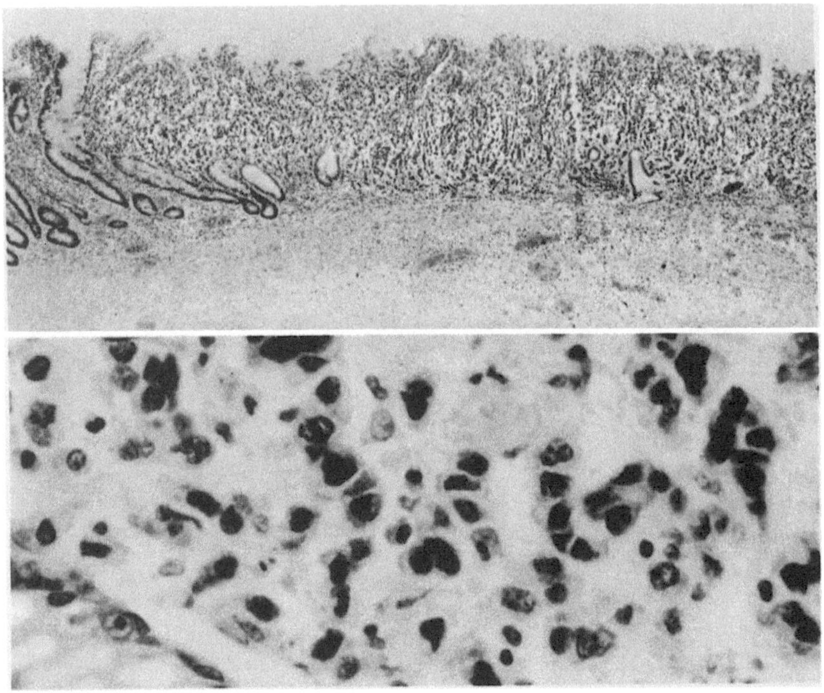

Fig. 14. In-situ anaplasia. Upper: The mucosa is virtually replaced by in-situ change that is limited by the muscularis mucosae. Fragments of residual crypts can be identified in the deep part of the mucosa (H & E x 30). – Lower: High power showing small cell very poorly differentiated adenocarcinoma (H & E x 480)

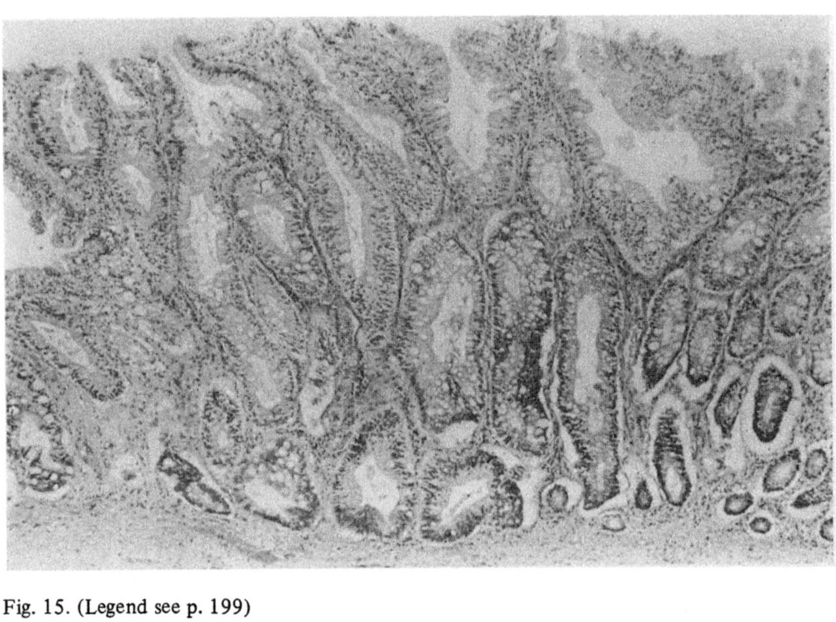

Fig. 15. (Legend see p. 199)

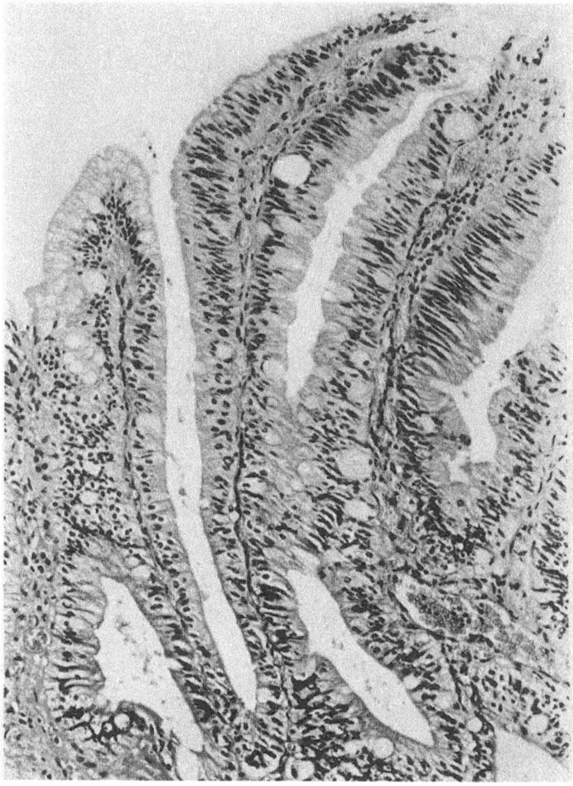

Fig. 16. Clear cell dysplasia. Superficial villi are present and the hyperchromatic elongated nuclei showing loss of polarity are better seen (H & E x 120)

but the other cell lines are invariably affected, albeit to a lesser degree. In the only tumour seen arising directly from it, argentaffin cells surrounded most of the crypts and infiltrated the lamina propria. However, the tumour present in the submucosa was a carcinoma with extracellular mucin pools in which there were signet ring cells and also cells with many argentaffin granules (Fig. 20). There were no metastases. It is clearly semantics as to whether this should be called a mucin secreting carcinoid tumour as described in the appendix (*Klein*, 1974; *Subbuswamy* et al., 1974) or a carcinoma with argentaffin cells.

Three macroscopic and five microscopic types of dysplasia occurring in ulcerative colitis are described. While the descriptions suggest that these are distinctive entities, it cannot be overemphasised that these are frequently mixtures, particularly of the two more common forms. Close examination of a proctocolectomy specimen for carcinoma in colitis will

---

Fig. 15. Clear-cell dysplasia. At first site this resembles an overgrown hyperplastic (metaplastic) polyp with more hyperchromatic nuclei in the basal part of the lesion and a suggestion of a "sawtooth" indentation of the upper crypts. (H & E x 75)

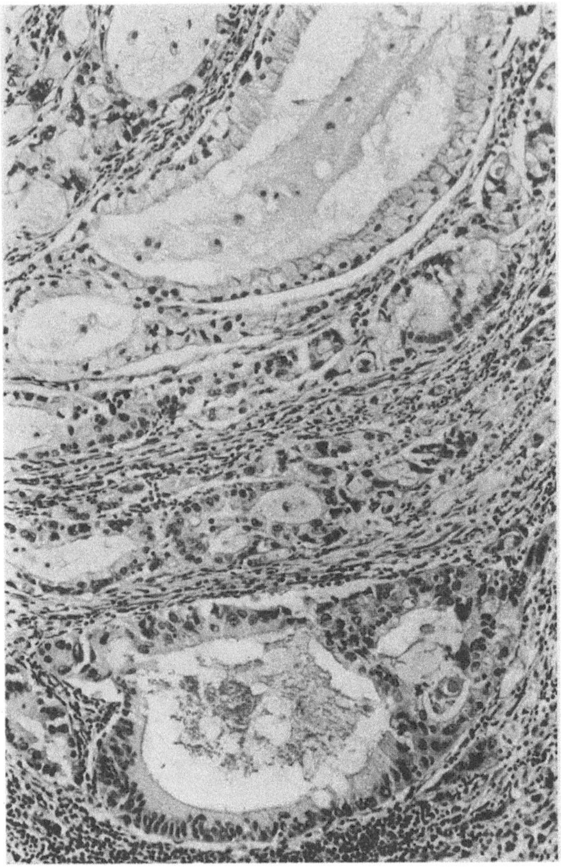

Fig. 17. Carcinoma arising from clear cell dysplasia. Note how parts of the tumour resemble the clear cell type of dysplasia while other areas resemble a more conventional well differentiated adenocarcinoma (H & E x 120)

often reveal a whole spectrum of changes, not only of the various types of dysplasia, but also of grades of any one type of dysplasia. The early phases of the two major types of dysplasia have been described in detail. Less attention has been paid to the early stages of the rarer types for several reasons. The early lesion of in-situ anaplasia is almost certainly the basal cell type of dysplasia, the early features of which have been described. In clear cell change, they may not have been recognised and those described are the earliest known, while the early stage of pancellular type is readily recongisable but is largely one of degree. It should also be remembered that because these changes are neoplastic, they tend not to conform, and while the changes described are the patterns most frequently encountered or the most distinctive, nevertheless, numerous subtle variations on all these themes can invariably be found. Because these changes tend to be zonal within the crypt in the initial stages, it is important that all biopsies are handled in a similar manner to jejunal biopsies so that the correct orientation of the biopsy can be maintained.

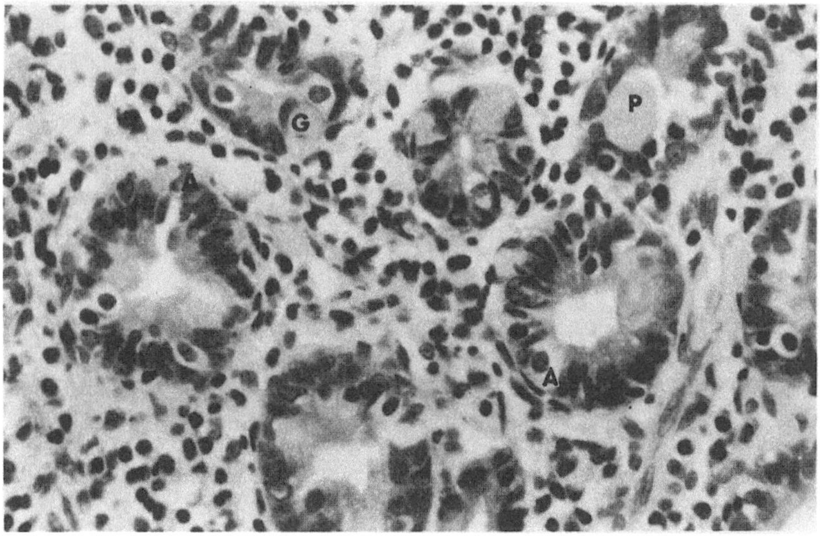

Fig. 18. Pancellular dysplasia. Lower part of mucosa showing atypical Paneth cells (P), argentaffin cells (A), and an atypical goblet cell (G). (H & E x 300)

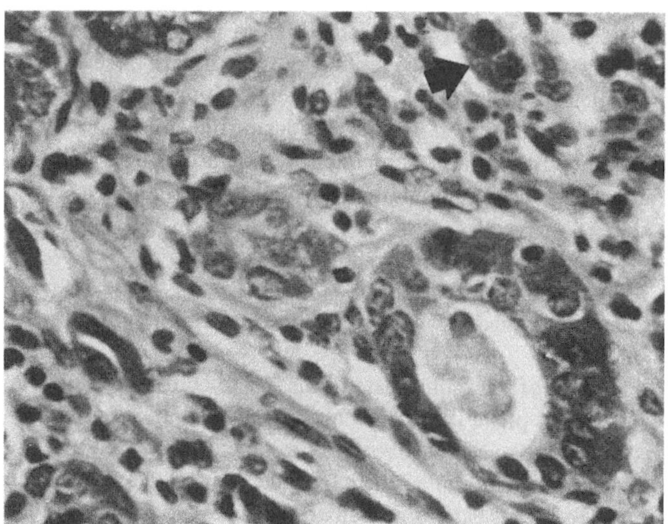

Fig. 19. Pancellular dysplasia and carcinoma. The largest crypt is almost surrounded by argentaffin cells and clusters of these cells can be seen infiltrating the lamina propria (arrowed, H & E x 480)

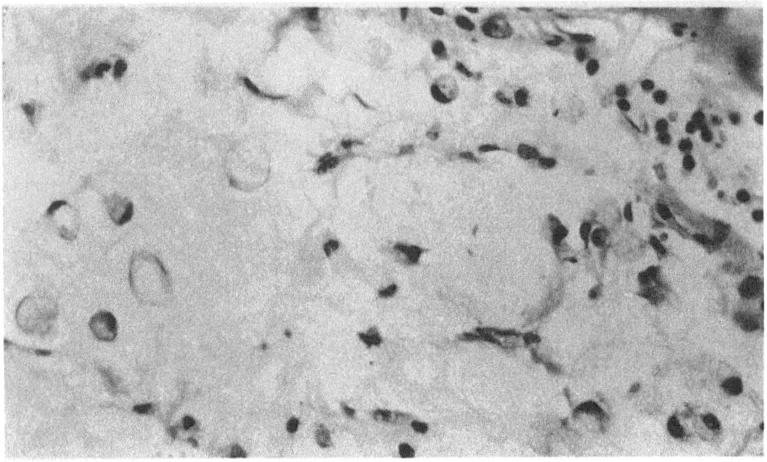

Fig. 20. Submucosal tumour of Figure 19. Note the mucous lake in which are floating typical signet ring cells. The more opaque of these have typical argentaffin granules in their cytoplasm. (H & E x 1200)

VII. The Relationship Between Inflammation and Dysplasia

The difficulty that can arise in the distinction between early neoplastic transformation and an intense reaction to inflammation has already been mentioned. It seems likely that these are part of a spectrum of changes so that in some patients the distinction can be almost impossible, particularly if repeat biopsies show no evidence of regression. The existence of this difficult, small group is undeniable, but it undoubtedly exists. However, it may be reduced to some extend by a knowledge of the appearances that can occur during an acute attack of colitis or in the subsequent regenerative phase as these should not be a source of confusion. The problem of co-existent inflammation and dysplasia must also be further explored.

1. Changes Associated with Acute Colitis or Regeneration

The features of the acute phase of ulcerative colitis are well described (*Price* and *Morson*, 1975). In this phase the nuclei become enlarged and vesicular with a light peripheral chromatin rim and the nucleolus becomes prominent. These features are seen throughout the mucosa and particularly in epithelium undergoing active regeneration (Fig. 21). Sequential biopsies from this patient demonstrated that it took almost a month for these changes to resolve and even then the nuclei were still distinctly enlarged when compared to the normal (Fig. 22). This is known as "epithelial hyperplasia".

Sometimes the regenerative phase is even more dramatic. Figures 23 and 24 are selected from the ascending colon of a 10 year old boy with only a three week history of ulcerative colitis which failed to respond to medical therapy, and there is little doubt that these features are regenerative. The presence of large vesicular nuclei with prominent nucleoli can, therefore, be a normal feature of regeneration following the acute phase of ulcerative colitis.

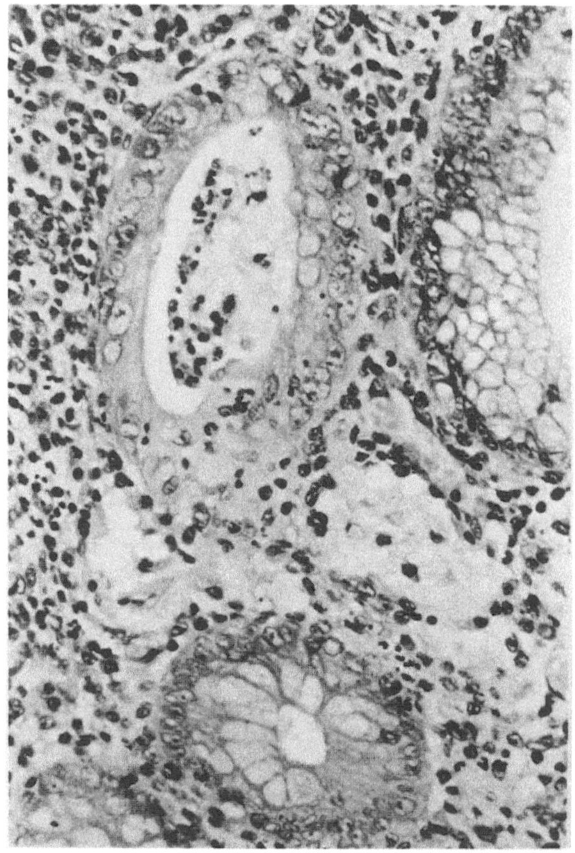

Fig. 21. Acute ulcerative colitis. The nuclei in the crypt abscess are enlarged, open and vesicular, some have prominent nucleoli and there is mucin depletion. Similar changes are apparent in the lower crypt. (H & E x 300)

It is slightly less surprising that children have such a high incidence of colitic carcinomas if they produce such exuberant reactive changes. These could be confused with the early phase of adenomatous type dysplasia and an early example of the latter with the variant showing open vesicular nuclei is shown in Figure 5. From this it is apparent that they have much in common and this is summarised in Table 2.

There is one other change where distinction from neoplastic dysplasia may be very difficult and that is the appearance which may be seen within 2 or 3 crypts of the edge of an ulcer and from which the ulcer base is being re-epithelialised. Because of the associated ulceration little attention is usually paid to it, but occasionally this change can be marked (Fig. 25). In the crypt selected differentiation from neoplasia would be very difficult if not impossible, yet there is little doubt that in this setting there is no indication that this is a premalignant lesion.

Table 2. Comparison of cytologic detail of regenerative dysplasia and neoplastic dysplasia

	Regenerative	Mild → Mod. Neoplastic	Severe Neoplastic
Cell size	↓ – ↑	↑ – ↑↑	↑ – ↑↑
N/C ratio	High	Low-Mod	High
Loss of polarity	+++	+ – +++	++ – +++
↑ nuclear size	+++	++	+++
Nuclear pleomorphism	++	+	++
No nuclei/unit area	↓ – sl ↑	↑↑	↑↑
Hyperchromatism of nuclei	↓ – sl ↑	↓ – ↑↑	↑ – ↑↑
Polychromatism of nuclei	±	+ – ++	+ – ++
Large eosinophic nucleoli	± – +++	+ – ++	+ – ++
Mitotic rate	0 – ±	± – ++	++ – +++
Mucin	0 – ±	+ – +++	0 – +
Inflammation	++ → +++	0 – ++	0 – ++
Adjacent crypts	variation ++	similar	similar

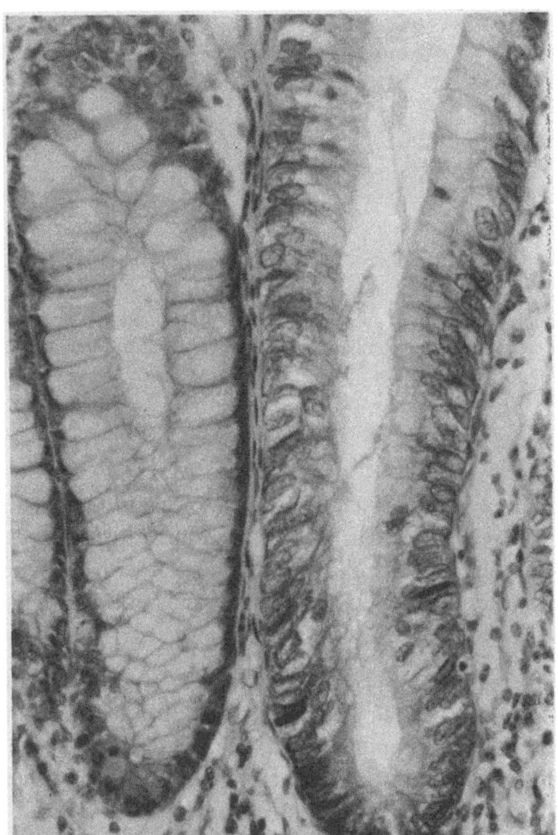

Fig. 22. (Legend see p. 205)

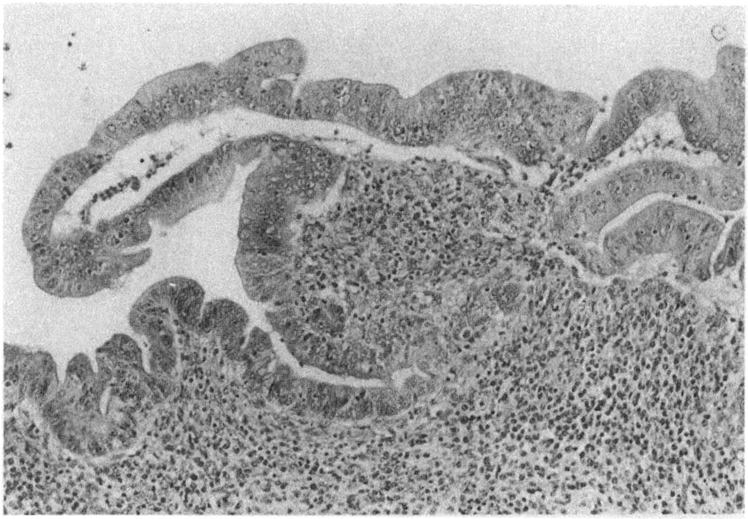

Fig. 23. Regenerative dysplasia from a 10 year old boy with a 3 week history of ulcerative colitis. At low power the nuclear disarray, homogenous cytpoplasm and lack of goblet cells is apparent. (H & E x 120)

2. Co-Existent Inflammation and Dysplasia

One of the great difficulties encountered by pathologists attempting to recognize the premalignant lesion as described by *Morson* and *Pang* (1967) is that inflammation can modify the appearances of the nuclei in the crypt, and there is uncertainty as to how much of this is genuine dysplasia and how much is the result of the inflammation. The recognition of changes associated with acute inflammation should reduce the number of difficult biopsies.

The interpretation of other biopsies may be facilitated when the following points are considered:

First, most pathologists will confidently diagnose an adenoma in the presence of severe inflammation and surface ulceration. These lesions are still very obviously either adenomas or possibly part of a carcinoma. It follows that a diagnosis of neoplasia can readily be made even in the presence of a heavy acute and chronic inflammatory infiltrate. The question then should not be whether a diagnosis of neoplasia can be made in the presence of inflammation, but rather how little dysplasia is required for a positive diagnosis of neoplasia when inflammation is present. Furthermore, in the absence of inflammation most pathologists will again be confident of making a diagnosis of dysplasia when only mild degrees of dysplasia are present.

Fig. 22. Epithelial hyperplasia. The crypt on the right shows the typical features of epithelial hyperplasia, the nuclei being enlarged and apparently increased in number, and this tends to occur predominantly in the base of the crypts. Here the hyperplasia is unusual in being focal, but this does allow comparison with an adjacent normal crypt. (H & E x 120)

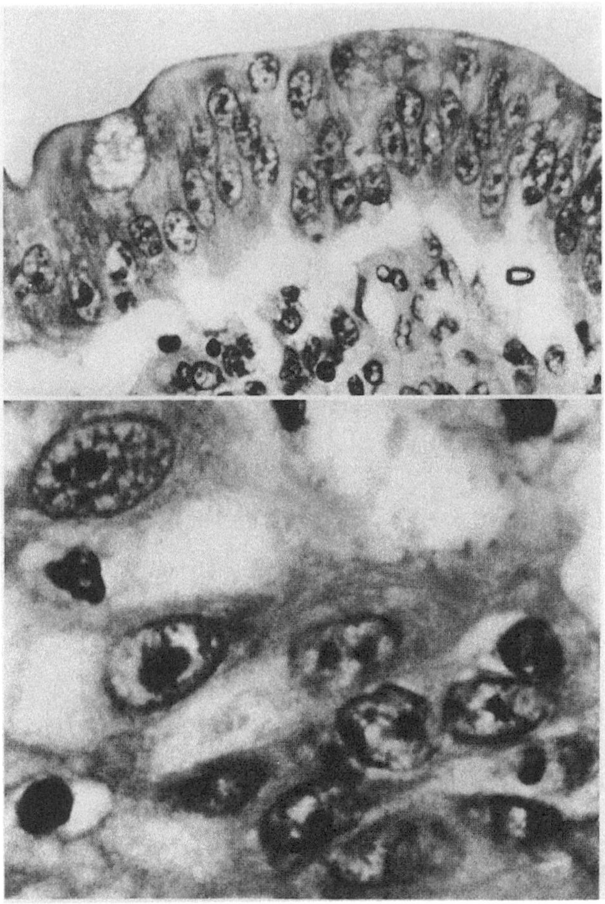

Fig. 24a. Higher power of regenerative epithelium. Note the enlarged, stratified, open vesicular nuclei with prominent nucleoli. (H & E x 480)

Fig. 24b. High power to show the nuclear features and the syncitial appearance of the cytoplasm (H & E x 1200)

Second, severe inflammation frequently occurs in ulcerative colitis with no evidence of dysplasia; indeed, dysplasia is the exception even during an exacerbation. This raises the question as to why there should be so much individual variation to inflammation and whether these merely represent different responses to inflammation or whether those patients that exhibit dysplasia in response to inflammation are the same patients that later are predisposed to develop carcinoma, although there is at present little evidence to support this concept.

Third, in some resected specimens for ulcerative colitis it appears that the dysplasia and the chronic inflammation are intimately related, for both cease abruptly at the same time. The question here is whether the inflammation produces the dysplasia or is a response to it. The latter is not unreasonable and is a well recognized pathological phenomenon, being

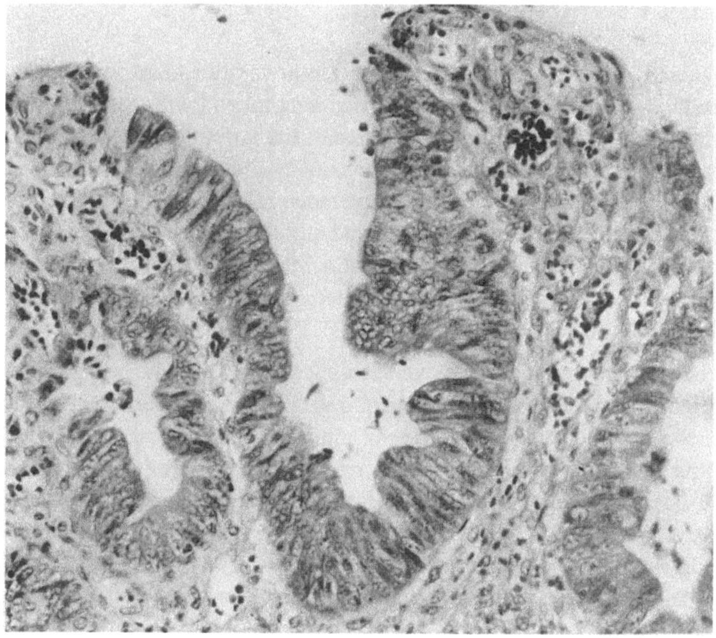

Fig. 25. Changes at the edge of a colostomy ulcer. The crypts are devoid of goblet cells and the nuclei are markedly stratified. (H & E x 100)

an integral feature of both Bowen's disease and lentigo maligna. In both of these lesions, it is always assumed that the chronic inflammatory infiltrate is a reaction to the neoplasia and not the reverse. It is, therefore, reasonable to extend this concept to the colon and postulate that a similar reaction may occur in a lamina propria as a reaction to dysplasia within the crypts. This is particularly applicable to those cases in which there is no evidence of acute inflammation and the inflammation present is crypt-sparing. Furthermore, the degree of chronic inflammation sometimes increases with the grade of dysplasia, and the fact that this is not reactive dysplasia is shown by dysplasia increasing until severe and a carcinoma developing in it. In control material studied, none of 11 patients with a history of less than 2 years had anything other than an inflammatory dysplasia while in 20 patients with a history of between 2 and 5 years, only 1 patient had a lesion categorized as genuine dysplasia. Although numbers here are small, this suggests that severe reactive changes may themselves be related to the length of history.

In conclusion, then, there are several reactions to inflammation that may be unusually exuberant and confused with neoplastic transformation, but there is little evidence that these are related to subsequent neoplasia and must be distinguished from it. However, there are occasions when true dysplasia and inflammation, particularly chronic inflammation, coexist without involving the crypts as occurs in the acute episode. It is suggested that this could be a host response to dysplasia rather than an epithelial response to the inflammation. This implies that if the inflammatory component is entirely mononuclear that it could be disregarded when dysplasia is being assessed.

VIII. The Reversibility of Dysplasia

It is generally held that one of the better methods of distinguishing inflammatory from neoplastic dysplasia is that the former is a reaction and will, therefore, regress when the stimulus producing it is withdrawn, whereas, the latter should be progressive. In ulcerative colitis, the resolution of the acute phase could be interpreted as a withdrawal of whatever initiated that exacerbation, but the persistence of exuberant epithelial hyperplasia, or the lack of its resolution, could be interpreted either as the persistence of the disease process or possibly early neoplastic transformation. Whatever its nature, this lesion is a problem only because of the uncertainty of its outcome, and dysplasia of this kind only requires careful follow-up.

The question of whether a true dysplasia ever resolves is a rather more difficult problem because of the lack of experience in following patients with rectal dysplasia in view of the high associated incidence of carcinoma and the possible focal nature of dysplasia so that a positive biopsy followed by a negative biopsy may not mean that the dysplasia has resolved, but that the second biopsy reflects a sampling error. To date, I have observed one patient who underwent total colectomy in 1971, and ileo-rectal anastomosis for ulcerative colitis in whom adenomatous dysplasia of villous type was present to the distal resection margin and a very early submucosal carcinoma was present in the transverse colon which infiltrated the submucosa only. The initial follow-up rectal biopsy revealed dysplasia, but numerous biopsies below the anastomosis line revealed decreasing grades of dysplasia and the last biopsies showed only minor changes which could at best have been interpreted as epithelial hyperplasia. Although the time interval is relatively short, this does suggest that dysplasia may occasionally be at least temporarily reversible.

IX. The Natural History of Dysplasia

It is desirable to know whether dysplasia inevitably progresses to invasive carcinoma. Ideally, this requires a control population of colitics with known dysplasia to be followed indefinitely. Only 3 patients, excluding that described in the previous section, have fallen into this category; one refusing operation in whom there was severe rectal dysplasia and two others in whom co-existent sclerosing cholangitis was sufficiently severe to preclude a prophylactic operation. To date, none are known to have developed carcinoma. However, a little more insight can be gained into this problem when patients with rectal dysplasia undergoing prophylactic proctocolectomy are considered. Earlier it was pointed out that this has been studied at several centers, and between them a total of 26 patients had proctocolectomies for rectal dysplasia, and of these, 15 had a carcinoma in the resection specimen which was usually an unsuspected finding. This suggests that dysplasia has at least a very high propensity to give rise to carcinoma.

X. The Frequency with which Colitic Cancers are Accompanied by Dysplasia

This remains a controversial topic, but there is evidence that a large proportion of colitic cancers are accompanied by dysplasia. *Hulten* et al. (1972) reviewed 25 colitics with cancer and found dysplasia in 22. In 12 of these the changes were in direct continuity with the carcinoma. The difficulty is that when tissue morphologically indistinguishable from an adenoma is found in a carcinoma, does this imply that the two merely co-exist, or that one preceded the other? *Morson* (1966) has shown that in non-colitic cancers the chance of finding an adenomatous component is inversely proportional to the degree of local spread, the incidence rising to 55% when only submucosal spread is present. In a series of 16 polyps excised colonoscopically which showed invasive carcinoma on the stalk on histological examination, 12 had evidence of such a component (*Williams* and *Riddell*, 1975). *Morson* (1973) has shown that when adenomas are excised the incidence of carcinoma is related closely to size and that almost 50% of polyps over 2 cm in diameter are accompanied by invasive carcinoma. These observations imply that as carcinomas grow, they tend to destroy evidence of their origin, assuming this to be an adenoma. As the presence of an adenomatous type of epithelium in carcinomas has been used as evidence of an origin in these lesions, it seems appropriate to use the same criteria when colitic cancers are considered.

In 80 carcinomas personally examined arising in ulcerative colitis treated by proctocolectomy, there was no evidence of a co-existing dysplastic lesion in 15 (19%). Many of these may have been due to destruction of any pre-existing lesion as occurs in non-colitic cancers; others may have been due to sampling error. The main difficulty in these patients is the possibility of the carcinoma arising independantly of the colitic process; 3 patients showed only the stigmata of longstanding ulcerative colitis, and no evidence of any other abnormality; 3 occurred in a patient with extensive basal cell type of dysplasia, but positive evidence of their having arisen from this mucosa was lacking. The remaining 9 showed a variety of minor degrees of dysplasia, a thickened mucosa and proliferation of tightly packed crypts, all of which suggested that there could well have been some relation to the carcinoma.

XI. "In-situ" Carcinoma in Ulcerative Colitis

This term is open to a variety of interpretations. It has been used synonymously with severe dysplasia, for a specific histological appearance such as a back to back arrangement of glands, and literally, as any lesion from which a carcinoma is directly arising can legitimately be called in-situ carcinoma irrespective of the grade of dysplasia present. In ulcerative colitis, as in non-colitic carcinomas, the likelihood of carcinoma increases with the severity of dysplasia, but some colitic cancers arise from mucosa showing surprisingly little dysplasia, although there is no real doubt that it is neoplastic mucosa. It is because carcinomas can occur in ulcerative colitis when relatively early neoplastic dysplasia is found that the presence of the latter on biopsy should lead to consideration of prophylactic surgery.

XII. The Relationship Between the Macroscopic Types of Dysplasia

It has been indicated above that in a resection specimen for carcinoma in colitis, a variety of microscopic forms of dysplasia may occur, but that the adenomatous type invariably produced carcinomas from a villous or polypoid macroscopic type, while the other major type of dysplasia (basal cell type) usually did so from a flat mucosa. The uncommon forms of dysplasia described were so few that no generalization could be made.

If the macroscopic (or low power) appearance of the dysplastic area actually giving rise to the carcinoma is considered, "flat" is very closely related to basal cell dysplasia, while "polypoid" and "villous" are closely related to adenomatous dysplasia. These are separated because the possible origin of the former from inflammatory polyps may indicate a different pathogenesis. Using these parameters, the different major types of premalignant change can be compared. A total of 99 carcinomas in 79 patients were available from a variety of sources (resection material, autopsy, referred patients, slides for opinion) in which it was possible to compare the types of dysplasia.

1. Relationship Between Macroscopic Type of Dysplasia and Multiple Carcinomas

The flat and villous type of mucosa have a similar propensity for producing multiple carcinomas (average 1.3/patient). In only 1/15 patients with a polypoid lesion were multiple carcinomas present.

2. Relationship of Type of Dysplasia to Histologic Type of Carcinoma

Almost half of the carcinomas produced by flat mucosa are of small cell undifferentiated or signet ring type while just over half of the carcinomas produced by villous mucosa are of colloid type. This can be further related to local spread.

3. Relationship of Type of Dysplasia to Local Spread

This is shown in Table 3. The potential for the flat dysplasia to produce carcinomas with extensive local spread is apparent. Conversely, the more polypoid lesions have a much greater proportion of cases where the carcinomas has not invaded through the muscularis propria (Dukes' A). The unexpectedly high proportion of Dukes' A cases is as difficult to explain as the apparent lack of patients with lymph node metastases.

Table 3. Relationship between type of dysplasia and local spread of carcinoma (Original Dukes' classification – C_1: highest lymph node uninvolved, C_2: highest lymph node involved.)

Dukes' classification:	A	B	C_1	C_2
Type of dysplasia				
Flat	13	14	10	2
Villous	18	21	5	0
Polypoid	10	2	4	0
Total	41	37	19	2

XIII. Relationship Between Length of History and the Precancer-Cancer Sequence

All evidence presented in this section is necessarily circumstantial and based on evidence from a large series of resections for ulcerative colitis and dysplasia both with and without carcinoma.

The length of history was well documented in 56 patients only and the average length of history from time of onset to the diagnosis of carcinoma in this group was 18.3 years. These 56 patients could be further subdivided into 10 who at the time of operation were considered to be inoperable (average length of history 22.5 years) and the remaining 46 with an average length of history of 17.7 years. The latter group could be further divided because in 6 patients the carcinoma was found unexpectedly in the resection specimen. The average length of history for this small group was 15.5 years, while that of the remaining 40 was 18.0 years.

In a further 36 patients in whom a diagnosis of definite neoplastic dysplasia had been made, but in whom no carcinoma could be found, the average length of history was 14.4 years. A possible chronological sequence in this group of patients is an average 14.4 years to reach neoplastic dysplasia, 15.5 years for early invasion to occur, 18.0 years for clinical detection and 22.5 years for an inoperable tumour to be present. From this it appears that the actual evolution of colitic carcinomas is surprisingly slow although it should be remembered that while most of the patients with occult carcinomas have early lesions that have not yet metastasised, many patients in the operable group will die of their tumour. This implies that the actual process of metastasising occurs over a relatively short period in the evolution of these tumours. The interval between dysplasia without carcinoma and dysplasia with carcinoma appears very short, and this may well correlate with the high incidence of unexpected carcinomas in those patients undergoing proctocolectomy because of dysplasia on biopsy.

An objection is that the vast majority of patients in the group with dysplasia only have severe dysplasia because the entire concept is relatively new and lesser grades of dysplasia will not result in proctocolectomy.

A further group of patients was, therefore, examined in whom early but definite neoplastic transformation was present on biopsy who had not undergone surgery (8 patients). These had a mean length of history of 13.1 years. This was compared with a further group of patients showing marked epithelial hyperplasia in whom a positive diagnosis of neoplastic transformation could not be made. The average length of history of this group was 12.1 years. Nevertheless, because of the relatively short time that regular rectal biopsies have become part of the routine management of longstanding colitis in the more specialised centres, coupled with the relative rarity of colitic cancers, only exceptionally is there an opportunity to observe the entire sequence of changes in a single patient. To date, only one patient has been observed to go trough the entire sequence from epithelial hyperplasia to an occult carcinoma. Until more data can be gathered to justify the existence of this spectrum of changes, it must remain largely speculative.

XIV. Misplaced Epithelium in Ulcerative Colitis

Misplaced epithelium is a well recognized feature of longstanding ulcerative colitis and may be seen as a localized form or as a more diffuse type when it is sometimes called generalized colitis cystica profunda. Characteristically, these form small mucin pools in the submucosa, are lined by normal epithelium, and these connect with the surface mucosa. Its pathogenesis is uncertain but probably arises as a result of deep submucosal ulceration when these are re-epithelialised. Occasionally this condition is misdiagnosed as carcinoma purely because of the presence of mucus cysts in the submucosa. In patients with a dysplastic mucosa, however, a more difficult situation is encountered because the overlying epithelium, being dysplastic, will re-epithelialize the same deep ulcers with dysplastic epithelium. The resulting colitis cystica profunda is then dysplastic and the distinction between an early invasive mucous secreting adenocarcinoma becomes very difficult (Figs. 26 and 27). In a personal study, 20 of the 55 patients with carcinoma undergoing total proctocolectomy had evidence of this condition.

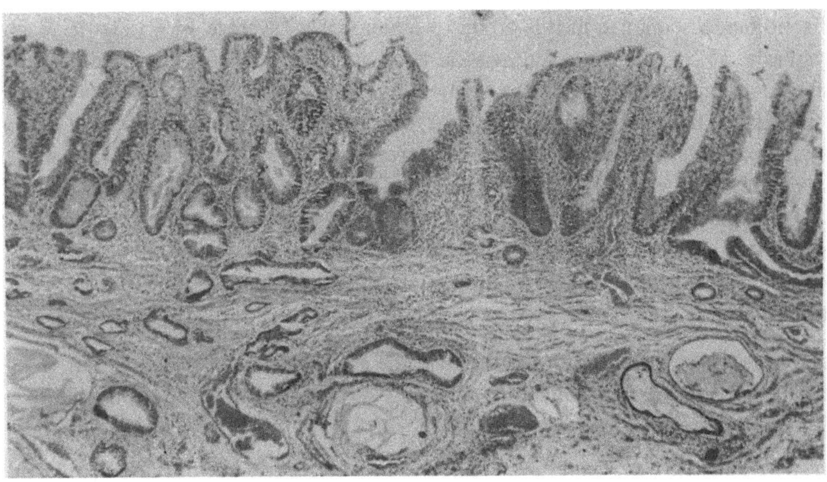

Fig. 26. Misplaced epithelium in longstanding ulcerative colitis. The distinction from early invasive adenocarcinoma when the glands are dysplastic can be difficult. (H & E x 48)

In 1945, *Dukes* drew attention to this as an important feature in the genesis of carcinoma in ulcerative colitis, while *Morson* and *Pang* (1967) concluded that it was sometimes impossible to decide whether the epithelium is just misplaced as a result of chronic inflammation or is really the early stage of invasive carcinoma. *Dyson* (1975) concluded that both misplaced epithelium and carcinoma were features of chronic ulcerative colitis but were otherwise unrelated. The major difficulties here are: a) whether misplaced glands by themselves are more prone to become carcinomatous and, b) whether it is possible to distinguish between an early well-differentiated carcinoma and misplaced glands lined by dysplastic mucosa because the overlying epithelium is also dysplastic which is the result of an episode of acute inflammation rather than true invasion.

In summary then there remains no easy way of distinguishing between dysplastic misplaced crypts in the submucosa and early invasive mucus secreting carcinoma. The lack of severe dysplasia in many of these lesions is no real criteria because many of the carcinomas arising in ulcerative colitis also frequently show surprisingly little dysplasia.

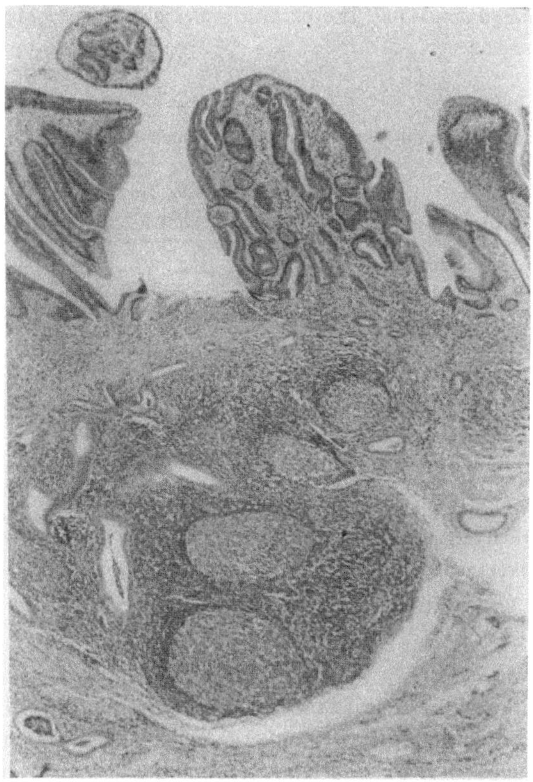

Fig. 27. Misplaced epithelium or early adenocarcinoma. The "misplaced" glands here are found in a submucosal lymphoid aggregate. (H & E x 30)

XV. The Extent of Dysplasia in the Rectum

This is important because if rectal biopsy is to be used to indicate which patients in the clinical high risk group are particularly prone to develop carcinoma, it is essential to know how often and to what extent the rectum becomes involved by dysplasia. To answer this question, a study was carried out on rectal mucosa from 41 patients with ulcerative colitis in whom proctocolectomy had been carried out for carcinoma. 26 of these had rectal and 15 had colon carcinoma. A further 22 patients had dysplasia in the large bowel but no carcinoma. These are perhaps the most important group of patients because if dysplasia in widespread and involves the rectum it is this group that should be detected and offered prophylactic surgery before carcinoma supervenes.

The slides of rectal mucosa were examined using an eyepiece micrometer so that the actual percentage of dysplasia could be estimated in each. In many patients, "swiss roll" sections had been taken allowing the examination of long strips of mucosa. The results are shown in Tables 4a and b. The major criticism of this approach is that the pathologist will obviously have selected his material from areas that look atypical. While this is valid, it is equally apparent that any clinician carrying out sigmoidoscopy would also biopsy an area that appeared abnormal. The pathologist might be in a better position to see any abnormality present.

Table 4a. Overall proportion of rectal mucosa affected by dysplasia and carcinoma

	No. of patients	Avg. No. slides	% Dysplasia	% Carcinoma
Rectal carcinoma	26	5.2	54	23
Colon carcinoma	15	2.2	69	0
Dysplasia only	22	3.1	59	0

Table 4b. Proportion of rectal mucosa affected by neoplastic transformation in 63 patients with dysplasia or carcinoma

	None	1-25%	26-50%	51-75%	76-99%	All	Total
Rectal carcinoma	0	4	7	9	4	2	26
Colon carcinoma	2	0	2	4	1	6	15
Dysplasia only	1	4	2	7	5	3	22

From this it is clear that while rectal dysplasia may involve the entire rectal mucosa, this is not usually the case, and even when a rectal carcinoma is present dysplasia in the residual mucosa may be focal or just around the tumour. It is also apparent that in those patients with a colon carcinoma or just dysplasia, there may be no evidence of rectal dysplasia in a small minority.

XVI. The Place of Biopsy in the Management of the High Risk Clinical Group

1. Rectal Biopsy

It has been stated above that approximately 40% of all colitic cancers occur in the rectum. Regular sigmoidoscopy should be able to detect virtually all of these at an early stage purely by observation. It is likely that if regular rectal biopsy is routinely added to this protocol then dysplasia could be detected in a pre-infiltrative stage. However, the purposes and limitation of rectal biopsy must be recognised, and in some instances further measures can be taken to minimise the disadvantages.

The objectives of rectal biopsy are, therefore:

1. To aid in the detection of the 40% of colitic cancers that will occur in the rectum.
2. To raise the index of suspicion of a proximal carcinoma or of proximal dysplasia by finding rectal dysplasia.

The limitation of rectal biopsy is basically that of the focal nature of rectal dysplasia. This is marginally less important in the case of rectal tumours as these should be detectable macroscopically at an early stage of their development even if a focal area of flat dysplasia remains undetected. However, it is rather more serious when rectal biopsy is used as an index of proximal carcinoma or dysplasia because a small focus of rectal dysplasia may be the only index of more severe proximal dysplasia or carcinoma and it is essential that every opportunity of detecting this is taken. In practice, this means that the sampling error must be reduced. This can be achieved by one of two methods:

1. Multiple biopsies can be taken at each sigmoidoscopy.
2. The biopsy sites can be deliberately varied.
3. A combination of these: both multiple biopsies and deliberate variation of the biopsy sites at subsequent visits.

Taking multiple biopsies will obviously reduce sampling error but the advantages to be gained from the accurate documentation of their sites of origin are several. If a suspicious or positive biopsy is obtained and the site of origin is known, it is easy to return to that precise area and take multiple biopsies at a subsequent visit. However, if all biopsies are negative, a further set of biopsies can be deliberately taken from sites other than those already biopsied and this will again reduce sampling error.

Using the technique of multiple rectal biopsies, it should be possible to detect all patients at risk from developing rectal cancer and, using Table 4b, approximately 87% (13/15) of patients with proximal carcinoma. This means that if all patients developing carcinoma in colitis are considered, multiple rectal biopsies could show evidence of dysplasia in 92%.

2. The Management of a Positive Rectal Biopsy

The detection of dysplasia on rectal biopsy should lead to serious consideration of proctocolectomy, but before a definite decision is made it is worth considering several other points. It should be remembered that the object of prophylactic surgery is to prolong the expected life span for the patient; this cannot be justified if in the short term the patient is likely to succumb to the operation itself or from a coexisting condition. If the health of the patient is good it can be difficult to justify proctocolectomy to the patient, particularly if symptomless, on the grounds of a single biopsy. For this reason it may be valuable to repeat the rectal biopsies, particularly if the site of the positive biopsy is known, because further more severe dysplasia may be encountered. Second, colonoscopy with multiple biopsies should be considered, for the patient may be one of the small group whose most marked dysplasia is proximal to the rectum. Furthermore, a small unsuspected carcinoma may be found and colonoscopy may, therefore, be useful in this respect.

If all of these investigations prove negative, management can be more difficult; however, as a working principle once a patient with ulcerative colitis has demonstrated the potential to produce a neoplastic lesion, that patient must be at increased risk from developing a carcinoma and should, therefore, be considered for proctocolectomy, On occasions, this is made even more difficult by the patient developing an adenoma. Theoretically, this could be treated solely by local excision. Provided there is no other evidence of dysplasia, local excision should be curative and the patient returns to his former dysplasia-free status. This problem is magnified if it occurs in a slightly older individual in the 5th or 6th decade, because it could always be argued that the adenoma might have arisen independantly of the colitis. Under these circumstances, it is feasible to treat the adenoma by local lesion, but the fact that the patient has produced an adenoma increases the risk that further neoplastic lesions will develop.

Sometimes dysplasia may be limited to one section of large bowel, for example, just the rectum, or just part of the colon. Under these circumstances, the temptation to limit resection to the affected bowel should be resisted. Patients undergoing local resection for carcinoma in ulcerative colitis are very likely to already have, or to develop, a further carcinoma in the residual colon (*Hulton* et al., 1971).

XVII. The Place of Colonoscopy

Table 4b shows that a small minority of patients in the high risk clinical group will develop proximal dysplasia and carcinoma in the absence of rectal dysplasia. Colonoscopy is at present the only method that is capable of visualising the whole colon and taking biopsies from all parts. It also has other advantages worthy of mention, and the place of colonoscopy in the management of a positive rectal biopsy has been discussed. It has a more subtle value in that some patients exhibit more severe dysplasia in the colon than the rectum. In this group of patients, colonoscopy and multiple biopsies are valuable in detecting the proximal dysplasia at an earlier stage than if rectal biopsy alone was used as an index of proximal malignancy. A further use for colonoscopy is in the actual definition of the high risk clinical group, or more precisely the accuracy of the extent of disease. There is no difficulty in patients in whom the disease is total radiologically, or in those in whom the upper limit of disease can be seen clearly sigmoidoscopically. However, in the intermediate group there will be some patients with left-sided disease radiologically who on colonoscopy or with multiple biopsies will be shown to have total colitis, and these patients should almost certainly be included in the high risk clinical group.

Finally, colonoscopy can be of value in patients in whom a stricture is present radiologically which is not causing symptoms. Multiple biopsies with or without cytology, especially if these can be obtained from within the stricture, can be of great value. If these show only the changes of longstanding colitis without dysplasia, it is reasonable to assume that the stricture is fibromuscular and not neoplastic, and in the absence of symptoms does not require further treatment. Positive biopsies or cytology, should lead to consideration for proctocolectomy.

Conclusion

An attempt has been made to put in perspective the reasons why clinicians have such difficulty in managing patients with ulcerative colitis who statistically are at greatest risk of developing carcinoma. The concept of a premalignant phase has been presented and its macroscopic and microscopic features discussed, together with the special relationship between inflammation and dysplasia. The value of using these criteria on both rectal and colonoscopic biopsies are described along with their limitations and methods to reduce these to a minimum.

The great difficulty that the practicing pathologist will experience is the relative rarity with which these changes will be encountered in biopsies in view of the relative rarity of colitic cancers at any single institution. However, there are several methods that the pathologist can use to familiarise himself with these changes:

First, he can familiarise himself with the changes described by examining material in his files from patients with carcinoma complicating ulcerative colitis, and should he receive such a specimen by paying particular attention to the mucosa as well as the tumour. Most of these specimens contain a vast range of changes, and it is only by making the best use of these that the more subtle changes will become apparent.

Second, the pathologist must remain familiar with the wide spectrum of features that are seen in ulcerative colitis. To this end the clinician can again be of value by providing regular biopsies from his colitic patients. It is virtually impossible for a pathologist to diagnose dysplasia unless absolutely obvious if he receives only a few rectal biopsies annually. Finally, the importance of having a slide containing well-oriented mucosa cannot be overemphasised. This is easily accomplished with rectal biopsies by treating them in a similar fashion to jejunal biopsies.

Acknowledgments: I wish to offer sincere thanks to Dr. *Basil C. Morson* for firing my initial interest into this fascinating problem and for his reliable assistance, advice and encouragement in this work, which was carried out at St. Mark's Hospital, London, also to the physicians and surgeons at that hospital, particularly Dr. *J.E. Lennard-Jones* and Mr. *P.R. Hawley* for their advice, support and interest, and Dr. *Jean Ritchie* for allowing me access to her files. I am grateful to Mr. *Lloyd Soodeen* and Mr. *Kenneth Glass* for their technical assistance, and to Mr. *Norman Mackie* at St. Mark's Hospital, *Larry Eisenstat* and *Craig Rosner* at The University of Chicago for their photographs, and Ms. *Betsy Hunt* for her secretarial assistance.

References

American Cancer Society (1974), '75 Cancer Facts and Figures

Bargen, J.A.: Complications and sequelae of chronic ulcerative colitis. Ann. Int. Med. 3, 335 (1929).

Counsell, P.B., Dukes, C.E.: The association of chronic ulcerative colitis and carcinoma of rectum and colon. Brit. J. Surg. 39, 485 (1952).

Crohn, B.B., Rosenburg, H.: The sigmoidoscopic picture of chronic ulcerative colitis (non-specific). Amer. J. med. Sci. 170, 220 (1925).

Dawson, I.M.P., Pryse-Davies, J.: The development of carcinoma of the large intestine in ulcerative colitis. Brit. J. Surg. 47, 113-128 (1959).

de Dombal, F.T. et al.: Local complications of ulcerative colitis-structure, pseudo-polyposis and carcinoma colon and rectum. Brit. med. J. 1966 I, 1442.

Devrode, G.J. et al.: Cancer risk and life expectancy of children with ulcerative colitis. New Engl. J. Med. Vol. 285, No. 1, 17-21 (1973).
Dilawari, J.B. et al.: Colonoscopy in the investigation of ulcerative colitis. Gut 14, 426 (1973).
Dilawari, J.B., Lennard-Jones, J.E., Mackay, A.M., Ritchie, J.K., Sturzaker, H.G.: CEA estimation in ulcerative colitis with and without malignancy. Gut 15, 828 (1974).
Dukes, C.E.: Surgical pathology of ulcerative colitis. Ann. roy. Coll. Surg. Engl. 14, 389-400 (1954).
Edwards, F.C., Truelove, S.C.: The course and prognosis of ulcerative colitis. Part IV. Gut 5, 15-22 (1964).
Evans, D.J., Pollock, D.J.: In-situ and invasive carcinoma of the colon in patients with ulcerative colitis. Gut 13, 566-570 (1972).
Felsen, J., Wolarsky, W.: Chronic ulcerative colitis and carcinoma. Arch. Int. Med. 19, 275 (1952).
Fenoglio, C.M., Pascal, R.R.: Adenomatous epithelium, intraepithelial anaplasia and invasive carcinoma in ulcerative colitis. Amer. J. dig. Dis. 18, 556 (1973).
Goldgraber, M.B., Kirsner, J.B.: Carcinoma of the colon in ulcerative colitis. Cancer 17, 657 (1964).
Goligher, J.C. et al.: Ulcerative colitis, Ch. 9. London: Balliere, Tindall, and Cassell 1968.
Hardy, T.L., Brooke, B.N., Hawkins, C.F.: Ileostomy and ulcerative colitis. Lancet 1949 II, 5.
Hinton, J.M.: Carcinoma in ulcerative colitis. Proc. roy. Soc. Med. 59, 632 (1966) and Gut 7, 433 (1966).
Hultén, L., Kewenter, J., Ahrén, C.: Precancer and carcinoma in chronic ulcerative colitis. A histopathological and clinical investigation. Scand. J. Gastroent. 7, 663-669 (1972).
Hulten, L., Kewenter, J., Koch, W.G.: The long term results of partial resection of the large bowel for intestinal carcinoma complicating ulcerative colitis. Scand. J. Gastroent. 6, 601-604 (1971).
Jackman, R.J., Barge, J.A., Helmholtz, H.F.: Life histories of 95 children with cronic ulcerative colitis. Amer. J. Dis. Child. 59, 459 (1940).
Klein, H.Z.: Mucinous carcinoid tumor of the vermiform appendix. Cancer 33, 770-777 (1974).
Lennard-Jones, J.E. et al.: Prospective study of outpatients with extensive colitis. Lancet 1974 I, 1065-1067.
Mac Dougall, I.P.M.: The cancer risk in ulcerative colitis. Lancet 1964 II, 655.
Morson, B.C.: The polyp-cancer sequence. Proc. roy. Soc. Med. 67, 451-457 (1974).
Morson, B.C., Dawson, I.M.P.: Gastrointestinal Pathology, London: Blackwell 1972.
Morson, B.C., Pang, L.S.C.: Rectal biopsy as an aid to cancer control in ulcerative colitis. Gut 8, 423-434 (1967).
Mottet, N.K.: Histopathologic spectrum of regional enteritis and ulcerative colits: Major problems in pathology, Vol. II. Toronto: W.B. Saunders 1971.
Myrvold, H.E., Kock, N.G., Ahrén, C.: Rectal biopsy and precancer in ulcerative colitis. Gut 15, 301-304 (1974).
Otani, S., Snapper, I.: On the incidence of carcinoma in chronic ulcerative colitis. J. Mt Sinai Hosp. 19, 275 (1952).
Rosenqvist, H. et al.: Ulcerative colitis and carcinoma coli. Lancet 1955 I, 906.
Svartz, N., Ernberg, T.: Cancer coli in cases of colitis ulcerosa. Acta Med. scand. 135, 444 (1949).
Swinton, N.W., Warren, S.: Polyps of colon and rectum and their relation to malignancy. J.A.M.A. 113, 1927 (1939).

Subbuswamy, S.G. et al.: Goblet cell carcinoid of the appendix. Cancer 34, 338-344 (1974).
Warren, S., Sommers, S.C.: Pathogenesis of ulcerative colitis. Amer. J. Path. 25, 657 (1949).
Williams, C.B., Riddell, R.H.: Chapter – Colonoscopic polypectomy – Topics in Gastrointestinal Fibre-endoscopy (eds. *K.F.R. Schiller, P.R. Salmon*). Heinemann (in press).
Yardley, J.H., Keren, D.F.: "Precancer" lesions in ulcerative colits, a retrospective study of rectal biopsy and colectomy specimens. Cancer (Philad.) 34, 835-8-4 (1974).
Yeaomans, F.C.: Carcinomatous degeneration of rectal adenoma. J.A.M.A. 89, 852-854 (1927).

The Endocrine Cells of the Gastro-Intestinal Tract and the Neoplasms which Arise from Them

I.M.P. DAWSON

PART 1 THE NORMAL CELLS

PART 2 TUMOURS AND HYPERPLASIAS OF ENDOCRINE CELLS

PART 1 THE NORMAL CELLS

I. Introduction

No-one, even as recently as 15 years ago, would have thought of the gut as the major endocrine organ which we now recognise it to be. The discovery and identification of a number of individual endocrine cell types each apparently secreting its own specific hormone, has been one of the most exciting aspects of gastro-intestinal pathology in the last decade. In this review I propose briefly to describe the historical development of the endocrine cell concept of the human gut, to discuss in more detail the techniques available for the recognition of normal endocrine cells in gut and pancreas and finally to relate these and other techniques and findings to our knowledge of the tumours which arise from them. The literature is now vast, and I propose to cite principally key papers of cardinal importance or adequate recent reviews wherein a more exhaustive literature can be found. The subject is advancing daily and it is likely that some statements made here will be superseded by the date of publication.

II. Historical Review

The recognition of individual mucosal cells in the small intestine and appendix which differed from absorptive cells (enterocytes), goblet and Paneth cells is usually attributed to Kultschitsky. These cells possess predominantly infranuclear acidophilic cytoplasmic granules about 300 mu in diameter, difficult to see in conventionally stained material and are still often eponymously referred to as Kultschitsky cells (see a good review by *Clara*, 1957). *Masson* (1914) recognised them as an endocrine type of cell and described in them a property, which has caused much confusion since, namely that after formaldehyde fixation many cells contained granules which would reduce neutral or alkaline silver solutions to metallic silver, a reaction which is usually called argentaffin. Argentaffin granules are also coloured brown by dichromate-formol mixtures and the cells have been alternatively called enterochromaffin. Chemical and early histochemical studies, combined with biochemical studies made to identify the reducing substance eventually determined it as 5-hydroxytryptamine (serotonin, enteramine) (*Erspamer* and *Asero*, 1952) which combines with formaldehyde to give a β-carboline (*Barter* and *Pearse,* 1955) which is actively reducing, fluorescent, will also couple with diazotates to produce coloured azo dyes (*Lillie*, 1961a, b, c) and, of course, take part in other reducing reactions such as Schmorl's ferric ferricyanide reaction. It was, perhaps, unfortunate that this particular cell within the endocrine family which secretes primarily an amine rather than a polypeptide hormone was the first to be discovered, since it concentrated investigation on the amine rather than the possible polypeptide nature of the granule component in endocrine cells.

Other studies using silver solutions with added reducing agents (so called argyrophil reactions) showed that a larger family of histologically similar cells contained granules which were argyrophil but not argentaffin and that the distribution of both types of cell was wider than had been first thought, extending from the stomach to the anus. The unsatisfactory terminology of silver staining reactions – argentaffin, argyrophil and ever argentophil – and the need for standardisation of silver techniques was not generally appreciated, and the hypothesis that argyrophil cells were precursors of argentaffin cells rather than being secretory cells in their own right was generally accepted. (See a comprehensive review of the earlier histochemical studies by *Dawson*, 1970). The stage was thus set for a cataclysm of new observations and research.

Paradoxically, the recognition of a family of endocrine cells in the normal gut other than those which contain 5HT began by their recognition in foregut derivatives not directly part of the alimentary tract, namely the bronchi, thyroid and pancreas. In the thyroid, cells containing argyrophil granules first described by *Nonides* (1931-2) – in the dog – were firmly linked with calcitonin secretion and labeled "C" cells (*Foster* et al., 1964; *Pearse*, 1966, 1968). In the pancreatic islets histologically similar cells were found to contain granules of at least three different types (*Brolin* et al., 1964; *Epple*, 1967; *Like* and *Orci*, 1972), separable on histochemical, ultrastructural and immunological grounds (Table 1). There has been little difficulty in linking A2 (α2 cells) with glucagon and B cells with insulin secretion, but the identification of A1 (α1), alternatively called D cells

Table 1. Histochemical features of normal endocrine cells

		5HT		Argyrophila					Metachromasia			Others							
Cell Type	Secretion	Argentaffin	Diazo	General	D + H.H.	Grimelius	Sevier Munger	Bodian	General	Tol. Blue	Acid hydrol	Lead H	PTAH	Chromalum H	Xanthydrol	Rosindole	DMAB nitrite	Pseudoisocyanin	Aldehyde fuchsin
Pancreas																			
A_2	Glucagon	–	–	?	–	+	+	+	±	±	+	+	+	+	+	+	+	–	–
B	Insulin	–	–	–	–	–	—	–	–	–	–	–	–	–	–	–	–	+	+
$D(A_1)$	? Gastrin ? Secretin	–	–	+	+	+	+	+	+	+	+	+	+	+	±	±	+	–	–
GI Tract																			
EC	5HT	+	+	+	+	+	+	+	+	+	+	+	0	0	0	0	0	0	0
EG	Entero-glucagon	–	–	+	+	+	+	+	±	±	+	+	0	0	0	0	0	0	0
G	Gastrin	–	–	? ±	? ±	? ±	0	–	–	–	±	+	0	0	±	0	0	0	0
S	Secretin	–	–	±	0	±	0	0	0	0	0	+	+	0	0	0	0	0	0
VIP	VIP	–	–	±	0	0	0	0	0	0	0	±	0	0	0	0	±	0	0
GIP	GIP	–	–	±	0	+	0	0	0	0	0	+	0	0	0	0	0	0	0

Notes: This table is compiled from a number of authors, all of whom are quoted in the text. Many have used different fixatives which tends to render at least some of the argyrophil techniques potentially non-comparable. The columns "general" are used to include papers where techniques are not precisely stated.

Key to Table: + = Positive staining; ± = Doubtful or faint staining; – = No staining; 0 = No reliable observations available; ? = Disagreement between workers as to whether staining is present or not.

with gastrin secretion is, though probable, less absolute. Concurrently a large number of histochemical, fluorescent, immunologic and ultramicroscopic techniques were developed for identifying and separating granules in apparently similar cells (see *Dawson*, 1970), and these were applied to the gastro-intestinal tract and bronchial epithelium as well as to pancreas and other endocrine organs. The concept now became one not of a single cell with a precursor which produced a single substance, 5HT, but of a family of histologically similar cells containing secretory granules within their cytoplasm capable of secreting a wide range of substances, each probably normally specific for a single cell. *Pearse* (1968, 1969) crystallised this concept by coining the term APUD (Amine Precursor Uptake and Decarboxylation) for the family, believing that all had the ability to synthesise or store biogenic amines, but the term has proved unsuitable since many of the cells cannot be shown to decarboxylate a demonstrable amine precursor while all but one, and possibly all secrete short chain polypeptide hormones; the more non-committal term "endocrine cell" is therefore preferable.

III. The Origin and Structure of Endocrine Cells

It is to be expected that cells within a common family will have a common ancestor, probably the neuroepithelial cell as suggested by *Pearse* (1969) and *Weichert* (1970). Working on mouse tissue injected with L-dopa and formaldehyde vapour fixed, *Pearse* and *Polak* (1971) also suggested that endocrine cells migrate from the neural crest, and later studies (*Gammill* and *Weichert*, 1973), have supported this suggestion, though it cannot be regarded yet as completely proven; it would certainly explain the widespread distribution of endocrine cells and the potential dual functions of polypeptide hormone secretion and amine precursor decarboxylation which are not otherwise obviously related to one another, and it would be practicable to postulate that multiglandular endocrine syndromes arose as a primary disturbance of neural ectoderm. There is a good recent review of the concept by *Bolande* (1974).

All cells within the family are broadly similar histologically. They tend to be triangular or pear shaped with their broad base lying on the basement membrane and their granules predominantly though not exclusively infranuclear. The apex of many reaches the lumen of gastric or intestinal glands and pancreas and is covered by modified microvilli. Ultrastructurally, with the exception of 5HT containing cells there is a conspicuous rough endoplasmic reticulum and Golgi apparatus presumably linked with the synthesis and packaging of the secretion product (*Toner*, 1964; *Forssmann* et al., 1969). Free ribosomes and mitochondria are numerous, and probably most if not all contain decarboxylases (*Aures* and *Håkanson*, 1968; *Pearse*, 1968) and non-specific and E-600 resistant esterases (*Carvalheira* et al., 1968). Individual cells have storage granules surrounded by a lipoprotein envelope and these vary in size, shape, electron density and the presence or absence of a "halo" between the core and the bounding membrane according to the product stored within them. There is evidence that large precursor molecules are synthesised in rough endoplasmic reticulum and transported to the Golgi apparatus where they are converted into smaller molecules and become enclosed within envelopes, prior to transport to the cell surface for release (*Lacy*, 1972; *Hammar* and *Sale*, 1975). This pattern of synthesis and packaging may explain the presence of large molecules such as "big" or "big-big" gastrin in certain gastrinomas in addition to the normal trideca- and heptadecapeptide forms.

5HT secreting cells have rather poorly developed rough endoplasmic reticulum and Golgi apparatus and are less rich in esterases; they are recognised by their amine content which, when reacted with aldehyde produces a reducing substance, which is also fluorescent; it is possible to recognise the presence of different biological amines, including histamine, adrenalin and nor-adrenalin by the use of freeze drying-vapour fixation techniques with different aldehyde or acid vapours and the subsequent measurement of fluorescent emission spectra (*Corrodi* and *Jonsson*, 1967; *Håkanson* et al., 1970; *Ewen* and *Rost*, 1972). They probably also secrete a polypeptide hormone of kinin type but this has not as yet been positively identified.

IV. The Polypeptide Hormones Present in Gastro-Intestinal Tract and Pancreas and their Distribution

The following hormones have now been identified in granules of endocrine cells in the gastro-intestinal tract; gastrin, enteroglucagon, secretin, motilin, vasoactive intestinal peptide (VIP), cholecystokinin-pancreozymin (CCK-PZ), gastro-inhibitory peptide (GIP) and possibly a growth hormone release-inhibiting factor. In the granules of islet cells in the pancreas insulin, pancreatic glucagon, probably gastrin and possibly secretin are also found. 5HT is present throughout the gastro-intestinal tract and probably also in pancreatic ducts. Brief details of the more recently identified hormones are appended; there is a good recent review by *Grossman* et al. (1974).

Gastrin exists in a number of forms, usually referred to by the number of amino acids in the polypeptide chain prefixed by the letter G. The classical form, G17 ("little" gastrin) was described in detail by *Gregory* et al. (1964) and synthesised by *Anderson* et al. (1964). Other forms are G34 ("big" gastrin), which contains the complete amino acid sequence of G17 gastrin linked to a sequence of 17 amino acids through the carboxyl of a basic amino acid, and a still larger "big big" gastrin, with an as yet undetermined number of amino acids in its sequence (*Yalow* and *Berson*, 1972; *Yalow* and *Wu*, 1973). There are also units smaller than G17 (*Rehfeld*, 1972; *Gregory* and *Tracy*, 1974) which appear to be G13 "little little" or minigastrins and to correspond to the 5-17 amino acid component of G17. Gastrin secreting cells are found in the midzone of the antral region of the stomach and in the crypts and basal glands of the duodenum and upper jejunum in decreasing numbers. The two normally secreted components are G17 and G34. G17 forms about 80% of the antral gastrin, about 50% of the duodenal gastrin and little of any jejunal gastrin formed, whereas G34 forms less than 20% of antral gastrin, about 50% of duodenal gastrin and probably nearly all of the jejunal gastrin (*Bloom*, 1974; *Berson* and *Yalow*, 1971). The larger and mini forms have been found in association with gastrinomas in the Zollinger-Ellison syndrome. G34 is approximately equally potent mole for mole with G17, but has a longer half life in the circulation and a longer duration of action (*Walsh* and *Grossman*, 1973). There seems fairly reliable evidence (*McGuigan*, 1973) that as one descends the gastro-intestinal tract from stomach through duodenum to upper jejunum there is a switchover from "little" to "big" gastrin secretion. Gastrin stimulates the secretion of hydrochloric acid and raised levels are found after meals, in old age, in patients with atrophic gastritis or pernicious anaemia

(*Polak* et al., 1971a), after vagotomy and in the Zollinger-Ellison syndrome. Some authors claim that gastritis affecting the antral region may reduce the functional G cell mass (*Kormann, Strickland* and *Hansky*, 1972).

Enteroglucagon shows immunological cross reactivity with pancreatic glucagon but has differing hormonal properties; it is found in dogs in the middle and deeper gland zones of the jejunum and ileum and in the fundus of the stomach (*Polak* et al., 1971b) and its release is stimulated by glucose or long chain triglycerides (*Unger* et al., 1968; *Bottger, Faloona* and *Unger*, 1972); its action seems to be to reduce bowel motility, perhaps to allow greater time for digestion (*Bloom*, 1972; *Gleeson* et al., 1971). There appear to be at least two forms of the hormone of differing molecular weight (*Valverde* et al., 1968) but its amino acid sequence is not yet known. *Makhlouf* (1974) doubts if it exists separately and links it with GIP and perhaps VIP, considering that it has a structure which can react with pancreatic glucagon antisera. There is a good recent review by *Whalen* (1974).

Secretin: The structure of secretin which has 27 amino acid residues has been known since 1961 (*Jorpes and Mutt*, 1961) and it was synthesised in 1964 (*Bodansky, Ondetti* and *Levine*, 1966). Its amino acid sequence bears a close similarity to that of pancreatic glucagon, enteroglucagon, gastroinhibitory polypeptide and vasoactive intestinal peptide (*Bodansky, Klausner* and *Said*, 1973), which is borne out by some overlap in their respective functions, though apart from pancreatic glucagon and enteroglucagon they are immunologically distinct, and suggests a cell of common ancestry (*Hubel*, 1972; *Bloom*, 1974). Secretin is formed in cells at bases of villi and in upper crypt of the duodenum and jejunum (*Polak* et al., 1971c; *Bussolati* et al., 1971) and is secreted in response to the introduction of acid gastric juice into the upper small intestine; it inhibits the secretion of gastrin, stimulates pyloric muscle, stimulates pancreatic and biliary electrolyte secretion and augments CCK-PZ activity; it may also stimulate pancreatic insulin release. It is thought by some to be the hormone responsible for the watery diarrhoea (pancreatic cholera, Verner Morrison) syndrome.

Motilin is probably secreted by cells in the duodenum and jejunum in response to an alkaline intestinal secretion and produces gastric contraction (*Brown*, 1967). Its amino acid sequence (22 residues) is now determined (*Brown, Cook* and *Dryburgh*, 1972) and is of interest in that it does not resemble that of other gastro-intestinal polypeptide hormones.

Vasoactive Intestinal Peptide (VIP): This polypeptide hormone was first discovered in 1970 (*Said* and *Mutt*, 1970a), purfied and its amino acid sequence established (*Said* and *Mutt*, 1970b). It has 28 residues and bears a close resemblance to glucagon and secretin (*Bodansky* et al., 1973), and besides dilating small intestinal arterioles it raises blood glucose and stimulates the exocrine pancreas to produce an alkaline juice. It may be the agent responsible for the pancreatic cholera syndrome. It is located in the fundus of the stomach and in the intestinal tract (*Polak* et al., 1974).

Cholecystokinin Pancreozymin (CCK-PZ): Colecystokinin pancreozymin has been recognised for many years but its complete amino acid sequence which is linear and has 33 residues is still undetermined; however, its C terminal octapeptide has been synthesised (*Rubin* et al., 1969) and appears to be as active biologically as the complete hormone. It produces gall bladder contraction.

Gastric Inhibitory Polypeptide (GIP): This hormone was first discovered as an "impurity" in cholecystokinin – pancreozymin preparation (*Brown* and *Pederson*, 1970) and its amino acid sequence was described in the following year (*Brown* and *Dryburgh*, 1971). It has 43 residues and has close similarities to glucagon, secretin and VIP. It is located in the middle zone of the glands of the duodenum and jejunum (*Polak* et al., 1973). It inhibits gastric acid and pepsin secretion and also stimulates insulin release (*Dupré* et al., 1973).

Growth-hormone release-inhibiting factor: This has recently been described as a hormone inhibiting membrane release of secretory granules (*Polak* et al., 1975) and is thought to be located in pancreatic D cells and in the D cells found in the midzone of gastric and in intestinal glands; however the authors do not describe how the antiserum which they used to identify it was produced and the identification of this factor must await further confirmation.

V. The Identification of Granular Contents

Endocrine cells can be separated from other intestinal mucosal cells by any technique which will delineate granules as such; individual endocrine cells can be classified only by techniques which distinguish between granules on a structural or functional basis (*Dawson*, 1970; *Pearse* et al., 1970). All granules have an enclosing lipoprotein envelope within which is the granule secretion which may be biological amine, short chain polypeptide hormone or both, with various enzymes necessary for amine or peptide synthesis or release. The following technical groups are therefore likely to be of value and will be briefly discussed in turn.

1. Techniques specific for biological amines or their precursors.
2. Techniques for short chain polypeptide hormones
   a) Specific immunological techniques using antisera raised against purified (usually synthetic) hormonal antigens.
   b) Semi-specific histochemical techniques which usually depend on detecting carboxyl or other iosinable side chain or terminal reacting groups. These may be common to a number of polypeptides but may also be a component feature of the lipoprotein envelope.
   c) Silver techniques: how, or with what, silver salts react is uncertain but variations in fixation and technique will delineate different granules. The subject is confusing but merits further study.
3. Electron microscopic studies of granule size, shape, appearance and electron density. Granules differ considerably in these features at ultrastructural level and carefully standardised techniques allow some granule separation.
4. Combination of these, especially immunocytochemical and cytohistochemical techniques.

1. Techniques for Biological Amines or their Precursors

Those endocrine cells in the gut whose granules contain 5HT synthesise it by decarboxylating a precursor, 5-hydroxy tryptophan (5HTP). A useful screening test for granules potentially containing biological amines might therefore be to demonstrate the presence of a decarboxylase. This cannot yet be done histochemically but biochemical investigations suggest a specific L-histidine decarboxylase in some gastric endocrine cells and a less specific L-amino acid decarboxylase, active on L-Dopa, 5HTP and L-histidine, in the small intestinal cells (*Aures* and *Håkanson*, 1968, see also the review by *Dawson*, 1970). Specific techniques for amines depend on condensing the amine with specified aldehydes or acids. This produces a series of compounds, different for each biological amine-aldehyde/acid condensate, which have the property of absorbing ultraviolet or blue violet light and emitting light at particular longer wave lengths. The combination of 5HT with aldehydes is also reducing, and forms the basis of the argentaffin and Schmorl reactions: the reducing compound also couples with diazonium compounds to produce insoluble coloured azo dyes. Under usual working conditions the only compound identified is the condensate of formaldehyde with 5HT, since other biological amines such as histamine, adrenalin, nor-adrenalin and dopamine diffuse rapidly in aqueous fixatives and are lost. For their detection freeze drying of absolutely fresh tissue is necessary, followed by vapour fixation in the appropriate aldehyde or acid, paraffin embedding and dry section mounting and the subsequent use of spectrofluorimetry. There appears to be a considerable future for this type of technique and *Ewen* and *Rost* (1972) have provided tables of results to be expected. Particularly hopeful is the use of O-phthaldialdehyde for the detection of histamine and there are special techniques including incubation of blocks in amine precursor solutions to demonstrate those cells which have decarboxylating potential but do not appear to store the amine in detectable amounts. Further details can be found in the papers of *Falck* (1962), *Falck, Hillarp, Thieme* and *Torp* (1962), *Corrodi* and *Jonsson* (1967), *Bjorklund* and *Falck* (1968), *Håkanson* et al. (1970), *Dawson* (1970). Although there is some evidence that some cells may also secrete histamine, there is so far little practical evidence to support the theoretical concept of Pearse that each cell within the family secretes both amine and polypeptide hormone.

2. Techniques for Short Chain Polypeptide Hormones

a) Specific Immunological Techniques

The primary amino acid sequences are now known for a number of polypeptide hormones including glucagon, gastrin, insulin, cholecystokinin-pancreozymin and others, and some can be synthesised. The successful inoculation of animals (usually rabbits) with synthetic or purified natural material results in the production of antibodies to the hormone which can be purified and used in direct or indirect fluorescent or peroxidase techniques. Currently studies are available in humans on the distribution of cells whose granules contain gastrin (*McGuigan*, 1968; *McGuigan* and *Greider*, 1971; *McGuigan*, 1973), glucagon (pancreatic and enteroglucagon) (*Polak* et al., 1971b), secretin (*Polak* et al., 1971c), motilin, vasoactive intestinal polypeptide (VIP) (*Polak* et al., 1974), insulin (*Lacy*, 1972), cholecystokinin-pancreozymin and gastric inhibitory polypeptide (*Polak* et al., 1973). Some polypeptide hormones, notably gastrin and enteroglucagon are apparently unaltered by formaldehyde fixation and the techniques can be performed on conventionally fixed and embedded material while others, e.g. secretin, require special fixatives such as carbodi-imide to preserve antigenicity. Penetration of the antiserum into the cell cytoplasm and across the granular envelope does not appear to be a problem. The use of peroxidase techniques may allow hormonal localisation at ultrastructural level (*Robinson* and *Dawson*, 1975).

b) Semi-Specific Histochemical Techniques

There are a variety of techniques, including those which use metachromatic and basophilic cationic stains with or without acid hydrolysis (masked basophilia or metachromasia) (*Solcia* and *Sampietro*, 1965a, b; *Solcia* et al., 1968; *Pearse*, 1969a, b), or metachromatic fluorochromes (*Bussolati* et al., 1969). All of these techniques are in fact demonstrating anionic amino acid side chains in the polypeptide under investigation; they given an indication of the number and siting of these available to react, but do not indicate their nature in a manner precise enough to infer the amino acid sequence of the polypeptide and hence its identification. The anionic groups in unhydrolysed material are probably carboxyl, sulphate and phosphate; hydrolysis removes the basophilia due to reactive groups in nucleic acids or acid polysaccharides and may both unmask further side chain carboxyl groups and convert carboxamido groups to carboxyls. *Pearse* (1969a, b) believes that metachromatic techniques are of most value in demonstrating secondary rather than primary protein structure. In summary, metachromatic techniques are of value in detecting the presence or absence of a polypeptide hormone, but are not necessarily specific for any one hormone and do not demonstrate all polypeptide hormones. In my view they have a definite but limited value and will probably be replaced by antibody techniques.

Lead haematoxylin is another semi-specific technique which is valuable as a screening agent: it will stain granules in many endocrine cells, but its mode of action is not precisely known.

c) Silver Techniques

Silver techniques in which no reducing agent is added (argentaffin) demonstrate an aldehyde/amine reducing complex and need no further discussion. There are a number of techniques available which use silver salts under different conditions with an added reducing agent (argyrophil); it is claimed that different techniques will demonstrate different granules (*Davenport,* 1930; *Bodian* 1936; *Hellerstrom* and *Hellman,* 1960; *Sevier* and *Munger*, 1965; *Grimelius*, 1964, 1968). The silver salts include silver proteinates, aqueous and alcoholic buffered and unbuffered silver nitrate. It is assumed that the silver salt links with amino acid side chains and is then reduced to metallic silver. There is no doubt that the fixative used has a profound influence on the result, presumably by preserving or blocking reactive groups; unfortunately formaldehyde is not the best fixative for many techniques, Bouin being in general preferable.

We (*Jones* and *Dawson*, unpublished) are investigating the whole range of solutions under varying conditions in normal human intestine in parallel with specific antibody studies. It seems proper at the moment to consider argyrophil techniques along with metachromasia as a useful screen for endocrine cell granules, though again some granules appear not to react with silver salts, to appreciate that certain techniques may be specific or semi-specific for certain polypeptide hormones, and to realise also that the lipoprotein envelopes of granules may themselves contain non-specific reactive groups.

3. Electron Microscopic Studies of Granules

Detailed electron microscopic studies of normal human and animal gastro-intestinal tract and pancreas have revealed that different endocrine cells possess granules of widely differing size, shape and density. The precise details of granule types, which need detailed and numerous photographs for their identification are outside the scope of this review, but an international classification of cells was agreed at a meeting in Wiesbaden in 1969 (*Solcia, Forssmann* and *Pearse*, 1970), and subsequently revised (*Solcia* et al., 1973), with a useful list of references.

Other helpful papers are those of *Kobayashi, Fujita* and *Sasagawa* (1970) (human duodenal endocrine cells); *Greider, Bencosme* and *Lechago* (1970), *Like* and *Orci* (1972), *Pearse, Polak* and *Heath* (1973) (human and mouse pancreas).

4. Combined Studies Using more than one Technique

This type of study is clearly likely to yield valuable results but presents the serious practical difficulty that one or more serial sections are likely to be necessary for each technique so that the same cell cannot be studied in more than one way. There are also problems in processing material which can be used for light and electron microscopic studies. These can be in part circumvented by the use of immunohistochemical techniques at electron microscope level which allows simultaneous observation of granule appearance with positive identification by a specific antiserum (*McGuigan* and *Greider*, 1973), by the use of semithin-thin sections (*Polak, Pearse* and *Heath*, 1975) or by the use of immune fluorescein labeled sera, photography and subsequent restaining using a histochemical technique.

VI. Summary

For the screening of gastro-intestinal material for the presence of endocrine cells of any type on formaldehyde fixed material I would use the lead haematoxylin and *Grimelius* (1968) silver techniques with perhaps a metachromatic technique; for absolute identification of 5HT containing cells I would use aldehyde-induced fluorescence and either a diazo or a silver reducing technique such as that of *Singh* (1964), while for absolute identification of polypeptide I would use specific antisera after appropriate fixation when available as a first choice, electron microscopy of granule appearances as a second choice and a combination of silver and metachromatic techniques as a third. There is room for careful comparative studies of these 3 types of technique on freshly obtained tumour material and on normal human gut, and such studies should always be linked with serum radioimmunoassay of any tumour material available.

PART 2 TUMOURS AND HYPERPLASIAS OF ENDOCRINE CELLS

Hyperplasias and benign or malignant tumours of virtually every known type of endocrine cell have now been described or postulated. It is practicable to classify them in terms of clinical behaviour, e.g. the presence of multiple peptic ulcers or a water diarrhoea syndrome; by the nature of their secretion as measured by radioimmunoassay of serum or analysis of tumour material (*Berson* and *Yalow*, 1972; *Bloom*, 1974); by their site of origin; by their structural histological pattern and histochemical reactions; and by the ultrastructure and immunochemistry of their contained granules. In practice as many of these aspects as possible need to be considered in every case, for the difficulties are formidable. Some neoplasms, especially those which are malignant, may contain few or no storage granules. Neoplasms with a similar function often have differing histological patterns, while those with similar patterns either have differing functions or no recognisable function at all; a number appear to secrete more than one hormone either simultaneously or sequentially. This section of the review seeks to explore how far tumour site, structure, ultrastructure, immunochemistry, and function can be related.

I. Histological Patterns

While there are a large number of reports of "carcinoid" tumours in the literature, many of which describe different histological patterns or variations in pattern, surprisingly few authors have set out to analyse and correlate tumours from different regions of the gastro-intestinal tract in terms of site, histological appearance and function (*Soga* and *Tazawa*, 1971; *Martin* and *Potet*, 1974; *Jones* and *Dawson*, in preparation). When this is done interesting facts are observed and the description which follows is based on the papers cited and on our own observations on patients with different forms of endocrine tumour.

Soga and *Tazawa* (1971) in an analysis of 62 cases recognised four basic patterns, which they classified as A – D and which *Martin* and *Potet* (1974) accept, but call types I – IV. Type A is the basic pattern which pathologists associate with appendiceal and ileal "carcinoids". In this there are solid nests of cells which when at the tumour edge often have a well developed peripheral rim of cells not unlike the basal cell layer of epidermis, but when central often lack the peripheral cell border (Figs. 1a and b). These tumours often incite a stromal desmoplastic reaction which may compress the nests into cords and trabeculae of cells (Figs. 1c and d). In our material the cell nests often appear to have a central vascular core producing a rosette appearance (Fig. 2) which is described also for type III tumours.

This pattern is commonly associated with 5HT production and the histochemical reactions and electron microscopic granule patterns to be expected of 5HT secreting cells; that is, positive argentaffin and diazo reactions, aldehyde induced fluorescence, and characteristically shaped basally situated, non-spherical, angulated, electron dense granules without haloes on e.m. examination. There is a recently recognised variant on this theme (*Klein*, 1974; *Subbuswamy* et al., 1974) of which we have seen examples in the appendix and duodenum. In this there is a differentiation of the solid nests towards a regular glandular mucus-secreting pattern, which is usually partial but may be complete so that part or all of the

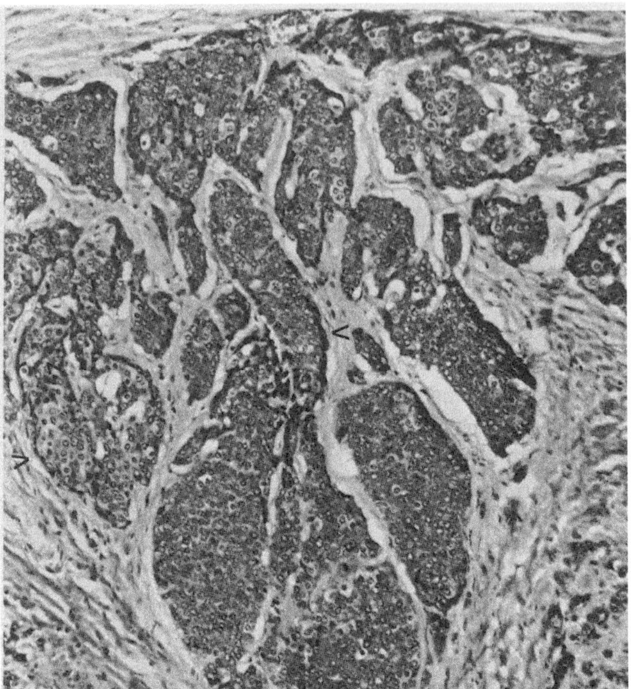

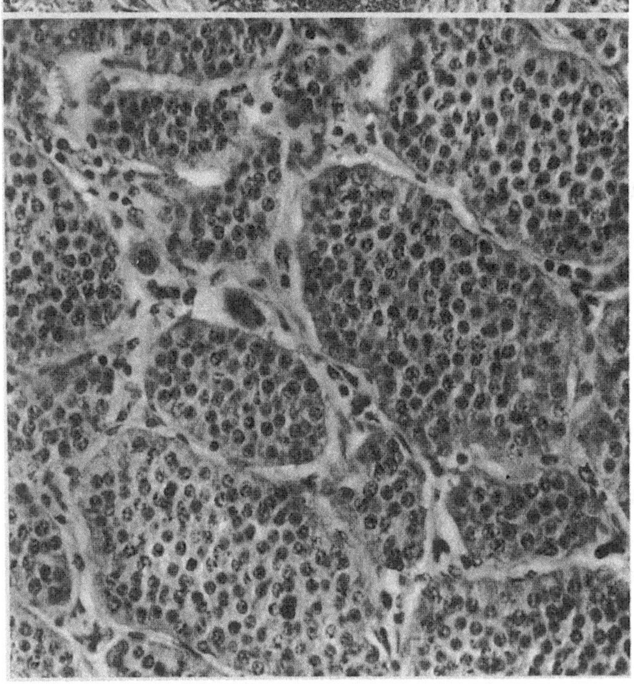

Fig. 1a. Type A ("carcinoid") tumour of ileum. Some nests of cells have a well developed peripheral rim (arrowed) while others either lack this feature or show it only in parts. Haematoxylin and eosin X 135.

Fig. 1b. Type A ("carcinoid") tumour of appendix. These solid nests of cells from the centre of the tumour do not have the peripheral rim of basal cell pattern cells. Haematoxylin and eosin X 335.

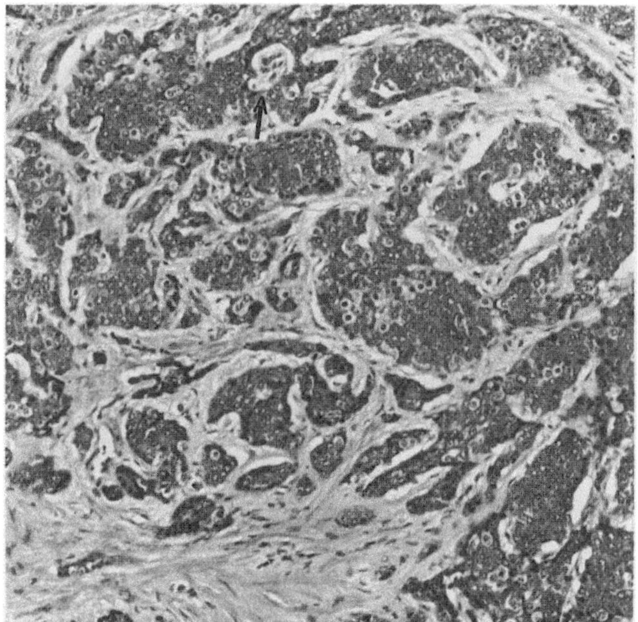

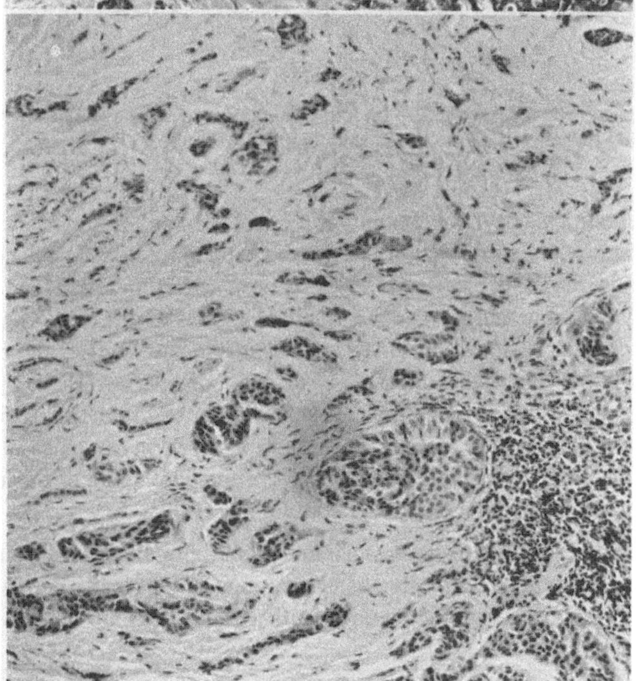

Fig. 1c. Type A ("carcinoid") tumour of ileum. Some desmoplastic reaction is present distorting the nests of cells. A so called "vascular core" is arrowed. Haematoxylin and eosin X 135.

Fig. 1d. Type A ("carcinoid") tumour of appendix. More severe desmoplastic reaction compressing the cell nests into columns of cells. Haematoxylin and eosin X 135

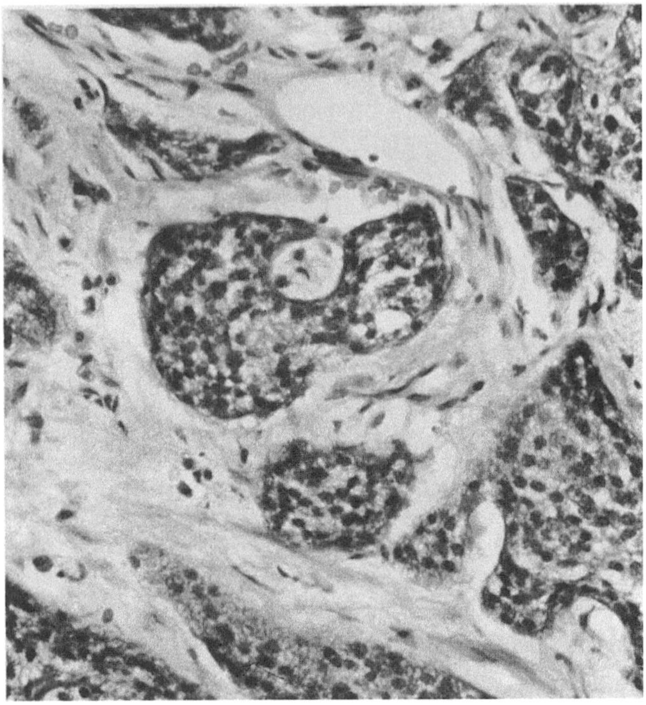

Fig. 2. Type A ("carcinoid") tumour of appendix to show a cell nest with a vascular core. Compare with Figures 10a and b. Haematoxylin and eosin X 335

tumour appears to be composed of small acini and is in pattern indistinguishable from a simple adenoma or well differentiated carcinoma (Fig. 3). Gland elements stain with PAS and with Alcian blue at pH 2.5. It is however, often possible to distinguish eosinophilic subnuclear granules on conventional H and E staining (Fig. 4) and the accepted techniques for 5HT are strongly positive throughout the basal part of the cytoplasm of apparently glandular cells, indicating their basic endocrine nature (Fig. 5). A similar pattern, of which we have also seen an example, has been described in the stomach (*Soga* et al., 1971) and in the pancreas (Figs. 6 a and b). As a corollary we believe that all apparent adenomas or adenocarcinomas occurring in the first part of the duodenum or the appendix should be investigated for the presence of 5HT containing cells.

Type B (II) tumours have a characteristic ribbon-like or trabecular pattern in which the ribbons form anastomosing bands or loops with a clearly defined vascular framework (Fig. 7). We have found that there are variants within this group on conventional histology, some cells

---

Fig. 3. Type A variant; so called mucus-secreting or goblet cell carcinoid of appendix. Granules are not visible at this magnification and appearances resemble a clear celled adenoma. Haematoxylin and eosin X 135.

Fig. 4. Type A variant; at higher power the granules can be seen in conventionally stained section. Haemotoxylin and eosin X 525

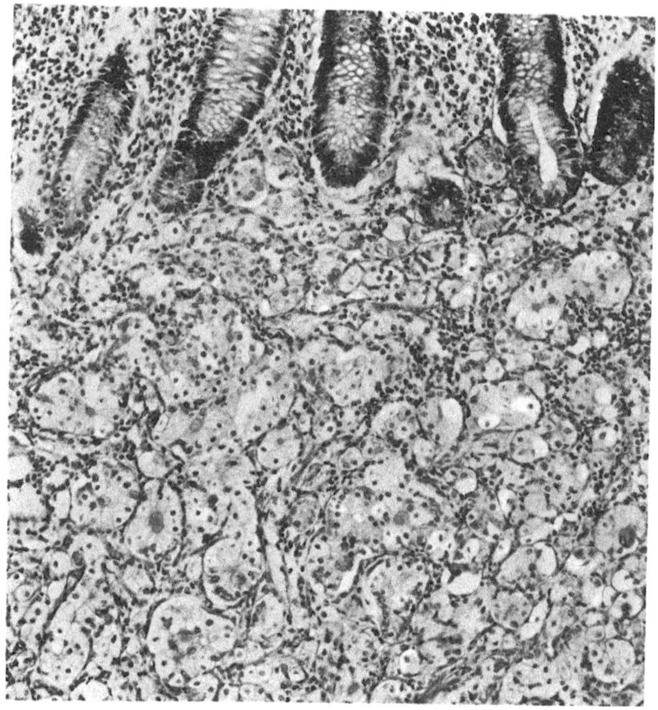

Fig. 3. (Legend see p. 234)

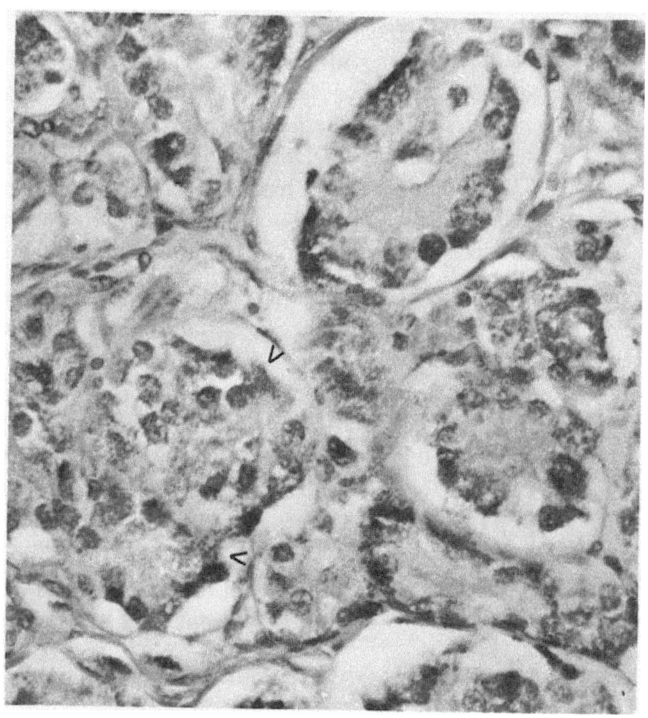

Fig. 4. (Legend see p. 234)

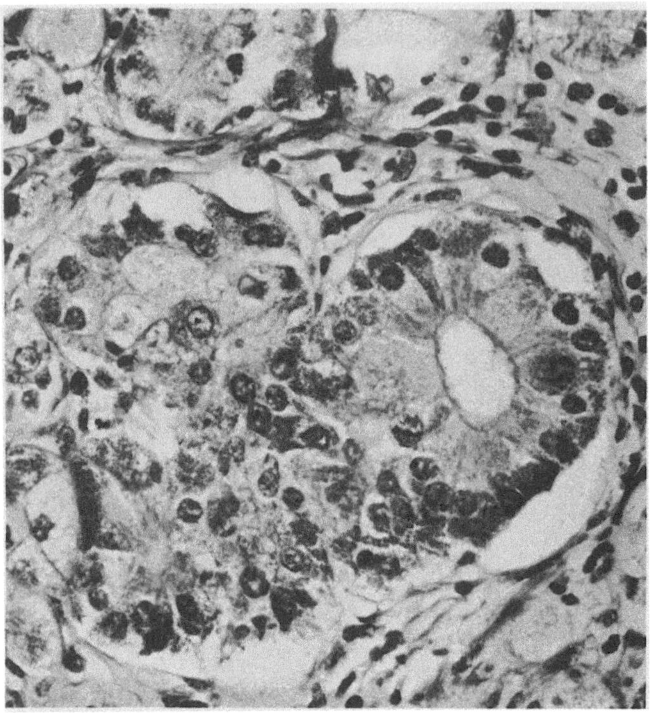

Fig. 5. Type A variant. Diazo technique clearly reveals positive staining granules. Diazo reaction X 525

having abundant cytoplasm with vesicular nuclei (Fig. 8a) while others, especially those of hindgut origin, are more compact with smaller cell size and less cytoplasm (Fig. 8b). *Soga* and *Tazawa* considered this pattern to be predominant in endocrine tumours of foregut origin – bronchus, stomach, duodenum and pancreas and to be largely non-reactive with silver stains (70% did not react). It has also been the pattern in the hindgut tumours we have seen and is described as a common hindgut pattern by other authors. In our experience the ribbon-like cells do not contain neutral or acid muco-substances.

Type C (III) tumours consist of plump rounded or angulated cells grouped in small irregularly-shaped masses and often showing central zones of PAS positive material which on low power examination seem to lie in gland acini (Figs. 9a and b). Closer inspection does not entirely confirm this impression; the acini are ill formed and may contain capillaries and the acinar cells often show no recognisable secretory activity; "rosettes" would be a more appropriate name for the majority, with the centre of the rosette sometimes containing PAS-positive material (Figs. 10a, b). *Soga* and *Tazawa* saw only two tumours of this pat-

---

Fig. 6a. Type A variant, stomach. Shows partial differentiation towards a glandular pattern: other areas, not shown, consisted of characteristic islands of cells giving reactions for 5HT. Haematoxylin and eosin X 135

Fig. 6b. Type A variant, stomach. Characteristic nests of type A cells and glandular elements. Haematoxylin and eosin X 135

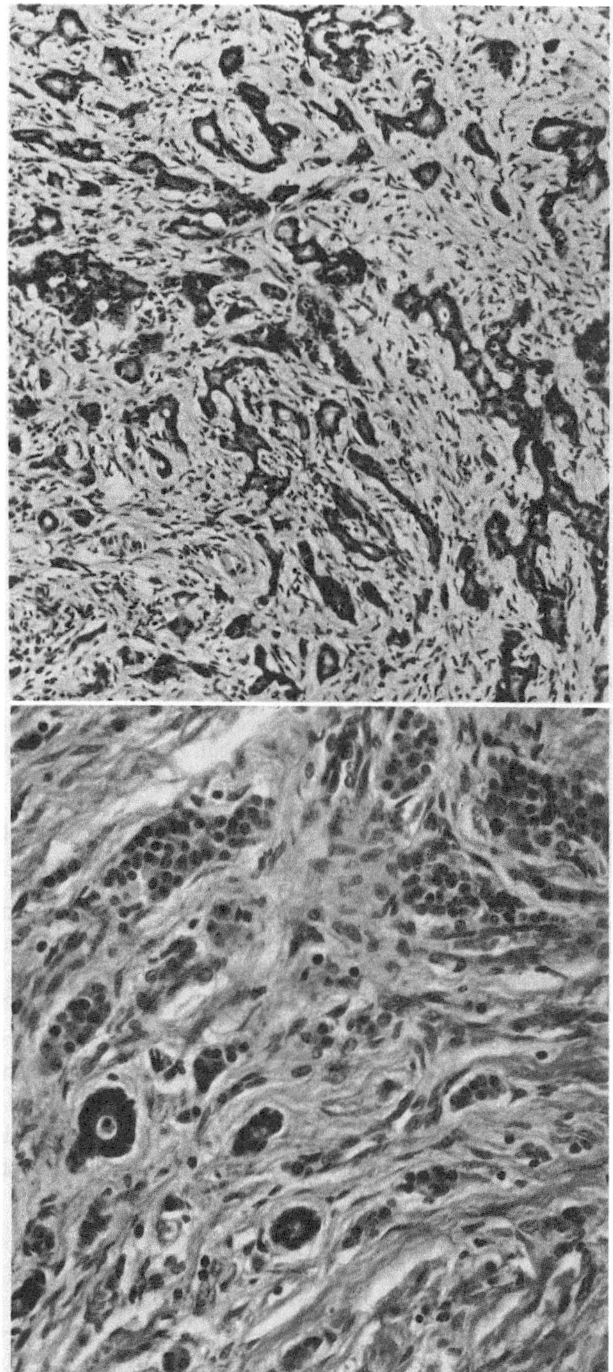

Fig. 6a and b. (Legend see p. 236)

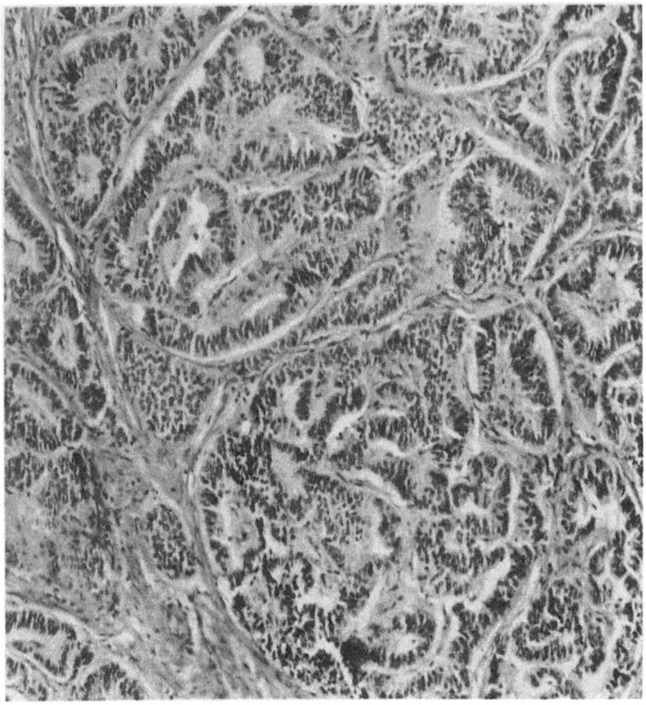

Fig. 7. Type B tumour of rectum. A looped ribbon pattern predominates with a delicate connective tissue stroma in which blood vessels are present. Haematoxylin and eosin X 135

tern, both in the pancreas; we have seen more examples in stomach, pancreas and hindgut; they are argyrophil or non-reactive and we have not seen an argentaffin example.

Type D is defined by *Soga and Tazawa* as "tumours with structures of lower or atypical differentiations" which though illustrated in a single photomicrograph are not defined further histologically. *Martin* and *Potet* (1974) use the term Type IV similarly for tumours with "an undifferentiated trabecular or medullary structure". There are undoubted tumours with a structure so anaplastic in some parts that a diagnosis of endocrine tumour cannot be made (Fig. 11) but with more differential zones which may be of A, B or C patterns or mixed pattern (E type). We prefer to group these under the primary (or mixed) pattern and not to use category D for them; an undifferentiated endocrine tumour can only be recognised histologically as endocrine by the differentiated zones which it contains and these are, by definition, classifiable.

The "mixed type" of *Soga* and *Tazawa* is also a feature of our material (Figs. 12, 13). The more thoroughly that endocrine tumours are sectioned, the more commonly can two or

---

Fig. 8a. Type B tumour of pancreas. A trabecular ribbon pattern with plump cells having abundant cytoplasm. Compare with Figures 7 and 8b. Haematoxylin and eosin X 135.

Fig. 8b. Type B tumour of rectum, showing looped ribbon pattern with small compact cells. Compare the cell size with Figure 8a. Haematoxylin and eosin X 135

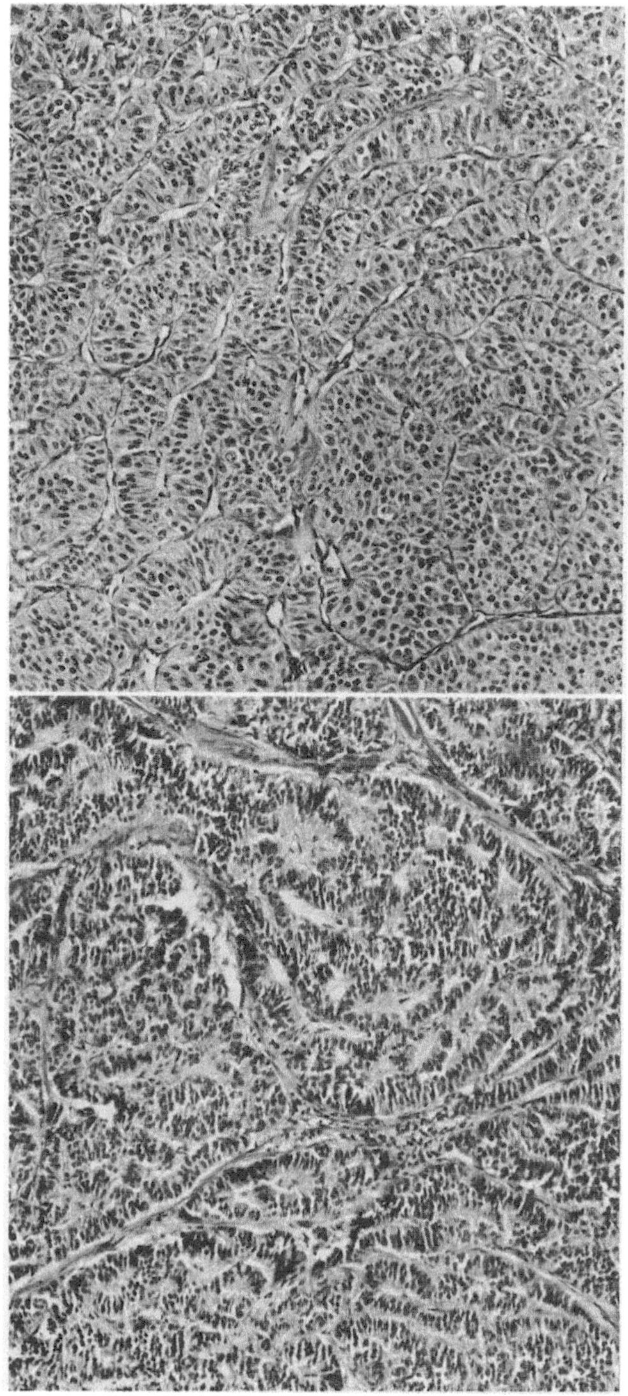

Fig. 8a and b. (Legend see p. 238)

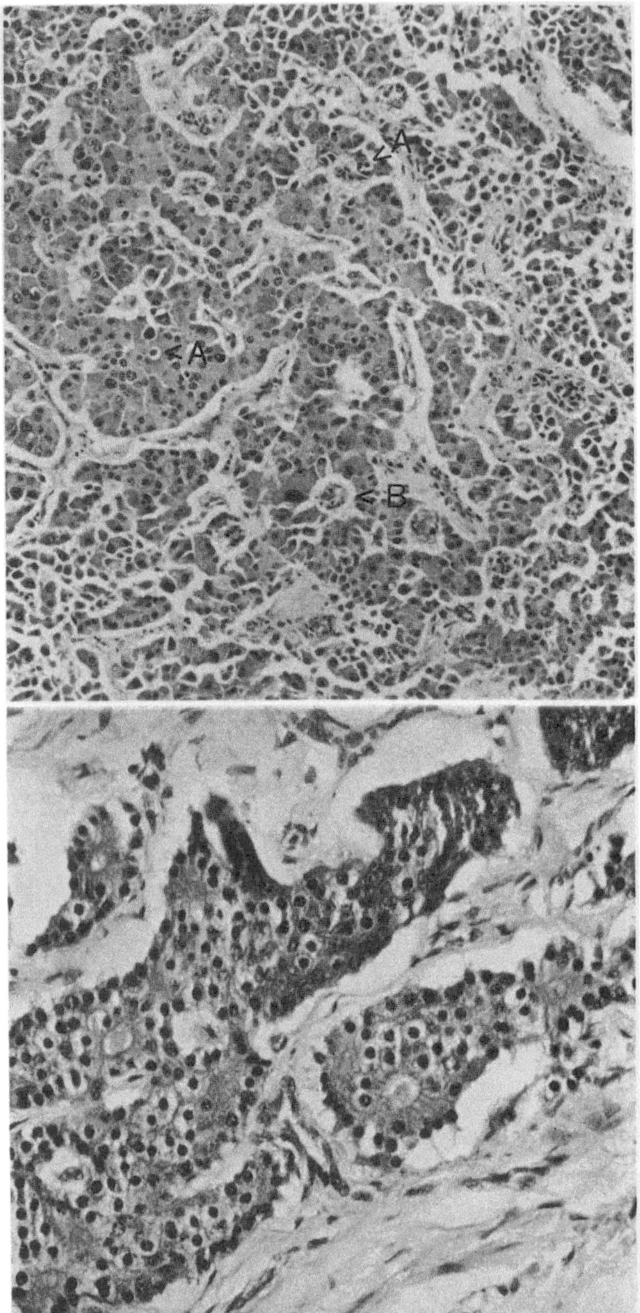

Fig. 9a. Type C tumour of pancreas. The pattern is partly solid, partly broad trabecular and two types of rosette are present; that arrowed "A" consists of PAS positive material (see Figure 10a), that arrowed "B" contains blood vessels (see Figure 10b). Haematoxylin and eosin X 135.

Fig. 9b. Type C tumour pattern in colon. The cells are more vacuolated than in Figure 9a, but rosettes are clearly visible. Haematoxylin and eosin X 335

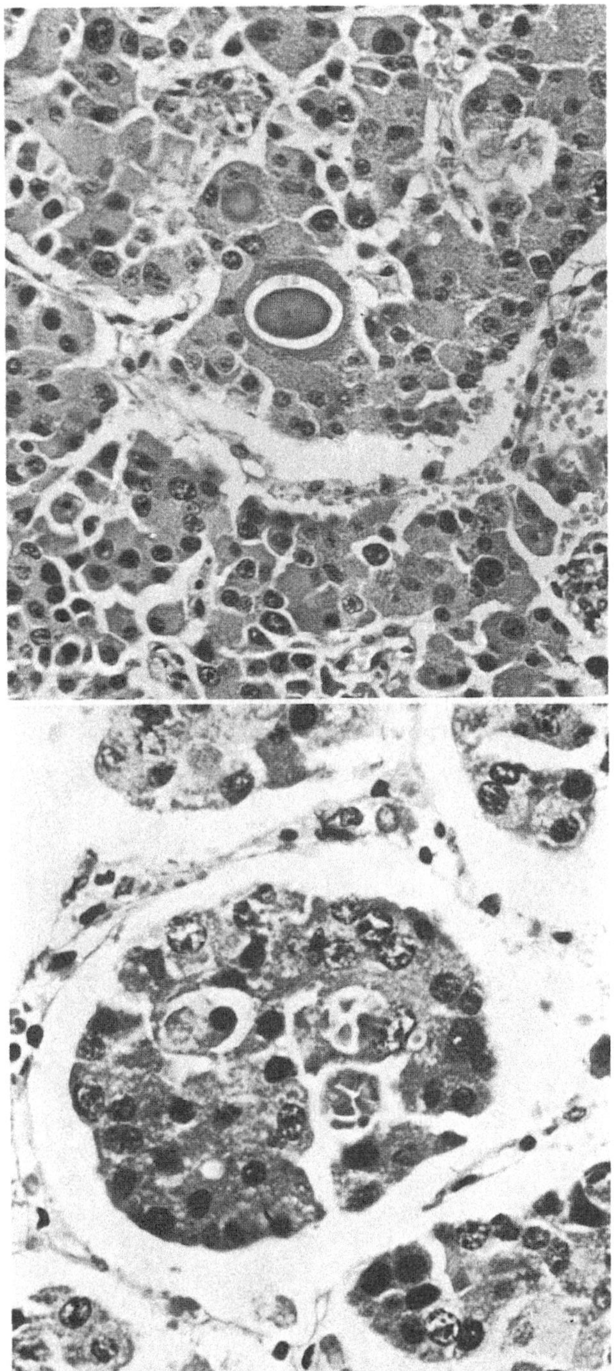

Fig. 10a. High power view of a "rosette" containing PAS positive material.Haematoxylin and eosin X 525.
Fig. 10b. High power view of a "rosette" containing two small capillaries. Haematoxylin and eosin X 735

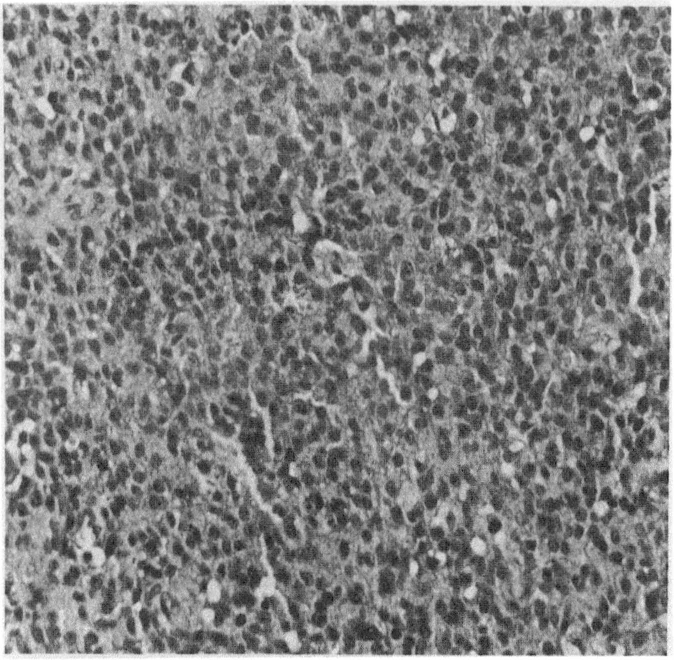

Fig. 11. So called type D (undifferentiated) endocrine tumour of pancreas. The diagnosis cannot be made on histological grounds from this photomicrograph, but other parts of the tumour showed a more definite type B pattern. Haematoxylin and eosin X 335

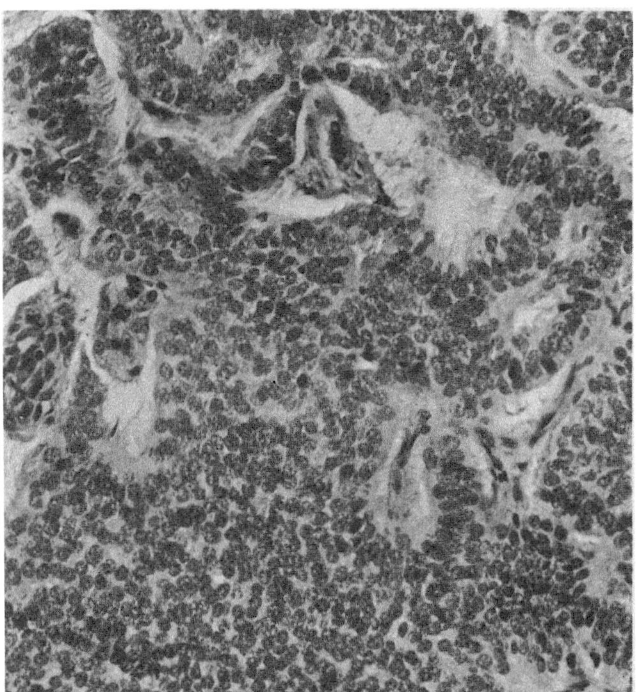

Fig. 12. (Legend see p. 243)

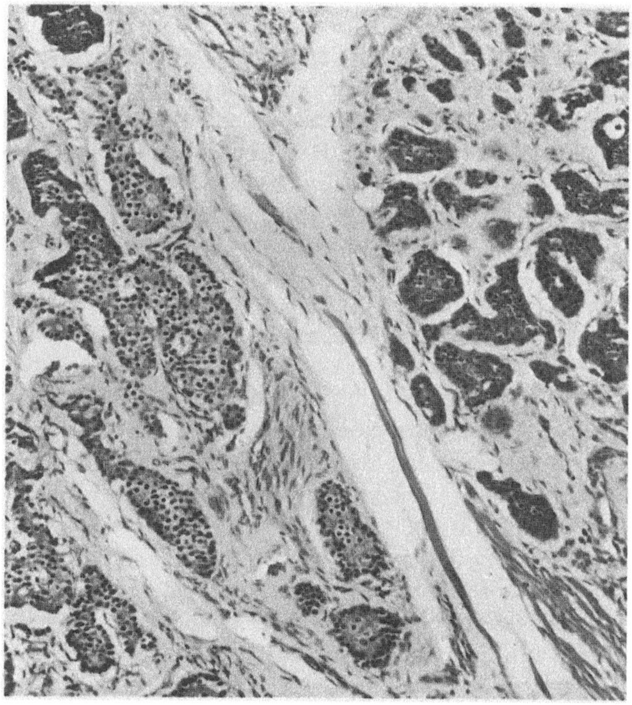

Fig. 13. Mixed A and C type C tumour of colon. There is a clear C type pattern with rosettes on the left, and a type A pattern which was positive for 5HT on the right. Haematoxylin and eosin X 135

three different but individually recognisable patterns of growth be distinguished from one another in a single tumour. These zones are, in our experience distinct and not usually intermingled. They give an appearance more suggestive of single or multiple tumours of one pattern growing independently alongside single or multiple tumours of another pattern to form a mosaic rather than an intimate intermingling of 2 or more patterns (Figs. 12, 13). A close study of the illustration of all patterns is recommended as, better than verbal description, they give an idea of the appearances seen.

We agree with various authors that it is usually impossible to designate a tumour as benign or malignant on cytological criteria alone; in our experience neoplasms of type A outside the appendix are likely to metastasise eventually but may take many years to do so, while those in groups B, C and E commonly metastasise in a shorter time.

II. The Relationship of Structure to Primary Site of Tumour

The first valuable observation in this field was when *Williams* and *Sandler* (1963) suggested that carcinoid tumours of bronchial, gastric and pancreatic, that is of foregut origin could

---

Fig. 12. Mixed A and B tumour of duodenum. A clearly recognisable ribbon B pattern is present in the upper parts, which merged below into a more solid A pattern, which was, however, negative for 5HT. Haematoxylin and eosin X 335 be separated from "classical" carcinoids of ileal or appendicular (midgut) origin on the basis of trabecular structure, negative diazo and argentaffin reactions, a tendency to metastasise to skin and bone and the secretion of 5-hydroxytryptophan; hindgut carcinoids were also commonly trabecular and metastasised similarly, but were non-functional. While this is still in general true apart from 5 HTP secretion, it is helpful to look at the distribution of the histological patterns as characterised above in terms of stomach, duodenum, upper jejunum, pancreas and gall bladder (broadly foregut), lower jejunum, ileum and appendix (midgut) and colon and rectum (broadly hindgut).

Foregut Tumours: These occur in the pancreas (*Sircus*, 1969), in which they are fairly uniformly distributed, and in the stomach and upper duodenum; in the latter they may be related to pancreatic rests. Most of them including those in the pancreas are small (under 2 cm in diameter) when first discovered. They are pinkish grey or tan rather than yellow in colour and when in the stomach or duodenum are primarily submucosal though they may later ulcerate the mucosa. In the pancreas they may be multiple. The vast majority fall into patterns B – C or are of mixed type E, often with a ribbon pattern predominating (*Schein* et al., 1973), and cell granules are either argyrophil or fail to stain with any silver technique; the reaction with metachromatic dyes and lead haematoxylin is variable. Neoplasms of pure pattern A are rare (*Patchefsky* et al., 1972, 1974; *Soga* et al., 1971), though 5HT secreting cells are present in stomach, duodenum, upper jejunum and in pancreatic ducts, and when pattern A is present it is usually in association with other patterns. *Weichert* et al. (1971) describe a pattern in the duodenum which they call "carcinoid islet cell" which they claim have morphological and functional features both of "carcinoids" and islet cell tumours, though they did not have the histochemical features associated with 5HT. We also have seen this "argentaffin negative carcinoid" pattern in the duodenum; it can be associated with the Zollinger-Ellison syndrome (Figs. 14a, b). Metastasis to liver is relatively common, but malignancy can rarely be foretold by the histological appearance. Functional aspects are discussed later: recently two such tumours have been described in the gall bladder one secreting 5HT (*Bernades* et al., 1972) and one ACTH (*Spence, Burns* and *Cox*, 1975).

Midgut Tumours: The appearance and distribution of these is too well known to warrant more than a brief description. In the appendix they are small and may not be visible naked eye; in our experience they are equally as common at the base as at the tip; the characteristic yellow colour described is more obvious after fixation. Infiltration of muscle coats is usual but metastasis rare. In the ileum they tend to be larger and though primarily submucosal may ulcerate, constrict the bowel or become pedunculated; infiltration and metastasis are common. They are virtually all of pattern A and true examples of patterns B – C are as far as I know undescribed. In the appendix some are argentaffin negative (*Dische*, 1968) and the pattern may vary towards that of adenoma or adenocarcinoma as already described but a typical pattern "A" is usually present in some part.

Hindgut Tumours: Endocrine tumours in the colon are most common in the caecum or ileocaecal region, but have not been well investigated as regards structure or staining reaction (*Berardi*, 1972). They tend to be large when first diagnosed and macroscopically often resemble carcinomas. Most appear to be argentaffin positive, and about half of Berardi's series had metastasised when first diagnosed, but the carcinoid syndrome is rare. Our own

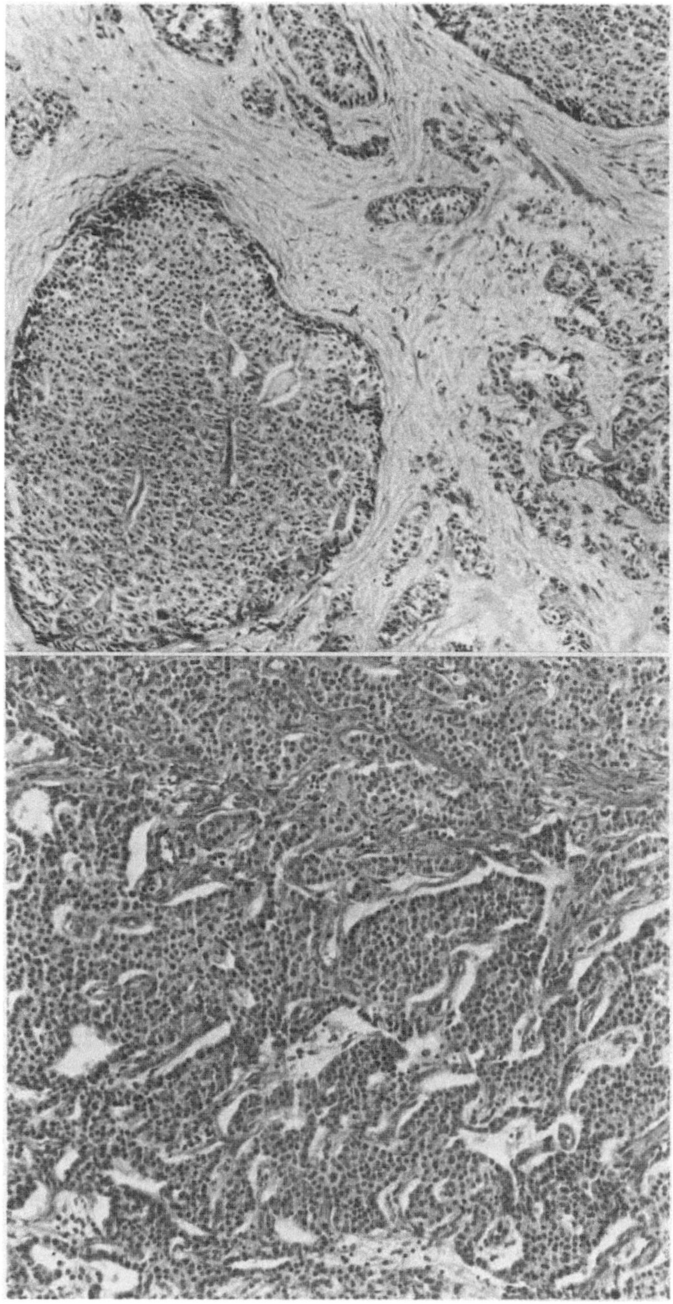

Fig. 14a. "Argentaffin negative carcinoid" pattern of tumour in duodenum. The islands are large, a rosette is present and the resemblance to a true type A is not really very close. Compare with Figures 1a and b. Haematoxylin and eosin X 135.

Fig. 14b. "Argentaffin negative carcinoid" pattern of tumour in duodenum. Again the resemblance to a type A is incomplete and some areas suggest a ribbon pattern. Haematoxylin and eosin X 135 experience in part confirms this but some tumours can certainly be of mixed pattern and we have seen one with type A and type C components (Fig. 13).

In the rectum endocrine tumours are usually small (less than 0.5 cm in diameter), submucosal without ulceration and pink or tan in colour (*Caldarola* et al., 1964; *Quan, Bader* and *Berg*, 1964; *Orloff*, 1971). Three histological patterns are described namely a typical "carcinoid" or pattern A though the diazo, argentaffin and even argyrophil stains are usually negative; a "scirrhous" in which a desmoplastic reaction surrounds columns of cells, and the well recognised type B ribbon pattern. We believe that there are in fact two types of ribbon pattern, one composed of small cells staining negatively with all histochemical techniques which we associate with rectal tumours, and one composed of plumper cells seen in pancreas and duodenum (and bronchus) which shows variable positive histochemical reactions (Figs. 7, 8).

Rectal endocrine tumours are in general non-functional; but there are occasional examples of carcinoid syndrome described (*Gross*, 1968; *Murray-Lyon* et al., 1972).

III. The Relationship of Structure, Ultrastructure and Immunology to Function

As we have seen, classification into tumour patterns on a histological basis is practicable, and is valuable in tumours which produce no overt clinical or laboratory evidence of functional hormone secretion. When a single clear function can be attributed to a tumour either on clinical grounds as in Zollinger-Ellison or Verner-Morrison syndromes, which is supported by laboratory investigations such as the finding of raised serum hormone levels on immunoassay or on tumour assay, it is permissable to speak of a gastrinoma, glucagonoma etc. irrespective of histological pattern. A study of the site as well as the histological, ultrastructural and immunological patterns of functional tumours is valuable, however, to see how far site, structure and function can be correlated. The problem is not made more simple by the observation that histologically more than one pattern may be present and that multiple hormone production by a single tumour is also not uncommon (*Gammill* et al., 1973). It is also insufficient to designate for example, a tumour of the pancreas secreting gastrin as merely "non β cell" in origin. What is needed, and will appear more frequently as superior techniques are elaborated, is a careful study, in each endocrine tumour in which the levels of the hormone or hormones secreted are known through serum immunoassay or tumour analysis, of the site, multiplicity, histological pattern, histochemical findings, electron microscopic appearance of granules and immunocytochemistry of granular content. Such reports are at the moment few, but it is these which I propose principally to review.

1. Gastrinomas

There are now a number of valuable reports on the structural and immunological aspects of gastrinomas (*Cavallero, Solcia* and *Sampietro*, 1967; *Tardini, Ansersa* and *Bordi*, 1969; *Schulte* et al., 1969; *Creutzfeldt* et al., 1971; *Royston* et al., 1972; *Vassallo* et al., 1972; *Bozymski* et al., 1973; *Creutzfeldt* et al., 1975), either proven by radioimmunoassay and/or tumour extraction, or firmly associated with a Zollinger-Ellison syndrome, which many authors would now prefer to call gastrinoma syndrome (*Isenberg, Walsh* and *Grossman*, 1973). I believe that the syndrome cannot be totally equated with a gastrinoma since there is evidence that it can also be associated with a non-neoplastic hyperplasia of antral gastrin cells (*Polak, Stagg* and *Pearse*, 1972; *Cowley* et al., 1973; *Robinson* and *Dawson*, 1976).

Tumours or hyperplasia are found in the islets of the pancreas or in the duodenum and have been variously described on special investigation as being either of non β cell or more positively of A1 or D cell origin. *Cavallero* et al. (1967) found normal A1 (D) cells and tumour cells positive with Bodian and Davenport silver techniques, with DMAB nitrite and with metachromatic techniques which they consider proof of identity. *Schulte* et al. (1969) believe that reactions with silver stains should be treated with reserve since tumour cells do not necessarily react in an identical way to their normal counterparts, though most A cell tumours do not have argyrophil granules, and *Royston* et al. (1972) in a single tumour were able to correlate argyrophil cells with positive immunofluorescence using an antigastrin serum. It is only fair to say, however, that in normal antral mucosa McGuigan has not been able to correlate argyrophilia with positive immunofluorescence (*Greider, Steinberg* and *McGuigan*, 1972). *Vassallo* et al. (1972) were able to stain some cells in all of 3 gastrinomas using antigastrin immunological techniques, but did not feel that in general the tumours reproduced the ultrastructural or immunological features of normal islet cells and suggest that they may arise from a primarily pathological type of D cell.

Creutzfeldt et al. (1975) have described 10 gastrinomas, seven pancreatic and three duodenal, all of which were malignant. Nine out of ten had positive staining of some granules with the 1968 Grimelius technique, which normally stains antral G cells and islet D cells. All gave a positive immunoperoxidase reaction with antigastrin antiserum, but the degree of immune staining did not correspond with the staining achieved with the Grimelius technique which in general stained more cells. Seven of the 10 contained granules similar to those of normal antral G cells, but all contained other cells with atypical granules, and all contained some agranular cells, suggesting a diminished storage capacity. *Creutzfeldt* et al. consider that a classification may be possible purely on ultrastructural grounds and suggest four groups.

I Tumours with cells containing granules which resemble normal antral G cells.

II Tumours with cells which contain typical G cell granules and other cells which contain atypical granules.

III Tumours with cells containing only atypical granules.

IV Multihormonal tumours containing secretory granules characteristic of other endocrine cells.

They do not, however, give a convincing account of the histological patterns found in the 10 tumours merely reporting them as similar to those of carcinoid tumours or insulinomas, with cells forming trabeculae, sheets or nests. The only authors really helpful here are *Schulte* et al. (1969) who stress that gastrinomas may have a histological pattern similar to type A "carcinoids" but with negative argentaffin type reactions, and that there is not a marked tendency to pure B or C type patterns, though these may appear as mixed patterns. Electron microscopically most tumours contain recognisable A cells.

Tumour analysis has shown the presence of both minigastrins (*Gregory* and *Tracy*, 1974) and big gastrins (*Dockray, Walsh* and *Passaro*, 1975) which may correlate with the idea that tumour cells can appear unlike the normal cell in ultrastructure because there is a defect in storage and release.

It appears in summary that gastrinomas are likely to contain argyrophil positive cells, especially after fixation in Bouin; to have a mixed histological pattern with usually at least a part resembling a "carcinoid" tumour but negative with techniques for 5HT-formaldehyde complexes; to react with specific immune sera at least as regards some cells, and to contain some cells with characteristic A (D) granules.

2. Insulinomas

A number of well authenticated reports of insulinomas are now extant (*Lacy*, 1961; *Golddenberg, Goldenberg* and *Benditt*, 1969; *Suzuki* and *Matsuyama*, 1971; *Arnold* et al., 1972; *Creutzfeldt* et al., 1973; *Marks* and *Samols*, 1974). They arise exclusively from B cells of pancreatic islets and may be benign or malignant. Histologically patterns B and C – ribbon or rosette – predominate and in our experience the ribbon patterns are composed of larger cells and are more convoluted than the ribbon patterns seen in rectal endocrine tumours (Fig. 7). Histochemically the granules are commonly positive with aldehyde-fuchsin or aldehyde thionin stains, as are normal B cells (*Arnold* et al., 1972) and usually also react positively with appropriate antisera, the latter technique being more reliable. There is some evidence that fuchsin/thionin-type reactions stain only normal insulin and that some tumours fail to react because the insulin is present in an abnormal form (*Arnold* et al., 1972). Ultrastructurally the granules in insulinomas have been said to resemble those of normal β cells (*Lacy*, 1961), but it has again been claimed that the presence of normal granules in tumours is related to the form of insulin present (*Goldenberg, Goldenberg* and *Benditt*, 1969), and also to the patterns, normal granular appearance correlating with a ribbon pattern (*Suzuki* and *Matsuyama*, 1971). *Creutzfeldt* et al. (1973) go further in relating positive thionin staining with immunoreactive insulin and negative staining with pro-insulin formation, and recognised four patterns of tumour, namely

a) Those containing typical B granules.

b) Those containing typical B and some atypical granules.

c) Those containing atypical granules only.

d) Those containing mainly agranular cells.

Groups (c) and (d) tend to be non-reactive with thionin type stains, are immunologically negative, do not have typical granules and therefore cannot be recognised structurally as insulinomas.

3. Glucagonomas

Glucagonomas are less likely to be recognised on clinical grounds than are other endocrine cell tumours and the literature on them, because many have been unsuspected, is less comprehensive (*Yoshinaga* et al., 1966; *McGavran* et al., 1966; *Lomsky, Langr* and *Vortel*, 1969; *Croisier, Lehy* and *Zeitoun*, 1971; *Gleeson* et al., 1971; *Bloom*, 1972; *Croughs*, et al., 1972; *Croughs*, 1974).

The patterns vary between B and C, with sometimes variation within the same tumour (*Yoshinaga* et al., 1966), and tumour cells commonly stain positively with Davenport or Hellerstrom and Hellman silver techniques, as do normal A cells (*McGavran* et al., 1966; *Crough* et al., 1972). Tumour cells can also be identified immunologically with appropriate antisera (*Lomsky, Langr* and *Vortel*, 1969). A recent example has been described in the kidney (*Gleeson* et al., 1971). It appears that this tumour may be more common than has been appreciated, and that it tends to reproduce the normal A cell to a greater extent than other endocrine tumours reproduce their normal cell counterparts.

4. A Cell Hyperplasias

There is some evidence that A cell hyperplasia is a significant feature in polyglandular syndromes (*Vance* et al., 1969; *Croisier, Lehy* and *Zeitoun*, 1971; *Croughs*, 1974).

5. Endocrine Tumours Associated with Water Diarrhoea and Hypokalaemia

A syndrome of refractory diarrhoea with hypokalaemia was first described in 1958 by *Verner* and *Morrison* and is now commonly known either by their eponyms or as pancreatic cholera or WDHA syndrome, and is associated with pancreatic islet cell tumours. These are recognised as being of non-B type (*Verner* and *Morrison*, 1974a), and suggestions have been made that the hormone responsible is glucagon, which is unlikely, vasoactive intestinal polypeptide (*Bloom, Polak* and *Pearse*, 1973), or a combination of gastrin and glucagon or secretin (*Greider, Rosai* and *McGuigan*, 1974). Describing 6 patients with the WDHA syndrome, *Bloom, Polak* and *Pearse* (1973) found that 4 had pancreatic tumours and one an islet cell hyperplasia; the latter has been a feature of other examples (*Sircus* et al., 1970; *Verner* and *Morrison*, 1974b). All of the tumour cells were said to be "argyrophil" and had granules positive with lead haematoxylin and both of the two studied immunologically were positive with anti VIP serum. The authors suggest the name VIPoma for this tumour, but in my view further evidence is needed on a larger series before VIP can positively be identified as the causative hormone, and more detailed studies on the histological and histochemical patterns are needed.

6. 5HT Secreting Tumours

These are so well recognised as to require little comment. They are all of type A, and when sufficient functional tumour tissue is present, may be detected by raised levels of 5 hydroxy indole acetic acid (5HIAA) in the urine. They may be associated, in the presence of hepatic metastases, with the carcinoid syndrome (*Davis, Moertel* and *McIlrath*, 1973). They probably all contain sufficient stored 5HT to condense with formaldehyde and give the characteristic histochemical reaction; failure to do so may be the result of diffusion prior to fixation when this has been delayed or to the fact that some endocrine tumours which are not of 5HT secreting type may have, at any rate in parts, a "carcinoid" or type A pattern.

7. Multiple Endocrine Syndromes

It is now well recognised that patients may present clinically with symptoms and signs suggesting hypersecretion of more than one hormone, or that evidence of such hypersecretion may be found on serum or tumour immunoassay. There are three main ways in which this may occur and each merits a short discussion.

a) Multiple Endocrine Adenomas or Hyperplasias

Adenomas or hyperplasias of more than one endocrine gland are well documented (*Wermer*, 1954; *Levin*, 1968) and are often inherited as an autsomal dominant (*Wermer*, 1954; *Ballard, Frame* and *Hartsock*, 1964). They usually affect one or more type of islet cell and commonly involve parathyroids; there is a group which tends to involve thyroid (medullary carcinoma) and adrenal medulla (phaochromocytoma) (*Shimke* et al., 1968). They are of importance in that when any endocrine tumour or hyperplasia is discovered the possibility of a multiple endocrine adenomatosis should be borne in mind, but they do not merit further discussion here as the adenomas or hyperplasias which occur are similar to those already described.

b) Single Endocrine Tumours Secreting more than one Hormone

There are well documented cases of apparently single tumours which produce more than one hormone either simultaneously or sequentially. Thus *Heitz* et al. (1971) describe an islet cell tumour in the head of the pancreas in a 12 year old boy with two distinct cell types, thought histochemically to be A and B cells, which produced both insulin and gastrin; *Belchetz* et al. (1973) an islet cell carcinoma in a 44 year old man which apparently produced ACTH, glucagon and gastrin; and *Hammar* and *Sale* (1975) review the available cases and add two of their own, one a 62 year old male with an islet cell carcinoma secreting gastrin, glucagon and insulin and a 44 year old woman with an islet cell carcinoma secreting ACTH, glucagon and insulin. Such histochemical and ultrastructural studies as are available do not always reveal different staining or granule patterns corresponding to the hormones secreted, and no definite histological pattern has been described, though mixed patterns are commonly present. Such multiple secretions may arise, in theory at least, either from simultaneous or sequential neoplasia in two different types of endocrine cell or by a single neoplastic pattern changing its function during tumour growth.

c) Inappropriate Hormone Secretion by other Tumours

There are occasional reports of gastro-intestinal or pancreatic hormones secreted by tumours outside the tract, such as the secretion of glucagon by a renal tumour (*Gleeson* et al., 1971) and 5HT by an oat cell carcinoma of lung (*Hattori, Matsuda* and *Tateisha*, 1968). There is a general review by *Omen* (1970).

IV. Conclusions

All neoplasms or hyperplasias of endocrine cells should be studied as fully as possible using a wide range of techniques. Serum radioimmunoassay and tumour extraction and assay are particularly important and serum and some fresh tumour material should always be preserved for this purpose. Adequate histological examination is essential since histological patterns vary within a single tumour and some material should be fixed in Bouin's fixative since many silver techniques depend upon it. Screening examination should attempt to define the histological patterns present and should include techniques for 5HT containing cells, metachromatic methods, silver stains, aldehyde fuchsin or thionin and lead haematoxylin. Material should be suitably preserved for immunochemistry which may indicate the use of special fixatives such as carbo-di-imide and for electron microscopy. Only when this is done on every suspected neoplasm will our knowledge of these fascinating tumours advance significantly.

Acknowledgements: My thanks are due to the many physicians, surgeons and pathologists who have supplied material for our own studies; to Dr. *K.D. Buchanan* who generously provides us with antisera; to my colleagues Dr. *Graham Robinson* and Dr. *Richard Jones*; to the technicians in our laboratory who have done most of the special staining needed for our studies; to Mr. *W. Brackenbury* for the photographs and to Miss *Colleen Peel* who typed the manuscript. Part of the costs were defrayed by a grant from the Cancer Research Campaign, and to them I am also grateful.

References

Anderson, J.C., Barton, M.A., Gregory, R.A., Hardy, P.M., Kenner, G.W., MacLeod, J.K., Preston, J., Sheppard, R.C., Morley, J.S.: The antral hormone gastrin. II. Synthesis of gastrin. Nature (Lond.) 204, 933 (1964).

Arnold, R., Deuticke, U., Frerichs, H., Creutzfeldt, W.: Immunohistologic investigation of human insulinomas. Diabetologia 8, 250-259 (1972).

Aures, D., Håkanson, R.: Amine formation in polypeptide-producing endocrine cells of the digestive tract. Europ. J. Pharmacol. 3, 316-321 (1968).

Ballard, H.S., Frame, B., Hartsock, R.J.: Familial multiple endocrine adenoma-peptic ulcer complex. Medicine (Baltimore) 43, 481-516 (1964).

Barter, R., Pearse, A.G.E.: Mammalian enterochromaffin cells as the source of serotonin (5 hydroxytryptamine). J. Path. Bact. 69, 25-31 (1955).

Belchetz, P.E., Brown, C.L., Makin, H.L.J., Trafford, D.J.H., Stuart Mason, A., Bloom, S.R., Ratcliffe, J.G.: ACTH, Glucagon and gastrin production by a pancreatic islet cell carcinoma and its treatment. Clin. Endocr. 2, 307-316 (1973).

Berardi, R.S.: Carcinoid tumours of the colon (exclusive of the rectum). Review of the literature. Dis. Col. Rectum. 15, 383-391 (1972).

Bernades, P., Bonnefond, A., Martin, E., Bonfils, S.: Syndrome de Zollinger Ellison avec tumeurs endocrines carcinoides insulaires de siège vesiculaire primitif. Arch. Françaises des Malads. de l'appareil Dig. 61, 759-766 (1972).

Berson, S.A., Yalow, R.S.: Nature of immunoreactive gastrin extracted from tissues of gastrointestinal tract. Gastroenterology 60, 215 (1971).

Berson, S.A., Yalow, R.S.: Radioimmunoassay in gastroenterology. Gastroenterology 62, 1061 (1972).

Bjorklund, A., Falck, B.: An improvement of the histochemical fluorescence method for monoamines. J. Histochem. Cytochem. 16, 717 (1968).

Bloom, S.R.: An enteroglucagon tumour. Gut 13, 520 (1972).

Bloom, S.R.: Progress report: radioimmunoassay of intestinal hormones. Gut 15, 502-510 (1974).

Bloom, S.R., Polak, J.M., Pearse, A.G.E.: Vasoactive intestinal peptide and watery-diarrhoea syndrome. Lancet 1973 II, 14-16.

Bodansky, M., Ondetti, M.A., Levine, S.D.: Synthesis of a heptacosapeptide amide with the hormonal activity of secretin. Chem. and Ind. 42, 1757 (1966).

Bodansky, M., Klausner, Y.S., Said, S.I.: Biological activities of synthetic peptides corresponding to fragments of and to the entire sequence of the vasoactive intestinal peptide. Proc. nat. Acad. Sci (Wash.) 70, 382 (1973).

Bodian, D.: A new method for staining nerve fibres and nerve endings in mounted paraffin sections. Anat. Rec. 65, 89 (1936).

Bolande, R.P.: The neurocristopathies: A unifying concept of disease arising in neural crest maldevelopment. Human Pathol. 5, 409-429 (1974).

Bottger, I., Faloona, G., Unger, R.H.: Response of islet cell and gut hormones to fat absorption: an 'enteroinsular axis' for fat. Clin. Res. 20, 542 (1972).

Bozymski, E.M., Woodruff, K., Sessions, J.T, jr.: Zollinger-Ellison syndrome with hypoglycaemia ssociated with calcification of the tumor and its metastases. Gastroenterology 65, 658-661 (1973).

Brolin, S.E., Hellman, B., Knutson, H.: The structure and metabolism of the pancreatic islets. Oxford: Pergamon Press 1964.

Brown, J.C.: The presence of a gastric motor stimulating property in duodenal extracts. Gastroenterology 52, 225 (1967).

Brown, J.C., Pederson, R.A.: A multiparameter study on the action of preparations containing cholecystokinin pancreozymin. Scand. J. Gastroenterol. 5, 537 (1970).

Brown, J.C., Dryburgh, J.R.: A gastric inhibitory polypeptide. II. The complete amino acid sequence. Canad. J. Biochem. 49, 867 (1971).

Brown, J.C., Cook, M.A., Dryburgh, J.R.: Motilin, a gastric motor acitivity-stimulating polypeptide: final purification, amino acid composition and C-terminal residues. Gastroenterology 62, 401 (1972).

Bussolati, D., Rost, F.W.D., Pearse, A.G.E.: Fluorescence metachromasia in polypeptide hormone-producing cells of the APUD series, and its significance in relation to the structure of the protein precursor. Histochem. J. 1, 517 (1969).

Bussolati, G., Capella, C., Solcia, E., Vassalo, G., Vezzadini, P.: Ultrastructural and immunofluorescent investigations on the secretin cell in dog intestinal mucosa. Histochemie 26, 218-227 (1971).

Caldarola, V.T., Jackman, R.J., Moertel, C.G., Docherty, M.B.: Carcinoid tumours of the rectum. Amer. J. Surg. 107, 844-849 (1964).

Carvelheira, A.F., Welsch, U., Pearse, A.G.E.: Cytochemical and ultrastructural observations on the argentaffin and argyrophil cells of the gastrointestinal tract in mammals and their place in the APUD series of polypeptide-secreting cells. Histochemie 14, 33-46 (1968).

Cavallero, C., Solcia, E., Sampietro, R.: Cytology of islet tumours and hyperplasia associated with the Zollinger Ellison syndrome. Gut 8, 172-177 (1967).

Clara, M.: Über die Morphologie und Histochemie der basalgekörnten Zellen. Acta neuroveg. 16, 294-312 (1957).
Corrodi, H., Jonsson, G.: The formaldehyde fluorescence method for the histochemical demonstration of biogenic monoamines. A review on the methodology.J. Histochem. Cytochem. 15, 65-78 (1967).
Cowley, D.J., Dymock, I.W., Boyes, B.E., Wilson, R.Y., Stagg, B.H., Lewin, M.R., Polak, J.M., Pearse, A.G.E.: Zollinger-Ellison syndrome Type 1. Clinical and pathological correlations in a case. Gut 14, 25-29 (1973).
Creutzfeldt, W., Arnold, R., Creutzfeldt, C., Feurle, G., Ketterer, H.: Gastrin and G cells in the antral mucosa of patients with pernicious anaemia, acromegaly and hyperparathyroidism and in a Zollinger Ellison tumour of the pancreas. European J. Clin. Invest. 1, 461-479 (1971).
Creutzfeldt, S., Arnold, R., Creutzfeldt, C., Deuticke, U., Frerichs, H., Track, N.S.: Biochemical and morphological investigations of 30 human insulinomas. Diabetologica 9, 217-231 (1973).
Creutzfeldt, W., Arnold, R., Creutzfeldt, C., Track, N.S.: Pathomorphologic, biochemical and diagnostic aspects of gastrinomas (Zollinger-Ellison syndrome). Human Pathol. 6, 47 (1975).
Croisier, J-C., Lehy, T., Zeitoun, P.: A2 cell pancreatic microadenomas in a case of multiple endocrine adenomatosis. Cancer 28, 707-713 (1971).
Croughs, R.J.M., Hulsmans, H.A.M., Israel, D.E., Hackeng, W.H.L., Schopman, W.: Glucagonoma as part of the polyglandular adenoma syndrome. Amer. J. Med. 52, 690-698 (1972).
Croughs, R.J.M.: Glucagonoma and A cell hyperplasia. Clinics in Gastroenterol. 3, 609-619 (1974).
Davenport, H.A.: Staining nerve fibres in mounted sections with alcoholic silver nitrate solution. Arch. Neurol. Psychiat. 24, 690-695 (1930).
Davis, Z., Moertel, C.G., McIlrath, D.C.: The malignant carcinoid syndrome. Surg. Gynec. Obstet. 137, 637-644 (1973).
Dawson, I.: The endocrine cells of the gastrointestinal tract. Histochem. J. 2, 527-549 (1970).
Dische, F.E.: Argentaffin and non-argentaffin carcinoid tumours of the appendix. J. Clin. Path. 21, 60-66 (1968).
Dockray, G.J., Walsh, J.H., Passaro, E., Jr.: Relative abundance of big and little gastrins in the tumour and blood of patients with the Zollinger-Ellison syndrome. Gut 16, 353-358 (1975).
Dupré, J., Ross, S.A., Watson, J., Brown, J.C.: Stimulation of insulin secretion by gastric inhibitory polypeptide in man. J. Clin. Endocrin. 37, 826 (1973).
Epple, A.: A staining sequence for A, B and D cells of pancreatic islets. Stain Technol. 42, 53-61 (1967).
Erspamer, V., Asero, A.: Identification of enteramine, the specific hormone of the enterochromaffin cell system, as 5-hydroxytyptamine. Nature 169, 800-801 (1952).
Ewen, S.B., Rost, F.D.W.: The histochemical demonstration of catecholamines and tryptamines by acid and aldehyde-induced methods. Microspectrofluorimetric characterisation of the fluorophores in models. Histochem. J. 4, 59-69 (1972).
Falck, B.: Observations on the possibilities of the cellular localisation of monoamines by a fluorescence method. Acta Physiol. scand. 56, Suppl. 197, 1-25 (1962).
Falck, B., Hillarp, N.A., Thieme, G., Torp, A.: Fluorescence of catecholamines and related compounds condensed with formaldehyde. J. Histochem. Cytochem. 10, 348-354 (1962).

Forssmann, W.G., Orci, L., Pictet, R., Renold, A.E., Rouiller, Ch.: The endocrine cells in the epithelium of the gastrointestinal mucosa of the rat. J. Cell. Biol. 40, 492-515 (1969).
Foster, G.V., McIntyre, I., Pearse, A.G.E.: Calcitonin production and the mitochondrion-rich cells of the dog thyroid. Nature 203, 1029-1030 (1964).
Gammill, S.L., Weichert, R.: Common origin for all endocrine tumours. Acta Radiologica (Therapy) 12, 321-326 (1973).
Gammill, S.L., Weichert, R., Smith, S.L., Font, R., Ingraffia, R.: Carcinoid-islet cell tumours. Acta Radiologica (Therapy) 12, 229-240 (1973).
Gleeson, M.H., Bloom, S.R., Polak, J.M., Henry, K., Dowling, R.H.: Endocrine tumour in kidney affecting small bowel structure, motility and absorptive function. Gut 12, 773-782 (1971).
Goldenberg, V.E., Goldenberg, N.S., Benditt, E.P.: Ultrastructural features of functioning α and β cell tumors. Cancer 24, 236-247 (1969).
Gregory, H., Hardy, P.M., Jones, D.S., Kenner, G.W., Sheppard, R.C.: The antral hormone gastrin: structure of gastrin. Nature (Lond.) 204, 931 (1964).
Gregory, R.A., Tracy, H.J.: Isolation of two minigastrins from Zollinger Ellison tumour tissue. Gut 15, 683-685 (1974).
Greider, M.H., Bencosme, S.A., Lechago, J.: The human pancreatic islet cells and their tumours. I. The normal pancreatic islets. Lab. Invest. 22, 344-354 (1970).
Greider, M.H., Steinberg, V., McGuigan, J.E.: Electron microscopic identification of the gastrin cell of the human antral mucosa by means of immunocytochemistry. Gastroenterology 63, 572 (1972).
Greider, M.H., Rosai, J., McGuigan, J.E.: The human pancreatic islet cells and their tumours. II. Ulcerogenic and diarrheogenic tumours. Cancer 33, 1423-1443 (1974).
Grimelius, L.: A modified silver protein method for studying the argyrophil cells of the islet of Langerhans. In: The Structure and Metabolism of the Pancreatic islets.(eds. *S.E. Brolin, B. Hellman, H. Knutson*). Oxford: Pergamon Press 1964.
Grimelius, L.: A silver nitrate stain for α_2 cells in human pancreatic islets. Acta Soc. Med. Upsal. 73, 243-270 (1968).
Gross, M.: Tumeurs carcinoides du rectum. Helvetica Chirurgica Acta 35, 239-248 (1968).
Grossman, M.I., Adelson, J.W., Rothman, S.S., Brown, J.C., Said, S.I., Lin, T-M., Chance, R.E., Gerring, E.L., Gregory, H., Glass, G.B.J., Andersson, S., Nasset, E.S., Sasaki, H., Faloona, G.R., Unger, R.H., Creutzfeldt, M., Kokas, E., Thompson, J.C.: Candidate hormones of the Gut. Gastroenterology 67, 730 (1974).
Håkanson, R., Juhlin, L., Owman, Ch., Sporrong, B.: Histochemistry of histamine: microspectrofluorimetric characterisation of the fluorophores induced by O-phthaldialdehyde. J. Histochem. Cytochem. 18, 93-99 (1970).
Hammar, S., Sale, G.: Multi-hormone-producing islet cell carcinomas of the pancreas. A morphological and biochemical investigation. Human Pathol. 6, 349-362 (1975).
Hattori, S., Matsuda, M., Tateisha, R.: Oat cell carcinoma of the lung containing serotonin granules. Gann 59, 123-129 (1968).
Heitz, Ph., Steiner, H., Halter, F., Egli, P., Kapp, J.P.: Multihormonal, amyloid-producing tumour of the islets of Langerhans in a 12 year old boy. Clinical morphological and biochemical data and review of the literature. Virchow's Archiv A 353, 312-324 (1971).
Hellerström, C., Hellman, B.: Some aspects of silver impregnation of the islets of Langerhans in the rat. Acta Endocrinol. 35, 518-532 (1960).
Hubel, K.A.: Secretin: a long progress note. Gastroenterology 62, 318 (1972).
Isenberg, J.I., Walsh, J.H., Grossman, M.I.: Zollinger-Ellison syndrome. Gastroenterology 65, 140 (1973).

Jones, R.A., Dawson, I.M.P.: The endocrine tumours of the human gastrointestinal tract and other foregut derivatives. In preparation (1976).

Jorpes, E., Mutt, V.: On the biological activity and amino acid composition of secretin. Acta chem. scand. 15, 1790 (1961).

Klein, H.Z.: Mucinous carcinoid tumour of the vermiform appendix. Cancer 33, 770-777 (1974).

Kobayashi, S., Fujita, T., Sasagawa, T.: The endocrine cells of human duodenal mucosa. An electron microscope study. Arch. Histol. (Japan.) 31, 477-494 (1970).

Korman, M.G., Strickland, R.G., Hansky, J.: The functional G cell mass in atrophic gastritis. Gut 13, 349 (1972).

Lacy, P.: Electron microscopy of Beta cells of the pancreas. Amer. J. Med. 31, 851 (1961).

Lacy, P.E.: The secretion of insulin. Diabetes 21 (Suppl. 2), 510 (1972).

Levin, M.E.: Endocrine syndromes associated with pancreatic islet-cell tumours. Med. Clin. N. Amer. 52, 295-312 (1968).

Like, A.A., Orci, L.: Embryogenesis of the human pancreatic islets: a light and electron microscopic study. Diabetes 21 (Suppl. 2), 511 (1972).

Lillie, R.D.: Investigations on the structure of the enterochromaffin substance. J. Histochem. Cytochem. 9, 184-189 (1961a).

Lillie, R.D.: Metal chelation reaction of enterochromaffin. J. Histochem. Cytochem. 9, 44-48 (1961b).

Lillie, R.D., Greco-Henson, J.P., Cason, J.C.: Azo coupling rate of enterochromaffin with various diazonium salts. J. Histochem. Cytochem. 9, 11-21 (1961c).

Lomsky, R., Langr, F., Vortel, V.: Demonstration of glucagon in islet cell adenomas of the pancreas by immunofluorescent technic. Amer. J. Clin. Pathol. 51, 245-260 (1969).

McGavran, M.H., Unger, R.H., Recant, L., Polk, H.C., Kilo, C., Levin, M.E.: A glucagon secreting alpha-cell carcinoma of the pancreas. New Eng. J. Med. 274, 1408-1413 (1966).

McGuigan, J.E.: Gastric mucosal intracellular localisation of gastrin by immunofluorescence. Gastroenterology 55, 315-327 (1968).

McGuigan, J.E., Greider, M.H.: Correlative immunochemical and light microscopic studies of the gastrin cell of the antral mucosa. Gastroenterology 60, 223 (1971).

McGuigan, J.E.: On the distribution and release of gastrin. Gasteroenterology 64, 497 (1973).

McGuigan, J.E., Greider, M.H.: The gastrin cell: characterisation by electron microscopy using specific immunochemical techniques. Clin. Research 20, 461 (abstract) (1973).

Makhlouf, G.M.: The neuroendocrine design of the gut. The play of chemicals in a chemical background. Gastroenterology 67, 159 (1974).

Marks, V., Samols, E.: Insulinoma: natural history and diagnosis. Clinics in Gastroenterol. 3, 559-573 (1974).

Martin, E.D., Potet, F.: Pathology of endocrine tumours of the G.I. tract. Clinics in Gastroenterol. 3, 511 (1974).

Masson, M.P.: La glande endocrinaire de l'intestine chez l'homme. Comptes rendus Acad. Sci., Paris 158, 59-61 (1914).

Murray-Lyon, I.M., Sandler, M., Cheetham, H.D., Watts, J.A.E., Williams, R.: 5 Hydroxy-indol secreting rectal carcinoid tumour. Gut 13, 385-386 (1972).

Nonidez, J.F.: The origin of the 'parafollicular' cell, a second epithelial component of the thyroid gland of the dog. Amer. J. Anat. 49, 479-505 (1931-2).

Omen, G.S.: Ectopic polypeptide hormone production by tumours.Ann. Int. Med. 72, 136 (1970).

Orloff, M.J.: Carcinoid tumours of the rectum. Cancer 28, 175-180 (1971).

Patchefsky, A.S., Solit, R., Phillips, L.D., Craddock, M., Harrer, W.V., Cohn , H.E., Kowlessar, O.D.: Hydroxyindole-producing tumours of the pancreas. Carcinoid islet cell tumour and oat cell carcinoma. Ann. Int. Med. 77, 53-61 (1972).

Patchefsky, A.S., Gordon, G., Harrer, W.V., Hoch, W.S.: Carcinoid tumour of the pancreas. Ultrastructural observations of a lymph node metastasis and comparison with bronchial carcinoid. Cancer 33, 1349 (1974).

Pearse, A.G.E.: Common cytochemical properties of cells producing polypeptide hormones with particular reference to Calcitonin and the thyroid C cells. Vet. Rec. 79, 587-590 (1966).

Pearse, A.G.E.: Common cytochemical and ultrastructural characteristics of cells producing polypeptide hormones (the APUD series) and their relevance to thyroid and ultimobranchial C cells and calcitonin. Proc. R. Soc. B. 170, 71-80 (1968).

Pearse, A.G.E.: The cytochemistry and ultrastructure of polypeptide hormone producing cells (the APUD series) and the embryologic, physiologic and pathologic implications of the concept. J. histochem. cytochem. 17, 303-313 (1969a).

Pearse, A.G.E.: Cytochemical evidence for random coil conformation in the protein precursors of polypeptide hormones. Nature 221, 1969 (1969b).

Pearse, A.G.E., Coulling, I., Weavers, B., Friesen, S.: The endocrine cells of the human stomach, duodenum and jejunum. Gut 11, 649-658 (1970).

Pearse, A.G.E., Polak, J.M.: Neural crest origin of the endocrine polypeptide (APUD) cells of the gastrointestinal tract and pancreas. Gut 12, 783 (1971).

Pearse, A.G.E., Polak, J.M., Heath, C.M.: Development, differentiation and derivation of the endocrine polypeptide cells of the mouse pancreas. (Immunofluorescence, cytochemical and ultrastructural studies). Diabetologia 9, 120-129 (1973).

Polak, J.M., Coulling, I., Doe, W., Pearse, A.G.E.: The G cells in pernicious anaemia. Gut 12, 319-323 (1971a).

Polak, J.M., Bloom, S., Coulling, I., Pearse, A.G.E.: Immunofluorescent localisation of enteroglucagon cells in the gastrointestinal tract of the dog. Gut 12, 311-318 (1971b).

Polak, J.M., Bloom, S., Coulling, I., Pearse, A.G.E.: Immunofluorescent localization of secretin in the canine duodenum. Gut 12, 605-610 (1971c).

Polak, J.M., Stagg, B., Pearse, A.G.E.: Two types of Zollinger Ellison syndrome; immunofluorescent, cytochemical and ultrastructural studies of the antral and pancreatic gastrin cells in different clinical states. Gut 13, 501 (1972).

Polak, J.M., Bloom, S.R., Kuzio, M., Brown, J.C., Pearse, A.G.E.: Cellular localisation of gastric inhibitory polypeptide in the duodenum and jejunum. Gut 14, 284-288 (1973).

Polak, J.M., Pearse, A.G.E., Garaud, J.C., Bloom, S.R.: Cellular localisation of a vasoactive intestinal peptide in the mammalian and avian gastrointestinal tract. Gut 15, 720-724 (1974).

Polak, J., Pearse, A.G.E., Grimelius, L., Bloom, S.R., Arimura, A.: Growth-hormone-release inhibiting hormone in gastrointestinal and pancreatic D cells. Lancet 1975 I a, 1220-1222.

Polak, J.M., Pearse, A.G.E., Heath, C.M.: Complete identification of endocrine cells in the gastrointestinal tract using semithin-thin sections to identify motilin cells in human and animal intestine. Gut 16, 225-229 (1975b).

Quan, S.H.Q., Bader, G., Berg, J.W.: Carcinoid tumours of the rectum. Dis. Col. Rect. 7, 197-206 (1964).

Rehfeld, J.F.: Three components of gastrin in human serum: gel filtration studies on the molecular size of immunoreactive serum gastrin. Biochim. biophys. Acta (Amst.) 285, 364 (1972).

Robinson, G., Dawson, I.: Immunochemical studies of the endocrine cells of the gastro-intestinal tract. J. Clin. Pathol. 28, 631-635 (1975).
Robinson, G., Dawson, I.M.P.: "So called Type I Zollinger Ellison syndrome". In preparation (1976).
Royston, C.M.S., Brew, D.St.J., Garnham, J.R., Stagg, B.H., Polak, J.: The Zollinger Ellison syndrome due to an infiltrating tumour of the stomach. Gut 13, 638 (1972).
Rubin, B., Engel, S.L., Drungis, A.M., Dzelzkalns, M., Grigas, E.O., Waugh, M.H., Yiacas, E.: Cholecystokinin-like activities in guinea pigs and in dogs of the C-terminal octopeptide (SQ 19, 844) of cholecystokinin. J. Pharm. Sci. 58, 955 (1969).
Rubin, W.: Endocrine cells in the normal human stomach. A fine structural study. Gastroenterology 63, 784 (1972).
Said, S.I., Mutt, V.: Potent peripheral and splanchnic vasodilator peptide from normal gut. Nature (Lond.) 225, 863 (1970a).
Said, S.I., Mutt, V.: Polypeptide with broad biological activity: isolation from small intestine. Science (Wash.) 169, 1217 (1970b).
Schein, P.S., Delellis, R.A., Kahn, C.R., Gorden, P., Kraft, A.R.: Islet cell tumours: current concepts and management. Ann. Int. Med. 79, 239-257 (1973).
Schulte, W.J., Hensley, G., Garancis, J.C., Wilson, S.D., Ellison, E.H.: Zollinger-Ellison syndrome: Clinical and histopathological manifestations. Amer. J. Surg. 117, 866-875 (1969).
Sevier, A., Munger, B.C.: A silver method for paraffin sections of neural tissue. J. Neuro. Path. Exp. Neurol. 24, 130-135 (1965).
Shimke, R.N., Hartmann, W.H., Prout, T.E., Rimoin, D.L.: Syndrome of bilateral phaeochromocytoma, medullary thyroid carcinoma and multiple neuromas. A possible regulatory defect in the differentiation of chromaffin tissue. New Eng. J. Med. 279, 1-6 (1968).
Singh, I.: A modification of the Masson-Hamperl method for staining of argentaffin cells. Anat. Anz. 115, 81-82 (1964).
Sircus, W.: Peptide-secreting tumours with special reference to the pancreas. Gut 10, 506-515 (1969).
Sircus, W., Brunt, P.W., Walker, R.J., Small, W.P., Falconer, C.W.A., Thomson, C.G.: Two cases of "pancreatic cholera" with features of peptide-secreting adenomatosis of the pancreas. Gut 11, 197-205 (1970).
Soga, J., Tazawa, K.: Pathologic analysis of carcinoid. Histologic re-evaluation of 62 cases. Cancer 28, 998 (1971).
Soga, J., Tazawa, K., Aizawa, O., Wada, K., Tuto, T.: Argentaffin cell adenocarcinoma of the stomach: an atypical carcinoid? Cancer 28, 999-1003 (1971).
Solcia, E., Sampietro, R.: On the nature of the metachromatic cells of pancreatic islets. Z. Zellforsch. 65, 131-138 (1965a).
Solcia, E., Sampietro, R.: Cytochemical observations on pancreatic islets with reference to some endocrine-like cells of the gastric mucosa. Z. Zellforsch. 68, 689-698 (1965b).
Solcia, E., Vassallo, G., Capella, C.: Selective staining of endocrine cells by basic dyes after acid hydrolysis. Stain Technol. 43, 257-263 (1968).
Solcia, E., Forssmann, W.G., Pearse, A.G.E.: In: *Creutzfeldt, W., Gregory, R.A., Grossman, M.I., Pearse, A.G.E.* (eds.). Origin, Chemistry, Physiology and Pathophysiology of the Gastrointestinal Hormones. Proceedings of International Symposium, Wiesbaden 1969, p. 95. Stuttgart: Schattauer 1970.
Solcia, E., Pearse, A.G.E., Grube, D., Kobayashi, S., Bussolati, G., Creutzfeldt, W., Gepts, W.: Revised Wiesbaden classification of gut endocrine cells. Rendiconti di gastro-enterologia 5, 13-16 (1973).

Spence, R.W., Burns-Cox, C.J.: ACTH-secreting "apudoma" of gall bladder. Gut 16, 473-476 (1975).
Subbuswamy, S.G., Gibbs, N.M., Ross, C.F., Morson, B.C.: Goblet cell carcinoid of the appendix. Cancer 34, 338 (1974).
Suzuki, H., Matsuyama, M.: Ultrastructure of functioning β cell tumours of the pancreatic islets. Cancer (Philad.) 28, 1302-1313 (1971).
Tardini, A., Anversa, P., Bordi, C.: Ultrastructure of multiple pancreatic tumours in a case of Zollinger Ellison syndrome. Amer. J. Clin. Pathol. 52, 25-36 (1969).
Toner, P.G.: Fine structure of argyrophil and argentaffin cells in the gastrointestinal tract of the fowl. Z. Zellforsch. 63, 830-839 (1964).
Unger, R.H., Ohneda, A., Valverde, I., Eisentraut, A.M., Exton, J.: Characterisation of the responses of circulating glucagon-like immunoreactivity to intraduodenal and intravenous administration of glucose. J. Clin. invest. 47, 48 (1968).
Valverde, I., Rigopoulou, D., Exton, J., Ohneda, A., Eisentraut, A., Unger, R.H.: Demonstration and characterisation of a second fraction of glucagon-like immunoreactivity in jejunal extracts. Amer. J. med. Sci. 255, 415 (1968).
Vance, J.E., Stoll, R.W., Kitabchi, A.E., Williams, R.H., Wood, F.C.: Nesidioblastosis in familial endocrine adenomatosis. J. Amer. Med. Assoc. 207, 1679-1682 (1969).
Vassallo, G., Solcia, E., Bussolati, G., Polak, J.M., Pearse, A.G.E.: Non G cell gastrin-producing tumours of the pancreas. Virchow's Archiv Abt. B. Zellpath. 11, 66-79 (1972).
Verner, J.V., Morrison, A.B.: Islet cell tumor and a syndrome of refractory watery diarrhoea and hypokalaemia. Amer. J. Med. 25, 374-380 (1958).
Verner, J.V., Morrison, A.B.: Non β islet cell tumours and the syndrome of watery diarrhoea, hypokalaemia and hypochlorhydria. Clinics in Gastroenterol. 3, 595-608 (1974a).
Verner, J.V., Morrison, A.B.: Endocrine pancreatic islet disease with diarrhoea: report of a case due to diffuse hyperplasia of non β islet tissue with a review of 54 additional cases. Arch. Int. Med. 133, 492-500 (1974b).
Walsh, J.H., Grossman, M.I.: Circulating gastrin in peptic ulcer disease. Mount Sinai J. Med. 40, 374 (1973).
Weichert, R.F. III: The neuroectodermal origin of the peptide-secreting endocrine glands. Amer. J. Med. 49, 232-241 (1970).
Weichert, R.F., Roth, L.M., Kremientz, E.T., Hewitt, R.L., Drapadas, T.: Carcinoid islet cell tumours of the duodenum. Report of 21 cases. Amer. J. Surg. 121, 195-205 (1971).
Wermer, P.: Genetic aspects of adenomatosis of endocrine glands. Amer. J. Med. 16, 363 (1954).
Whalen, G.E.: Editorial: Glucagon and the small gut. Gastroenterology 67, 1284 (1974).
Williams, E.D., Sandler, M.: The classification of carcinoid tumours. Lancet 1963 I, 238.
Yalow, R.S., Berson, S.A.: And now "big big" gastrin. Biochem. biophys. Res. Commun. 48, 391 (1972).
Yalow, R.S., Wu, N.: Additional studies on the nature of big big gastrin. Gastroenterology 65, 19 (1973).
Yoshinaga, T., Okuna, G., Shinji, Y., Tsujii, T., Mishikawa, M.: Pancreatic A cell tumour associated with severe diabetes mellitus. Diabetes 15, 709 (1966).

Immunological Aspects of Gastro-Intestinal Pathology

J.M. SKINNER and R. WHITEHEAD

The bulk of the investigations into the immunological status of patients with gastro-intestinal disease have concerned evaluation of changes in circulating antibodies. In ulcerative colitis and Crohn's disease for example antibody formation to food antigens (*Taylor* and *Truelove,* 1961; *Wright* and *Truelove*, 1965, 1966) to bacterial antigens (*Lagercrantz* et al., 1968; *Thayer* et al., 1969) and to colonic epithelial cell antigens (*Broberger* and *Perlmann,* 1959, 1962; *Harrison,* 1965; *Marcusson* and *Nerup*, 1973) have been described. Similarly, in coeliac disease serum antibodies against gluten, fractions of it, and against reticulin and other proteins have been identified (*Seah* et al., 1971). There have also been studies of peripheral blood lymphocytes in a variety of disorders. Although lymphocyte numbers do not alter, changes in function have been recorded. Lymphocyte cytotoxicity for colonic epithelium has been described in ulcerative colitis and Crohn's disease (*Watson* et al., 1966; *Shorter* et al., 1968). Transformation of the lymphocyte to a blastoid form in response to non-specific antigens, for example, phytohaemaglutinin and to specific fractions of bacterial and colonic cells has been noted (*Hinz* et al., 1967; *Stefani* and *Fink*, 1967). Other lymphocyte functions such as the skin response to application of dinitrochlorobenzene (DNCB) (*Verrier-Jones* et al., 1969) to injections of Tuberculin (*Fletcher* and *Hinton*, 1967), and Kveim reagent (*Mitchell* et al., 1970; *Siltzbach* et al., 1971) have also been studied. The results have often been contradictory and have not added significantly to our understanding of the immunological mechanisms concerned in gastro-intestinal diseases. In some instances, however, the study of antibodies actually in the gut secretions themselves have resulted in useful diagnostic information, for example, pernicious anaemia (*Wright* et al., 1966) in others, e.g. coeliac disease they have once more produced largely unhelpful information (*Fry* et al., 1967; *Douglas* et al., 1970).

Little attention has been given to the detailed morphological examination of the gut lymphoid tissue or the mesenteric lymph nodes until recently. Following the work of *Cottier* et al. (1972) it is now possible for example to apply strict criteria to the histological examination of lymph nodes which are meaningful in terms of immunological function. In addition, by the application of immunohistochemical methods the exact secretory function of gut immunocytes can be defined in terms of antibody production and immunoglobulin type. Moreover, by using morphometric methods the number of immunocytes can be accurately counted and their changes monitored in sequential studies. In order to be able to recognise changes of this sort in disease processes it is necessary first to define the limits of normality in both its anatomical and physiological aspects.

I. The Anatomy of the Gut Lymphoid System

In the adult gut the immunocytes are distributed along its entire length. In addition to the discrete lymphoid follicles there are immunologically competent cells scattered diffusely

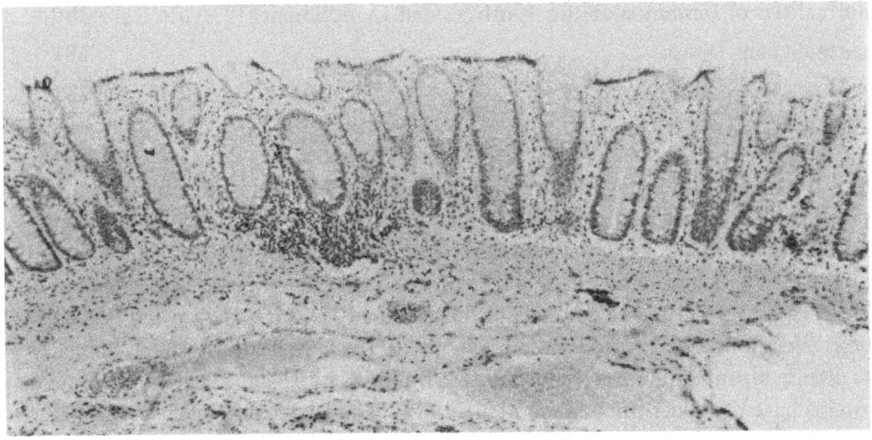

Fig. 1a. A section of normal human colon (H + E). In the epithelial layer (E) there are a few intra epithelial lymphocytes, rather more would be found in the small intestine. In the lamina propria are lymphocytes and plasma cells. The lymphoid follicle is shown in contact with muscularis mucosa and is in the unstimulated state. When stimulated a germinal centre appears, as is the case in follicles within lymph nodes

throughout the lamina propria (Fig. 1) and to a lesser extent in the submucosa. This tissue constitutes 25% of the mass of the gastro-intestinal tract (*Ferguson*, 1972). The lymphoid follicles have a germinal centre when stimulated and a surrounding cuff of small lymphocytes similar to the cortical follicles in lymph nodes. In comparison with other tissues, the permanent population of lymphocytes and plasma cells in the gut wall is almost unique. For in other situations they only appear in significant numbers in response to a specific stimulus. The situation in the bronchial tree is somewhat similar but the numbers of cells is much smaller and it is pertinent that this is also a foregut derivative. An important part of the diffuse gut immunocyte system is formed by those cells which actually appear between the surface epithelial cells. They have been designated "theliolymphocytes" by *Fichtelius* (1968) and occur in a ratio of up to 1 for every 6 epithelial cells.

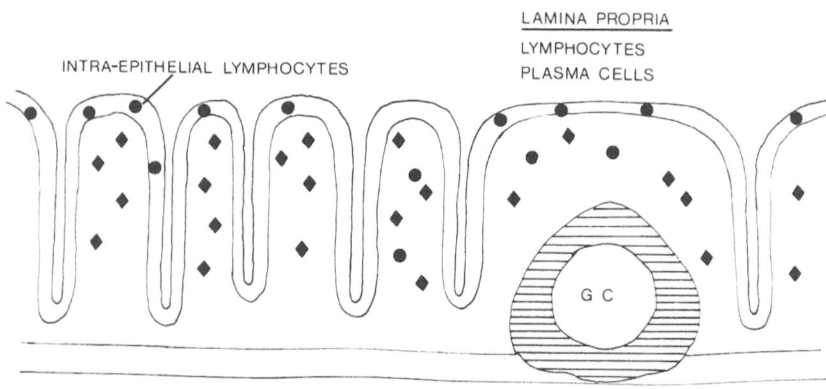

Fig. 1b. A diagramatic representation of the distribution of lymphoid tissue elements in the human colon

1. Development

There is little quantitative information available concerning the development of the gut immune system and most of it is the result of animal observations (*Perey* and *Good*, 1968), which cannot necessarily be extrapolated to man. In the most detailed yet qualitative study by *Kyriazis* and *Esterly* (1970, 1971) it was noted that recognisable lymphocytes appeared in the thymus at the 9 mm (6 weeks gestation) stage of embryonic development but not in the gut. By the 80 mm stage (10 weeks gestation) lymphocytes were recognisable in the tonsils and possibly also in the lamina propria of the bowel. Lymphoid follicles were not seen until the 14 week stage of gestation and recognisable plasma cells not until around 40 weeks and then they were present only in small numbers. In a study of fresh autopsy material *Cornes* (1965) recorded an average of 45 Peyer's patches at the 24 weeks stage of gestation in each gut rising to about 240 patches in the gut at puberty, the patches becoming larger after birth. Neonatal studies indicate that plasma cells in significant numbers are not seen until about the month after birth (*Kyriazis* and *Esterly*, 1971). However, it should be remembered that the observations have been made on post mortem material and the results need not necessarily reflect the normal situation. It would seem possible, however, that the arrival of immunocytes in the lamina propria and the colonisation of the gut by bacteria and other organisms are connected.

2. Functional Anatomy

The lymphoid tissue of the gastro-intestinal tract has an important immunological role as part of the peripheral lymphoid system (*Ferguson*, 1972). It has been shown, for example, that in the absence of a thymus in experimental animals or in DiGeorge's syndrome in humans the tight lymphocyte cuff of the lymphoid follicles is absent (*Perey* and *Good*, 1968). Moreover when the bone marrow is ablated in animals or there is congenital agammaglobulinaemia in man plasma cells are absent from the lamina propria (*Good* et al., 1968). The plasma cells in the lamina propria are concerned in the formation of secretory immunoglobulins (*Tomasi*, 1972) as well as some which circulate. The secretory antibodies are the most important component of the "antiseptic paint" (*Heremans* et al., 1968) which lines the bowel and acts as a layer protecting the body from the intestinal contents. The plasma cells which produce these antibodies are part of the B cell system (*Nossal* and *Ada*, 1971; *Ferguson* and *Parrott*, 1972). "Theliocytes" on the other hand, are part of the T cell system and the strongest evidence for this is their decrease in number in thymectomised animals (*Fichtelius* et al., 1968; *Nossal* and *Ada*, 1971).

There have been suggestions that part of the lymphoid tissue of the gut, e.g. the central parts of Peyer's patches and the lymphocytes closely associated with the overlying epithelium, together with the appendiceal lymphoid tissue have a central lymphoid role analogous to the bursa of Fabricius in birds (*Perey* and *Good*, 1968; *Gatti* et al., 1970), i.e. they are responsible for the origin of B cells. A similar role in man has been suggested but as yet there is no evidence for it. There is no congenital defect comparable to the DiGeorge syndrome, an absence of B cells, in which Peyer's patches and the appendiceal lymphoid tissue are entirely absent.

II. The Circulation of Gut Lymphoid Cells

A diagrammatic representation of the circulation of gut lymphocytes is shown in Figure 2. Lymphocytes arrive in the mucosa via the blood stream and some pass out through the capillary walls into the lamina propria, where a proportion differentiate into plasma cells (*Hall* et al., 1968; *Halstead* and *Hall*, 1972). The differentiation may, however, be initiated before the cells reach the lamina propria (*Hall* et al., 1968). Some lymphocytes return to the main circulation via the central lacteal and other pass thsrough the basement membrane to appear between the epithelial cells (*Andrew*, 1965). These "theliocytes" are carried in the stream of migration of epithelial cells towards the surface and are finally shed in the bowel lumen. This enteric loss has been measured by a radioactive technique (*Weetman* et al., 1974) and amounts to a normal daily loss of about 0.05% of estimated total lymphocytes.

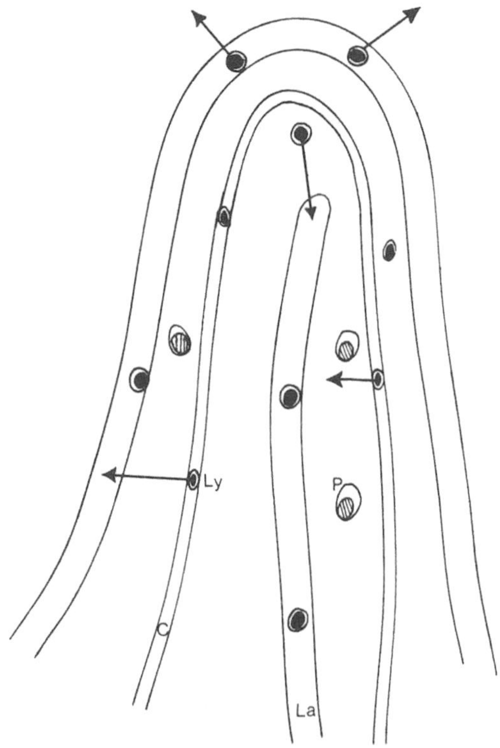

Fig. 2. Diagram to illustrate the circulation of lymphoid cells in the gut. Lymphocytes reach the mucosa via the blood stream and pass out of the capillaries into lamina propria. Some pass the basement membrane into the epithelial layer, some remain in the lamina propria, some recirculate, first leaving the mucosa via the central lacteal. The precursors of plasma cells arrive in the lamina propria via the capillaries

Plasma cells are not thought to recirculate to any great degree and only very small numbers appear in the thoracic duct lymph, and the small numbers of immunoblasts found in the thoracic duct lymph "home" to the gut on reinjection and do not reappear there (*Gowans* and *Knight*, 1964). There is evidence that intracellular immunoglobulin is degraded by proteases and cathepsin D from lysozymes (*Menninger*, 1974) and it is likely that a combination of the "ecotactic" mechanism attracting and keeping plasma cells in the lamina propria (*De Sousa*, 1971) and proteolytic activity causes a local destruction and disappearance of plasma cells.

III. The Secretory Immune System

The concept of a separate secretory immunological system followed a demonstration that the immunoglobulin content of certain external secretions, mainly saliva, colostrum and jejunal juice had a different immunoglobulin composition from serum or internal secretions such as synovial fluid. The most notable difference was that the main component of external secretions was IgA where as this immunoglobulin amounts to only 10% or 15% of total serum immunoglobulins. Clearly simple exudation of serum immunoglobulins cannot explain the composition of the external fluids. This subject has been extensively reviewed by *Tomasi* (1972). Secretory IgA of molecular weight 400,000 has a sedimentation coefficient on ultracentrifugation of II Svedberg units. This 11S IgA is different from serum IgA (7S) which has a molecular weight of 150,000. It has been shown that secretory IgA is a dimer (10S) of two 7S molecules which is produced in the plasma cells of the lamina propria and is then attached to the secretory component (SC) and secreted into the lumen as 11S secretory immunoglobulin (Fig. 3). The secretory component is formed in the epithelial cells

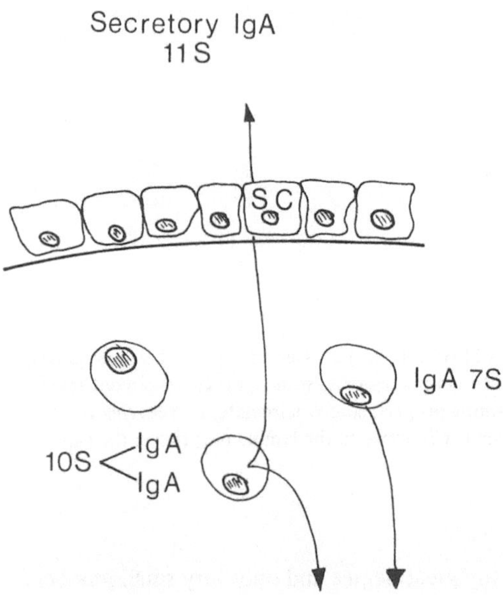

Fig. 3. A diagramatic representation to illustrate the site of production of IgA in plasma cells of the lamina propria and its transport into the gut lumen (10S dimer plus secretor component (SC)) or blood vessels (10S and 7S types)

and it is likely that 10S dimeric IgA is attached to the secretory component in these cells though it is possible that the combination occurs in the lamina propria just below the basement membrane. The secretory IgA probably reaches the lumen by reversed pinocytosis. The secretory component has an affinity only for the dimeric form of IgA. This is produced within plasma cells as such and not by combination of 7S molecules in the interstitium as is shown by the fact that a single molecule of secretory IgA contains either Kappa or Lambda light chains but never both. Indeed it has been possible to show that 2 types of IgA producing cells can be detected in the lamina propria using fluorescein labeled secretory component as a marker. A few cells make 7S IgA but the majority make 10S IgA (*Brandtzaeg*, 1973). It has further been suggested that it is another component, the "J" chain which helps in the polymerisation of IgA to which secretory component attaches. This has also been used to explain the avidity of IgM (a 5 component polymer with J chain) for secretory component and also explains the presence of IgM attached to secretory component in external secretions.

Secretory IgA has some unique biological properties. It has a chemical structure which is particularly stable and resists enzyme degradation (*Brandtzaeg*, 1972), an obvious advantage in the proteolytic environment of the gut lumen. The secretory IgA molecules has 4 antigen combining sites and is more efficient in agglutination reactions than either 7S IgA or IgG. It has been shown to have antibody affinity to viruses as well as bacteria and to a wide variety of other antigens (*Bienenstock*, 1974). Current opinion is weighted against its ability to opsonize for phagocytosis (*Zipursky* et al., 1973) and it will not activate complement via the classical pathway (*Colten* et al., 1973) or via the alternative pathway as in the case of 7S IgA. Secretory IgA blocks bacterial adherence to mucosal surfaces (*Williams*, 1972) and may inhibit bacterial growth or alter their growth characteristics (*Brandtzaeg*, 1968). By combining with various food antigens it may well interfere with their absorption and their ability to initiate possible harmfull systemic immune responses of various types. IgA deficient infants for example frequently become atopic in later life.

The main functions of the gut immune system appear to be to provide a barrier to the absorption of antigens in the gut. In this capacity it appears to be extremely efficient because after oral ingestion only small amounts of dietary protein can ever be detected in the circulation (*Walker* et al., 1972).

Whereas the main barrier to absorption of antigens is mechanical, i.e. the surface epithelium, inevitably some penetration occurs (*Warshaw* et al., 1971). This is dealt with either by locally sensitised lymphocytes, or by a combination with preformed antibodies, or by the ingestion of complexes by macrophages. The secretory immunoglobulins give local protection and generally are formed in greater amounts following local are opposed to systemic immunisation (*Crabbé* et al., 1969; *Werner* et al., 1971; *Brandtzaeg*, 1972). Moreover immunisation at a single site will result in antibody producing cells throughout the whole bowel (*Ferguson* and *Parrott*, 1972). However, parenteral immunisation can stimulate the production of bowel secretory antibody. The importance of this is seen in the work of *Hall* and *Smith*, (1970). They showed that in rats tritiated thymidine labeled immunoblasts harvested from antigen stimulated lymph nodes when reinjected into syngeneic strains localised in a regular and reproducible manner. Twenty per cent of the injected cells were found in the small gut lamina propria, 2.8% in the spleen, 2.7% in the large gut and only 2.5% in the rest of the lymphoid tissue as a whole. In the bowel most were recognisable as plasma cells and in some instances it was possible to demonstrate antibody activity against the injected antigens, for example Brucella abortus. In passing it has been shown that T immunoblasts also show a non-specific gut localisation, in this case to Peyer's patches (*Sprent* and *Miller*, 1972; *Parrott* and *Ferguson*, 1974). In short, the gut associated lymphoid system forms an extremely important part and arguably the most important part of the body's peripheral immune system.

IV. Morphological Methods in the Study of the Gut Immune System in Man

1. Immunochemical Methods

From the above it is clear that the normal morphological parameters have yet to be defined and much has still to be done in this field. Abnormalities are best shown by objective techniques, for example the presence or absence of a single feature, but when changes involve similar cells or tissues to a different degree then quantitative methods are required. Most work to date has concentrated on plasma cells rather than lymphocytes because it is this cell which produces immunoglobulin, making a positive identification of the cell easy.

There are a number of histochemical methods that can be used to identify plasma cells, e.g. the Methyl green/Pyronin technique, but they are non-specific and give positive results with any cell which is actively synthesizing protein, e.g. the erythroblast. More specific methods have been developed which utilise the fact that plasma cells produce immunoglobulin and this large molecule is itself antigenic. The immunofluorescence method of *Coons* (1942, 1958) can thus be applied. Antibodies raised in other animals against the specific immunoglobulin classes ($\alpha\ \gamma\ \mu\ \delta\ \epsilon\ \kappa\ \lambda$) can be conjugated with fluorescein isothiocyanate and then can be used to specifically identify the plasma cells in the tissues which contain the immunoglobulin providing that suitable control experiments are incorporated in the tests (*Nairn*, 1969). This method, known as the direct immunofluorescence method is easy to control but gives a less intense fluorescence in general than the recently more widely used indirect method (Fig. 4). Both techniques are usually applied to frozen unfixed tissue sections but have the defect that cell outlines are indistinct because of diffusion of

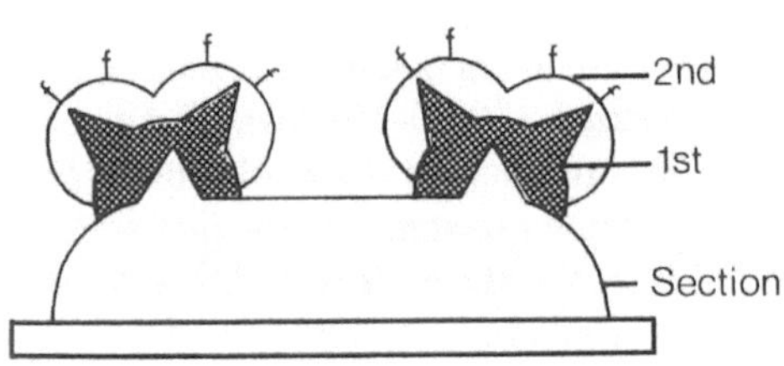

Fig. 4. Diagram to illustrate the layers of the indirect immunofluorescence "sandwich". The working dilutions of reagents used in each layer are determined by previous titration experiments. The second layer shows the fluoresceinated antibody – f

the proteins in the aqueous solutions employed. Counting of positive cells thus becomes difficult and tedious as *Crabbé* et al. (1965) noted in their original study. The use of cold alcohol fixation (4°C) followed by a cold paraffin embedding technique (*Ste Marie*, 1962), was an improvement in that cell outlines were better preserved and surrounding structures more easily identified (Fig. 5) and until recently this was the method of choice. For the purpose of quantitation, however, fluorescence techniques have a further drawback. Fluorescence fades rapidly and the time available for accurate cell counting is limited. It is thus

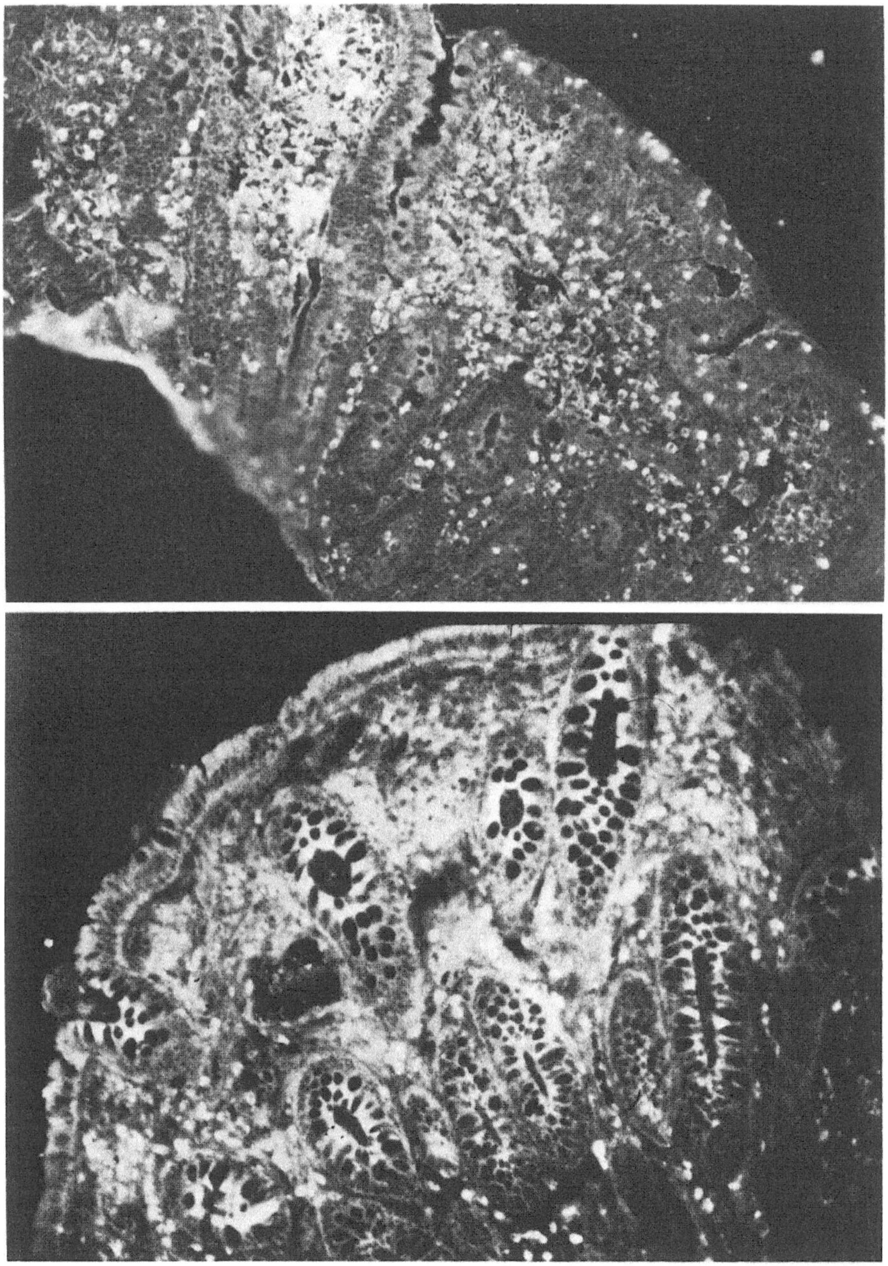

Fig. 5a and b. Colon, processed by the Ste Marie method and stained using the indirect immunofluorescence method to demonstrate IgA in plasma cells in the lamina propria and in the superficial epithelial cells

necessary to photograph many different fields so that permanent preparations, in photographic form, can be used for quantitation. This is in itself time consuming and expensive,

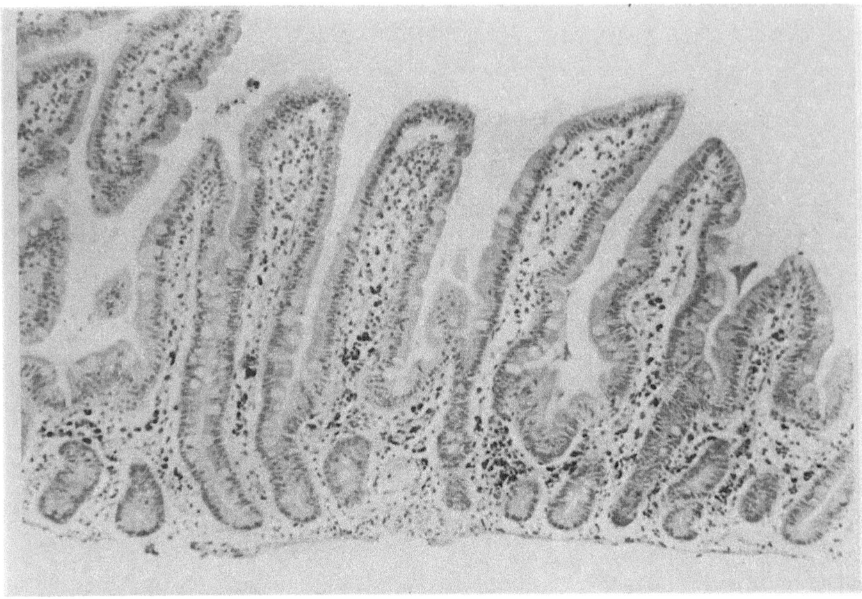

Fig. 6a-c. Sections of bowel, fixed by formalin and processed in the routine manner, and stained by the indirect method using horseradish peroxidase as the label instead of fluorescein. The preparation obtained is permanent and easily quantified. The photographs show cells stained with antibody raised in rabbits to α, γ, μ heavy chain components (Dakopatts A/S) followed by swine anti-rabbit IgG conjugated to horseradish peroxidase.
Section (a) is of normal jejunum and shows the IgA cells clustered mainly at the base of the villi. There is a light degree of staining of the epithelial cells and brush border

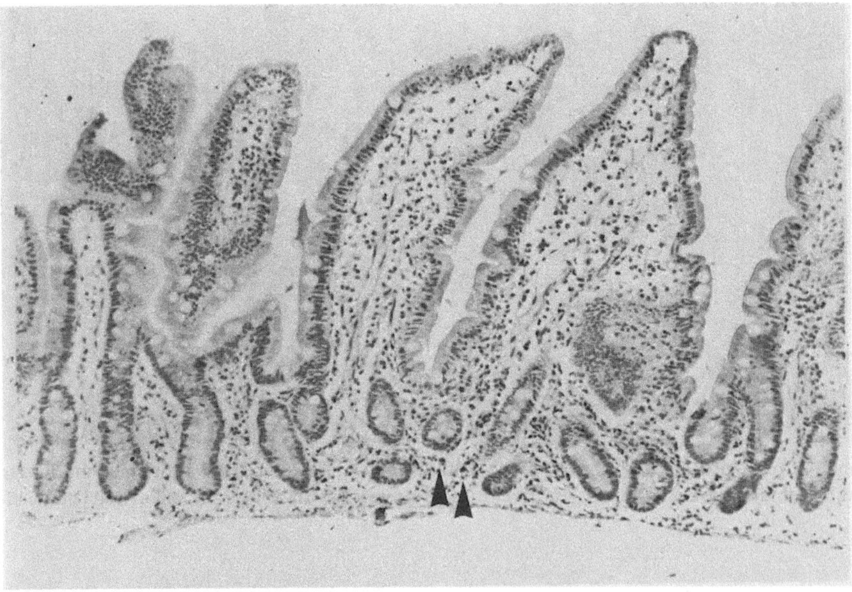

Fig. 6b. Section (b) is of normal bowel stained to show IgG. Very few cells are positive and the staining is faint (arrow)

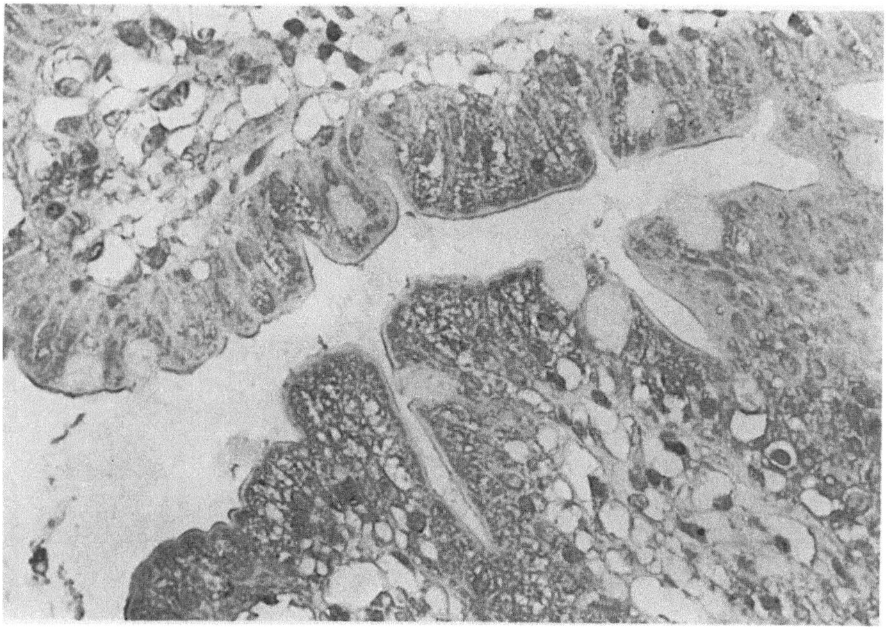

Fig. 6c. Section (c) – high power to show IgM staining. Note the staining of the brush border and epithelial cell cytoplasm similar to the distribution of IgA

making large scale surveys difficult. More recently an alternative immunohistochemical method using the enzyme horse-radish peroxidase as a label rather than fluorescein has been available (*Nakane*, 1966) and has been further developed (*Taylor* and *Burns*, 1974) (Fig. 6).

The technique depends on the same principle as the fluorescence method but the site of the immunological reaction is identified by developing the peroxidase activity using a suitable substrate (e.g. diaminobenzidine), which gives a brown precipitate. The preparation is permanent, can be visualised with a routine light microscope, and because the surrounding tissues are clearly outlined the positive cells can be accurately quantified. There is a further advantage in that routine formalin-fixed paraffin embedded sections can be used (*Burns*, 1975a, b) and providing it is not too old material collected in previous years, can be examined. The criticism of using fixed tissues is that complement is said to be destroyed and thus cannot be demonstrated. However, even in frozen material complement could only be visualised unequivocally if it lay within the blood vessels of gut tissues.

2. Quantitative Methods

The first attempt to quantify the plasma cells of the gut wall was by *Crabbé* et al. (1965), using what was basically a planimetric method (Fig. 7) (*Søltoft*, 1969, 1972). This was extremely time consuming and the authors noted a pronounced fatigue which has an inherent tendency to cause considerable observor error. A second method and one which is still widely

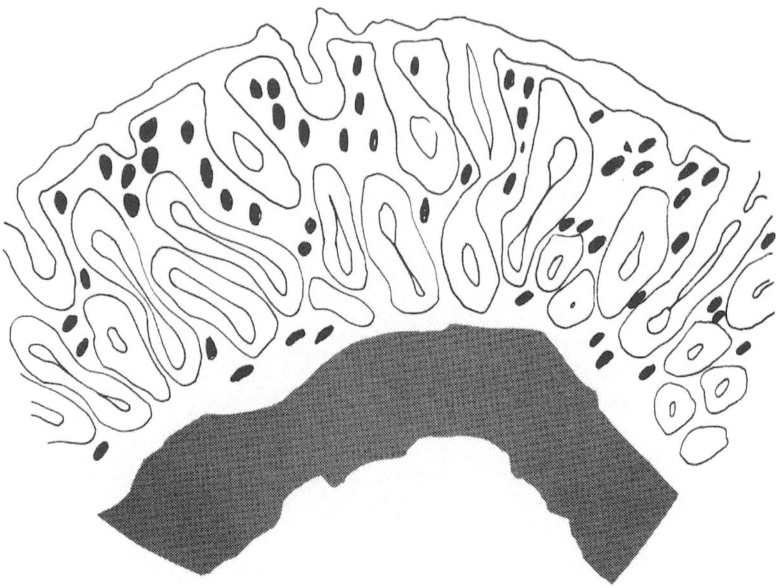

Fig. 7. Diagram of colon showing plasma cells in the lamina propria (black dots), epithelium (white) and muscularis mucosa (grey). Cell densities can be estimated by defining the area of lamina propria using a planimetric method and counting the number of cells within the same field of view. (See text)

favoured is based upon the use of counting grids incorporated into the microscope eyepiece (*Binder*, 1970). An area of lamina propria is estimated by counting the number of small squares of known size which lie on it, and in this area the number of plasma cells is evaluated and expressed as number per unit area, or, if the section thickness is known as number per unit volume (Fig. 8). Because of the structure of the gut mucosa difficulty is met due to squares falling partially on epithelium, particularly in the normal situation, and errors arise because of the need to guess the proportion of the small square which lies on epithelium rather than lamina propria. This can be overcome in two ways, firstly by examining only squares which fall on lamina propria, but this imposes limitations of sampling. Secondly it can be overcome by using extremely small squares but this then introduces the same drawback as planimetry, namely observor fatigue, due to the necessity to count large numbers of squares.

The method of choice is based upon the principle of point counting (*Weibel*, 1963). A grid composed of a number of regularly dispersed points is cast at random onto the tissue to be assessed. The number of points falling on any component of the tissue is proportional to its volume (Fig. 9). It follows that if a particular number of points is counted this will always correspond to a fixed tissue volume. In this volume it is then possible to count the number of plasma cells, the results being expressed as cells per unit volume (for example, number of cells per 1,000 points on lamina propria). This method clearly is not an attempt to derive absolute figures but does allow an accurate and reproducible comparison between specimens. If, in a given study, there is a gross alteration of a particular histological component by a disease process a simple assessment of cell density may be misleading. For ex-

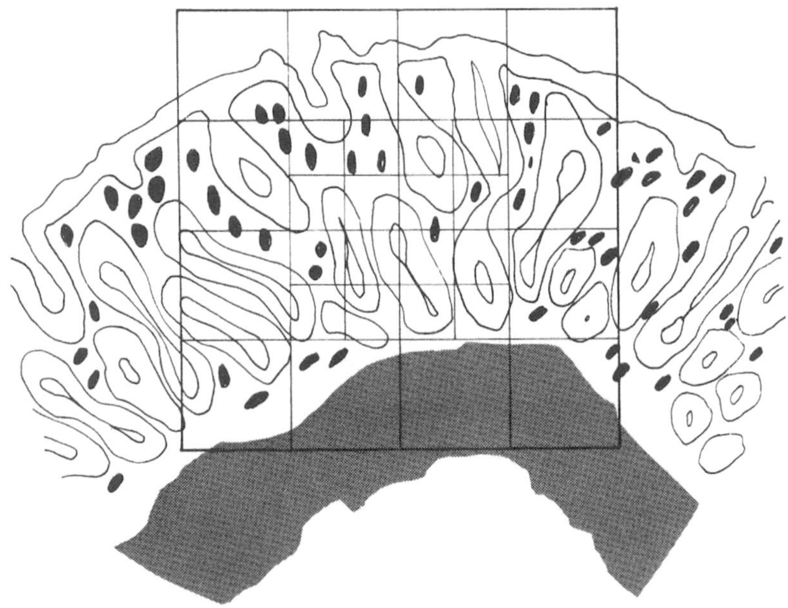

Fig. 8. Diagram to show the principle of cell density estimations using an eyepiece grid with squares of known size. Unless the squares are small large errors can occur in estimating the amount of epithelium present in relation to lamina propria within each square of the grid

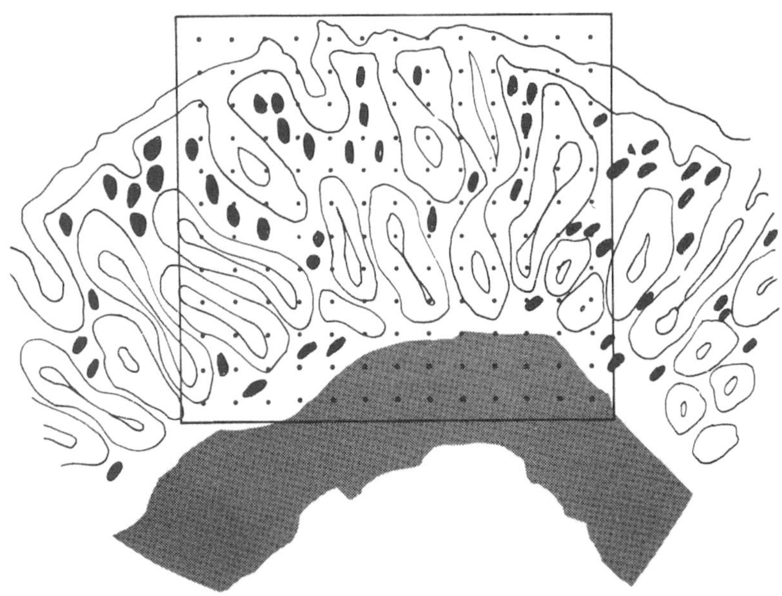

Fig. 9. Diagram to show the principle of point counting in estimating plasma cell density. The number of points falling on lamina propria is proportional to its volume. The number of cells in a given volume can then be calculated and a density figure derived. This can be used to compare normal and abnormal specimens

ample, if in a comparison of ulcerative colitis cases, the mucosa is extremely thin and atropic in one and of normal thickness or thickened in another, a measurement of cell density may be the same but it is clear that the number of cells will be different. In order to account for this it is necessary to include a further morphometric principle, that is the linear intercept. In this instance the aim is to count the number of cells overlying a given surface area of muscularis mucosa or other histological structure not affected by the disease process. This area is determined by counting the number of intercepts through the surface of the muscularis or similar structure made by randomly placed lines of known length (*Weibel*, 1963). Thus a given area is defined by a fixed number of intercepts and cell counts are related to this. The point or line density used in the grid is determined empirically choosing a density which gives the greatest accuracy within the amount of tissue available for examination. The accuracy is easily tested using the principle of summation averages (*Chalkley*, 1943).

It can usefully be stressed again that these methods do not purport to give absolute values. To assign absolute values to the measurements obtained by any of these techniques requires a knowledge of section thickness, which must be of low order in comparison to the size of cells counted, the exact area of the grid used, and the precise magnification. Most of all the tissue shrinkage between the time of biopsy and examination on the slide must be known. This requirement is almost impossible to meet. Sections have to be cut at random angles throughout the block (*Hennig*, 1956) a factor which of itself is wasteful of the tissue to be examined. Consequently, non-absolute techniques are the choice methods for any studies involving more than a few specimens. Abnormal tissue should ideally always be compared with normal control material. Sometimes as already stated there will be some difficulty in the choice of method because of alteration of the histological structure by the disease process. When choosing a reference point for comparison of cell density counts it is imperative, therefore, that the reference point itself is not involved in the disease process. The counting of lymphocytes in small bowel epithelium can be used as an example to illustrate this point. In Figure 10 it is plain that using a given number of epithelial cells as a reference point the ratio of lymphocytes to epithelial cells, in b as opposed to a, has increased. However, the area of epithelium has decreased, and a fixed area of epithelium as defined by linear intercepts would be a better fixed point for comparison (*Skinner* et al., 1971) (see Fig. 11). Better still would be to use a fixed point which is not subject to variation, in this case the muscularis mucosa. In the above example using this reference point the number of cells does not alter. In fact only decreases in number or enormous increases would be meaningful using epithelilal cell numbers as a reference point. Much of the recent literature concerning lymphocyte numbers in the superficial epithelium in relationship to coeliac disease can be criticised from this point of view.

The normal levels for plasma cells in the gut were recorded by *Crabbé* et al. (1966) and their findings have been confirmed in subsequent work (*Gelzayd* et al., 1968; *Søltoft*, 1969; *Chen* and *Tobe*, 1974a). *Crabbé* et al. (1965) showed that in the jejunal mucosa IgA cells numbered 181,000 (± 19,000) per c. mm, IgM cells 30,000 (± 4,5000) per c. mm and IgG 18,000 (± 3,000) per c. mm. As stated above the use of absolute figures in this way is

---

Fig. 11. Diagram to show the principle of linear intercepts used to define surface area. The number of times a line crosses a surface (cuts) is proportional to its area. In this way the area of epithelial surface or the upper surface of muscularis mucosa can be determined for the purpose of comparison

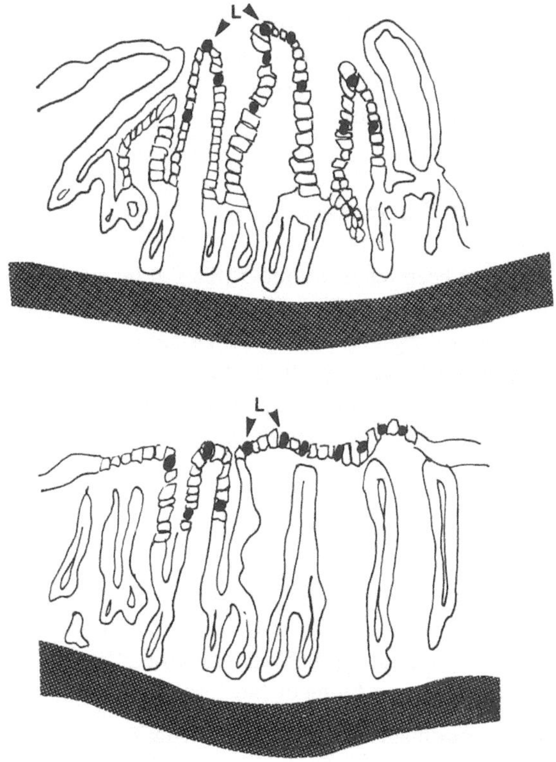

Fig. 10. Diagram to illustrate the counting of cells within epithelial surfaces. (See text)

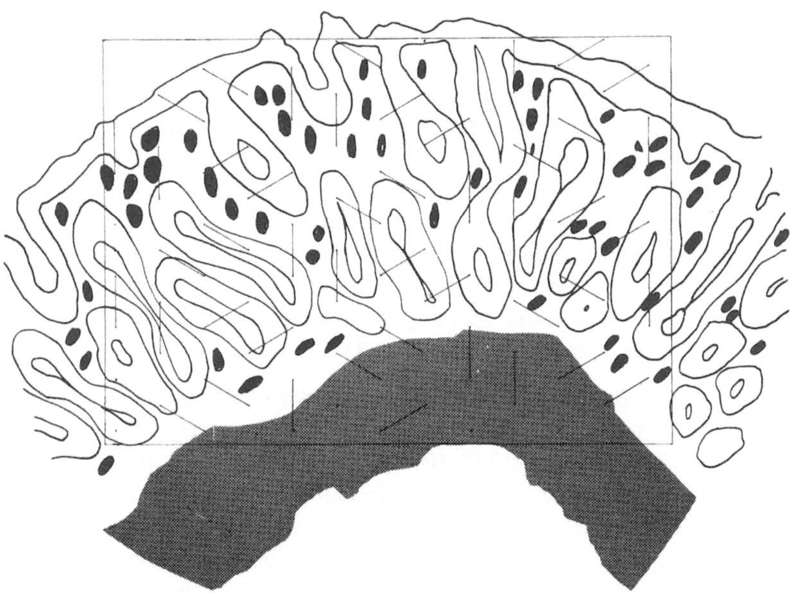

Fig. 11. (Legend see p. 272)

questionable and the most important point is the ratio of cells IgA:IgM:IgG which is 10:1.6:1. Most workers have shown that IgA cells compose 80% or slightly more of the plasma cell population throughout the gut and that IgD and IgE cells are even fewer in number than IgG cells.

V. Disease Processes

There have been relatively few studies of immunological mechanisms involved in gastrointestinal disease processes which have not been based upon changes in circulating immunoglobulins or lymphocytic function. What follows is a review of the information at present available which has arisen from study of the immunological factors operating at a local level which may be concerned in bowel pathology and which have been derived by the more recent methods of approach.

1. Infections

Immune processes prevent the invasion of the mucous membranes by pathogens only if active at the mucosal cell outer surface and it is at this level of course that large amounts of secretory immunoglobulin are present in the glycocalyx of the microvillous layer and the adjacent mucus lining of the bowel.

Cholera is probably the best understood infection of the small bowel and although circulating antibody responses have been investigated, little is known of local gut immunological responses. The organisms colonise the bowel lumen but do not penetrate the wall. They multiply very quickly and produce an exotoxin which damages epithelial cells and causes the loss of massive amounts of isotonic fluid into the lumen of the bowel. Little is known of factors affecting host susceptibility and morphologically there is said to be no abnormality of the bowel structure. The exotoxin has not been demonstrated beyond the epithelial barrier, and it is in this situation that secretory antibodies to the organism or toxin could play a protective role. In one study (*Pierce* et al., 1971) it was shown that patients with Cholera secreted more than 8 gms of IgA in their stools per day and that this had some antibody activity against organisms but did not prevent their growth. Fifty per cent or more was secretory IgA and presumably produced by the plasma cells of the gut wall, and with secretion of such large amounts it is highly unlikely that the number of IgA cells was not increased. Indeed in the earlier literature there is one report (*Fresh* et al., 1964) which does refer to an increase in mononuclear cells in cholera.

The induction of diarrhoea in other infections due for example to E. coli, some Shigellae, Clostridia, etc., is possibly by a mechanism similar to that in Cholera, at least in part (*Du Pont* et al., 1971; *Carpenter*, 1972; *Gemski* et al., 1972). It might be expected that local antibody formation would be stimulated and afford some protection. Work to date indicytes, however, that it is the circulating agglutinating antibodies of 7S IgA class induced by parental immunisation, which are the ones that confer some limited protection albeit short lived (*Carpenter*, 1972). In a study of the enteritis caused by Yersinia enterocolitica infection it was shown that regional lymph nodes contained large pyroninophilic cells (presumably plasma cells) in high numbers and similar cells were seen in the lamina propria of the appendix and at the base of ulcers (*Ahlqvist* et al., 1971). A passing reference was made to an increase in mononuclear cells, including plasma cells, in the lamina propria away from Peyer's patches in Typhoid (*Søltoft* and *Soeberg*, 1972a).

Though cell mediated immune reactions appear to be unimportant in protection against Cholera and some other bacterial infections, they are probably of great value in other instances. In experiments on "nude" mice, for example, which have a gross deficiency of T dependent intra mucosal lymphocytes, an enhanced susceptibility to Salmonella infections can be shown in the presence of a normal resistance to Vibrio Cholera (*Bjerregaard*, 1974).

Recently a great deal of interest has focused on acute sporadic enteritis in children and its possible viral aetiology (*Davison* et al., 1975; Lancet editorial 1975) and abnormality of the local cell mediated immune reactions have been implicated by some in their aetiology (*Ferguson* and *Jarrett*, 1965). However, in a study of acute diarrhoeal diseases of presumed viral aetiology, *Søltoft and Soeberg* (1972a) showed that the jejunal mucosa contained raised numbers of IgA and IgM cells during the course of the disease, which returned to normal levels on recovery, which at least implies that humoral mechanisms are involved. The same authors (1972b) found an increase of IgA and IgD cells in the jejunum during attacks of epidemic viral hepatitis. This suggests that whatever the original portal of entry that gut produced antibodies may play a protective role against further infection in this condition.

Increased mononuclear cells, including plasma cells have been noted in giardiasis (see*Søltoft* and *Soeberg*, 1972a). Infections with Giardia lamblia have often been reported in individuals with agammaglobulinaemia, hypogammaglobulinaemia or selective IgA deficiency (*Brown* et al., 1972; *Ament* and *Rubin*, 1972; *Ochs* et al., 1972) and have almost invariably been found in cases of Nodular Lymphoid Hyperplasia associated with combined immunoglobulin deficiency (*Hermans* et al., 1966). Deficiency of IgE has also been raised as a possible pathogenetic mechanism in these infestations (*Brown* et al., 1972).

Selective deficiency of IgA has been noted in association with coeliac disease (*Mawhinney* and *Tomkin*, 1971) and recurrent gut and chest infections (*Tomkin* et al., 1971). It is also present in about 1 in 500 of seemingly normal people.

There are other unusual and possibly infective disorders such as Whipple's diesease in which a study of immunocytes may throw light on pathogenesis and in some cases of Whipple's disease agammaglobulinaemia has been described (*Maizel* et al., 1970).

2. Pernicious Anaemia

In pernicious anaemia there is a loss of parietal cell mass with an associated gastritis in which at some stage large infiltrates of lymphocytes and plasma cells are seen, morphlogical features which suggest the possibility of an immune mediated destructive process. Circulating antibodies, usually of IgA or IgG class, have been shown against the microsomal component of parietal cells (*Irvine*, 1965; *Fisher* et al., 1967) and against intrinsic factor (*Fisher* et al., 1967). Antibodies to intrinsic factor are less common than antibodies to parietal cells and are associated with the more severe grades of gastritis. They are usually found in patients with pernicious anaemia or latent pernicious anaemia. When present in other conditions such as thyroid diseases (*Wright* et al., 1966) they appear in the serum. In pernicious anaemia, however, antibodies to intrinsic factor are found in the gastric juice (*Fisher* et al., 1966; *Schade* et al., 1966; *Rose* and *Chanarin*, 1968, 1969) and to intrinsic factor and parietal cells in extracts of gastric mucosa (*Brus* et al., 1968). Local immunological changes in the gastric mucosa have received little attention though an IgA cell increase and IgG cell decrease was noted in one study (*Odgers* and *Wangel*, 1968). Somewhat similar changes in the plasma cells were noted in the jejunum of patients with pernicious anaemia by *Søltoft* (1974). *Bauer* et al. (1968) noted antibody activity against microsomal component of parietal cells and against intrinsic factor in the plasma cells of gastric biopsies but studies were limited to a few cases. In general little quantitative work has been done and observations on lymphocytes in the lamina propria and epithelium are absent.

In patients with chronic gastritis not associated with pernicious anaemia all immunoglobulin containing cells appear to be increased in number but with a preservation of normal IgA/IgM/IgG ratios (*Chen* and *Tobé*, 1974b). Similar findings were also noted in patients with gastric ulcer and with gastric adenocarcinoma.

3. Coeliac Disease

Gluten sensitive enteropathy has been regarded as due either to a mucosal enzyme defect possibly permitting the accumulation of toxic peptides or an immune reaction to certain fractions of gluten, and an extensive literature on immunological phenomena in coeliac disease has accumulated. Studies of serum immunoglobulins have shown a fairly consistent decrease in the circulating IgM levels (*Fry* et al., 1967; *Hobbs* and *Hepner*, 1968; *Douglas*, 1970). Reports concerning changes in serum IgG levels have been inconsistent and the changes in the serum IgA levels have been variable also some showing a raised level (*Asquith* et al., 1969; *Watson*, 1969; *Kenrick* and *Walker-Smith*, 1970), and some decreased level (*Crabbé*, 1967; *Mawhinney* et al., 1970). This latter finding is usually interpreted as meaning that patients with selective IgA deficiency are more likely to develop coeliac disease. In the early stages of investigation serum antibodies against gluten were demonstrated (*Rubin* et al., 1962), but these have since also been found in normal individuals, and in fact, antibodies to other food components including the lactolbumen in milk have also been found. It is of interest that more recently *Amman* and *Hong* (1971) demonstrated serum antibodies to reticulin or to a particular fraction of basement membrane which occurred more frequently in individuals with coeliac disease than in other cases of inflammatory bowel disease or in normal individuals, and this finding has been confirmed by others (*Seah* et al., 1971; *Wright*, 1972). In another study *Doe* et al. (1973) demonstrated the presence of immune complexes in the serum of individuals with coeliac disease, and suggested that these complexes when deposited in the small bowel may initiate some of the pathological changes. Moving closer to the site of damage, some investigations have been done on antibodies in jejunal juice, the socalled copra antibodies. *Herskovic* et al. (1968) demonstrated antibodies in jejunal juice to fraction 3 of gluten and *Douglas* et al. (1970) has shown that the levels of jejunal juice IgM are constantly raised. In an investigation of the immunoglobulin producing cells of the mucosa of the jejunum in coeliac disease *Rubin* et al. (1965) demonstrated a relative increase of IgA cells, though their method of quantitation was not very precise. More recent work has demonstrated fairly consistent increases of IgM containing cells in the lamina propria (*Savilhati*, 1972) and more usually a relative decrease in IgA cells (*Douglas* et al., 1970) but the findings have always been open to the interpretation that though they may be important in the pathogenesis of the disease it is also possible that they are secondary effects following on the exposure of the gut associated lymphoid tissue to a wide variety of new antigens once the mucosa has been damaged. With the knowledge that lymphocytes, usually T lymphocytes, can exert their own cytotoxic effects independent of antibody production, interest has turned to the study of the lymphocytes within the lamina propria and within the epithelial layer (*Bayless* et al., 1970; *Ferguson* and *Murray*, 1971; *Fry* et al., 1972). Their studies have usually shown an increase of epithelial lymphocytes during the active phase of the disease, and a fall in the number when the patients have been put on a gluten free diet, though the levels did not become normal. In a similar study *Holmes* et al. (1974) showed an increase of intra-epithelial lymphocytes associated with a decrease of lymphocytes within the lamina propria and it was suggested that the lymphocytes were perhaps causing the epithelial cell damage. The changes in epithelial lymphocyte numbers which have been a fairly consistent feature of recent reports, have been based on quantitative methods which, as already stated, are open to criticism and many of the changes described could easily have been due to faulty technique. Nevertheless, it has been argued that cellular immune mechanisms of the delayed hypersensitivity type are important in the evolution of the lesion of coeliac disease. The changes in plasma cell numbers in the lamina propria would then be secondary to an increased exposure to antigens following the epithelial damage. However, in a recent rather elegant study using organ cultures *Strober* et al. (1974) have produced evidence indicating that an antibody being produced during the active phase of the disease is important in causing the tissue damage. It only damages a mucosa from coeliac patients and does not affect a normal mucosa. Therefore, it would appear that in the coeliac patient a certain receptor mechanism for gluten antibody complex is important and this is absent in the normal individual. More recently *Ferguson* et al. (1965) using similar techniques demonstrated cell mediated immunity to gliadin in coeliac patients. In this context it is interesting that over 80% of patients with coeliac disease have the immunocompatibility antigen HLA8 (*Asquith* et al., 1974) and it has been suggested that either this gene in combination with others, or a closely linked gene is important in explaining this host susceptibility to gluten induced damage.

4. Tropical Sprue

Tropical Sprue is a chronic diarrhoeal disorder with many clinical similarities to both adult coeliac disease and the stagnant loop syndrome (BMJ 1972). There have been many reports of the morphological changes in the jejunal mucosa in tropical sprue, including the increased cellularity of the lamina propria which decreases on treatment (*Swanson* et al., 1965, 1966), but there have been no studies on local antibody formation either in jejunal juice or in the mucosa. Quantitative studies on immunocytes in the gut wall similar to those in coeliac disease have not been performed, but it may also be that individual body variations in immunity are important in its development. There are strong indications that it is an infective or related condition and its pattern of occurrence suggests that some individuals are more prone to develop the damage than others. In this context there is one interesting report of dysgammaglobulinaemia in Tropical Sprue (*Jarnum* et al., 1968) in which decreased levels of IgG were noted. It is important to stress that from the point of view of assessing changes in cellularity in Tropical Sprue that the control group is defined in the same population because of the well recognised racial differences in jejunal morphology (*Sprinz* et al., 1962).

5. "Temperate Sprue"

A condition similar to Tropical sprue in its clinical manifestations and first called "Acute Sprue" by *Drummond* and *Montgomery* (1970) has been reported in Western countries and has variously been termed acute non-tropical sprue, temperate sprue, or post infective malabsorption syndrome. Jejunal biopsy shows minor abnormalities with an increase in cellular infiltrate of the lamina propria (*Whitehead*, 1971) but again no specific attempts to define antibody activity in the mucosa or to look at the immunocytes in detail appears to have been performed.

6. Ulcerative Colitis and Crohn's Disease

Immunological studies of ulcerative colitis and Crohn's disease have been extensive and they have largely concentrated on studies of circulating antibodies, lymphocyte transformation and cytotoxicity tests and skin tests of delayed hypersensitivity. The results have in general been contradictory and inconclusive and the source of much confusion (see reviews *Thayer*, 1970; *Kirsner*, 1970; *Kraft* and *Kirsner*, 1971).

Of late attention has focused more strongly on the local immune response in the gut and a number of quantitative studies have been made (*Kraft* et al., 1966; *Gelzayd* et al., 1968; *Søltoft* et al., 1973; *Skinner* and *Whitehead*, 1974; *Brandtzaeg* et al., 1974). The results of these surveys have been somewhat variable though all show an increase in plasma cells in the lamina propria. Increased numbers of IgG and sometimes IgM have been found and apart from the isolated report of *Gelzayd* (1968) it was usual to find an increase in IgA cells also. The degree of increase of cell types in the various studies have been slightly different and the conclusions drawn have varied from report to report. In our own investigations of inflammatory disease of the large bowel (Figs. 12 and 13) it can be seen that IgG, IgA and IgM cells are increased in active disease, both ulcerative colitis and Crohn's disease, the degree of increase being greatest for IgG and IgM cells, a feature in agreement with the most recent work of *Brandtzaeg* (1974). There is, however, a significant difference in the IgA cells between Crohn's disease and cases of active ulcerative colitis and it is possible that this increase may be of some importance in the pathogenesis. *Brandtzaeg* (1974) suggests that the large increase in IgG cells with consequent production of immunoglobulin G could represent a mechanism causing chronicity. It is known, for example, that certain IgG antibodies can induce non-specific lymphocyte mediate cytotoxicity (*Eden* et al., 1973) and it is true that lymphocytes are a feature of the infiltrate in Crohn's disease and to a lesser extent ulcerative colitis. Others (*Jensen* et al., 1973; *Doe* et al., 1973) have suggested that in ulcerative colitis immune complexes are important either by initiating Arthus type reactions or by stimulating lymphocyte cytotoxicity. It may well be that these mechanisms occur in both Crohn's disease and ulcerative colitis. Our own study, however, indicates that the different morphological appearances seen in Crohn's disease may be the result of the large increase in IgA cells. It is known that large immune complexes with antibody

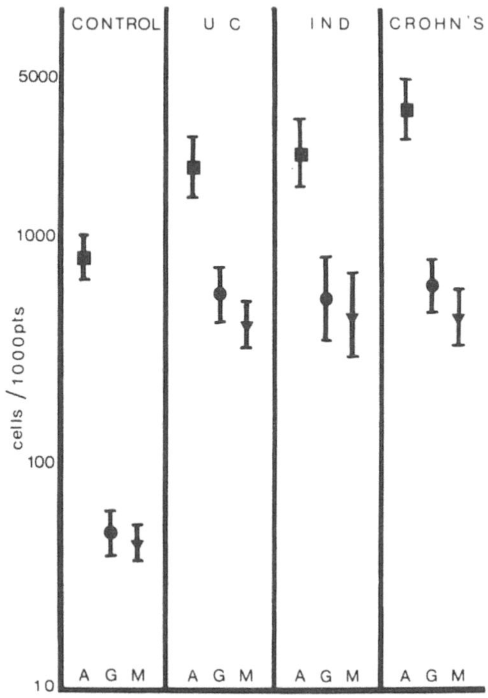

Fig. 12. The number of plasma cells/unit volume in each immunoglobulin class IgA, IgG, IgM, in control cases (normals and patients with irritable colon syndrome) ulcerative colitis cases (U.C.), in Crohn's disease and a group which would not be categorised as either ulcerative colitis (U.C.) or Crohn's disease and called indeterminate (IND)

excess stimulate granuloma formation (*Spector* and *Heesom*, 1969) and the large amounts of IgA produced in the patients with Crohn's disease could well result in large antibody excess complexes being formed. Granuloma formation requires an intact T lymphocyte system (*Warren* et al., 1966) and the appearances of lymphoid follicles with the surrounding cuff of small lymphocytes and a lymphocyte infiltrate which is so common in the deeper tissues in Crohn's disease could be a manifestation of stimulation of this system. These phenomena are probably important in the pathogenesis of the chronic lesions rather than in the initiation of the disease. Evidence is lacking for an autoimmune origin for either ulcerative colitis or Crohn's disease despite the findings of circulating antibodies to colonic epithelium.

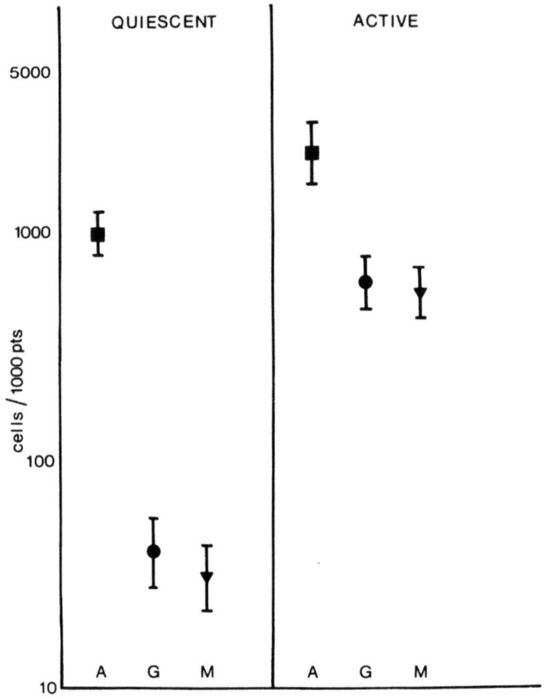

Fig. 13. The number of plasma cells/unit volume in quiescent and active colitis. The classes IgA, IgG, IgM are shown separately

It has been suggested (*Green* and *Fox*, 1974) that abnormalities in the secretory mechanism for IgA and possibly IgM are important in the pathogenesis of Crohn's disease as distinct from ulcerative colitis, but it is interesting that in our own study and in the others referred to no abnormality in secretory component was shown. It is also of interest that immune complexes containing the C3 component of complement have not been detected so that it is unlikely that abnormalities of the secretory mechanism are important in pathogenesis. Similarly there is no evidence that local complement fixation occurs, a further point against the involvement of small immune complexes initiating an Arthus reaction. One reason for the variation in cell numbers detected in the different series can be ascribed to variations in sampling. In our study the sections examined were at least five in number from separate areas and they included the complete mucosa and avoided ulcerated areas or the immediately adjacent mucosa where IgG cells are seen in vast numbers. Other zones may obviously not be free from the influence exerted by a large number of luminal antigens.

VI. Abnormalities of Immunoglobulin Synthesis and Lymphomas

The occurrence of malignancy in immunodeficiency diseases has been reviewed by *Gatti* and *Good* (1971), but one group is of especial interest. Cases of malabsorption due to lymphomatous disease of the small bowel are reported in the Eastern Mediterranean and because of similar clinical and pathological findings the condition has been called Mediterranean lymphoma (*Ramot*, 1965). However, similar cases are described (*Rambaud* et al.,

1968), in which there is a characteristic production of the heavy chain fragment of immunoglobulin (α chain disease) similar to the original cases of "heavy chain" disease described by *Franklin* et al. (1964) in which IgG was involved. A portion of the immunoglobulin A, i.e. part of the alpha chain can be detected in urine. There is involvement of the gastro-intestinal tract by pronounced proliferation of plasma cells which distorts the mucosa. Though it is clear that the plasma cells are the source of this immunoglobulin fraction there has been little investigation of the cells concerned in the lamina propria (*Manousos* et al., 1974). It is assumed that in alpha chain disease the plasma cells are dedifferentiated and produce only the alpha chain. Studies of biopsies from the intestinal tract have not shown any strong evidence of a particularly malignant process. Indeed, recently it has been suggested that the cause of the disease is an unusual and sustained stimulus to local immune reactions in which the capacity of the IgA producing cells to produce the complete immunoglobulin has been exhausted. It has even been suggested that some infectious agent may be responsible and evidence was presented (*Manousos* et al., 1974) of a patient having been cured by antibiotic treatment and cyclophosphamide. This group of diseases obviously lends itself to further investigation using the immunohistochemical methods available as outlined above and recently it has been shown that tumours arising in one individual with alpha chain disease contained a fairly high proportion of cells producing not only alpha chain but also some Lambda light chain (*Skinner* et al., 1976) raising the possibility that these abnormalities in the gut are similar to plasmacytomas (*Heenan* et al., 1975) and multiple myeoloma.

It is also of interest that patients with coeliac disease can acquire, as a late complication, a primary lymphoma of the gut which first appears as a progressive hyperplasia and then proceeds to a recognisable sarcomatous stage (*Whitehead*, 1968). Recently, using the immunoperoxidase technique it has been shown (*Taylor*, 1974) that many cases of gut lymphoma previously classified as reticulosarcoma were, in fact, poorly differentiated plasma cell tumours. Where heavy chain was present it was most frequently of the alpha type but often only light chain either kappa or lambda but never both were detected. It is highly likely that, in view of this work, the tumour seen in coeliac disease is of a similar nature for the advent of tumour in the bowel is preceeded in some cases by a rise in the circulating levels of IgA in the serum.

VII. Other Malignant Disease

It is of interest that cancers elsewhere and in the bowel are often surrounded by large numbers of immune competent cells mainly lymphocytes but also including plasma cells. The plasma cells are often of IgG or IgM class and in some instances specific activity against tumour cell has been shown (*Chen* and *Tobé*, 1974b). Quantitative analysis on such material may allow us in future to predict whether a particular tumour is likely to have a good or poor prognosis.

References

Ahlqvist, J. Ahvonen, P., Räsänen, J.A., Wallgren, G.R.: Enteric infection with Yersinia Enterocolitica. Acta path. microbiol. scand. A 79, 109-122 (1971).

Ament, M.G., Rubin, C.E.: Relation of giardiasis to abnormal intestinal structure and function in gastrointestinal immunodeficiency syndromes. Gastroenterology 62, 216-226 (1972).

Amman, A.J., Hong, R.: Unique antibody to basement membrane in patients with selective IgA deficiency and coeliac disease. Lancet 1971 I, 1264-1266.

Andrew, W.: Lymphocyte transformation in the epithelium. J. nat. Cancer Inst. 35, 113-237 (1965).

Asquith, P., Mackintosh, P., Stokes, P.L.: Histocompatibility antigens in patients with inflammatory bowel disease. Lancet 1974 I, 113-115.

Asquith, P., Thompson, R.A., Cooke, W.T.: Serum immunoglobulins in adult coeliac disease. Lancet 1969 II, 129-131.

Bauer, S., Fisher, J.M., Strickland, R.G., Taylor, K.B.: Autoantibody containing cells in the gastric mucosa in pernicious anaemia. Lancet 1968 II, 887-890.

Bayless, T.M., Rubin, C.E., Topping. T.M., Yardley, J.A., Hendrix, T.R.: Morphologic and functional effects of gluten feeding on jejunal mucosa in coeliac disease. In: Coeliac Disease (eds. *C.C. Booth, R.H. Dowling*). Edinburgh: Churchill-Livingstone 1970.

Bienenstock, J.: The physiology of the local immune response and the gastrointestinal tract. In: Progress in Immunology II, vol. 4 (eds. *Brent* and *Holborrow*), pp. 197-207. North Holland Publishing Co. 1974.

Binder, V.: Cell density in lamina propria of the colon. A quantiative method applied to normal subjects and ulcerative colitis patients. Scand. J. Gastroent. 5, 485-490 (1970).

Bjerregaard, P.: Quoted by *A.C. Wardlaw, P.J. Watt,* "Immunity to Mucosal Infections". In: Progress in Immunology II, vol. 4 (eds. *Brent* and *Holborrow*). North Holland Publishing Co. 1974.

Brandtzaeg, P.: Intestinal aspects of local immunity. Scand. J. Gastroent. suppl. 16, 7-9 (1972).

Brandtzaeg, P.: Two types of IgA immunocytes in man. Nature New Biol. 243, 142-143 (1973).

Brandtzaeg, P., Baklien, K., Fausa, M.D., Hoel, P.S.: Immunohistochemical characterisation of local immunoglobulin formation in ulcerative colitis. Gastroenterology 66, 1123-1136 (1974).

Brandtzaeg, P., Fjellanger, I., Gjeraldsen, S.T.: Adsorption of Immunoglobulin A onto oral bacteria in vivo. J. Bacteriol. 96, 242-249 (1968).

Broberger, O., Perlmann, P.: Autoantibodies in human ulcerative colitis. J. exp. Med. 110, 657-674 (1959).

Broberger, O., Perlmann, P.: Demonstration of an epithelial antigen in colon by means of fluorescent antibodies from children with ulcerative colitis. J. exp. Med. 115, 13-26 (1962).

Brown, W.R., Burns, F.A.: Application of peroxidase-labelled antibody methods to identification of immunoglobulin containing cells in gastrointestinal tissues. J. Immunological Methods 2, 303-307 (1973).

Brown, W.R., Butterfield, D., Savage, D., Tada, T.: Clinical microbiological and immunological studies in patients with immunoglobulin deficiencies and gastrointestinal disorders. Gut 13, 441-449 (1972).

Brus, I., Seigel, H., Yamaguchi, S.N., Jerzy-Glass, G.B.: Immunoglobulins IgA and IgG in gastric mucosa of patients with atrophic gastritis and pernicious anaemia. Scand. J. Gastroenterol. 3, 43-57 (1968).

Burns, J.: An appraisal of immunocytochemical methods in routine histology. Proc. roy. Micro. Soc. 10, 97 (1975a).

Burns, J.: Background staining and sensitivity of the unlabelled antibody enzyme (PAS) method. Comparison with the peroxidase labelled antibody sandwich method using formalin fixed paraffin embedded material. Histochemistry (1975b) in press.
BMJ Editorial. BMJ 1, 2-3 (1972).
Carpenter, C.J.: Cholera and other enterotoxin related diarrhoeal diseases. J. Infectious Diseases 126, 551-564 (1972).
Chalkley, H.W.: Method for the quantitative morphological analysis of tissues. J. nat. Cancer Inst. 4, 47-53 (1943).
Chen, S.-T., Tobé, T.: Cellular sites of immunoglobulins IV. Studies of antral mucosa of human stomachs. Digestion 10, 117-183 (1974).
Colten, H., Bienenstock, J.: Proceedings of International symposium on IgA. Birmingham (Ala) (Plenum NY) 1973.
Cottier, H., Turk, J., Sobin, L.: A proposal for a standardised system of reporting human lymph node morphology in relation to immunological function. Bull. Wld Hlth Org. 47, 375-408 (1972).
Coons, A.H.: In. General Cytochemical Methods (ed. *J.F. Danielli*), pp. 400-422. New York: Academic Press 1958.
Coons, A.H., Creech, H.J., Jones, R.N., Berliner, E.: The demonstration of pneumococcal antigen in tissues by the use of immunofluorescence. J. Immunol. 45, 159-170 (1942).
Crabbé, P.A., Carbonara, A.O., Heremans, J.F.: The normal mucosa as a major source of plasma cells containing IgA immunoglobulin. Gastroenterology 14, 235-248 (1965).
*Crabbé, P.A., Heremans, J.F.:*The distribution of immunoglobulin containing cells along the human gastrointestinal tract. Gastroenterology 51, 305-316 (1966).
Crabbé, P.A., Heremans, J.F.: Selective IgA deficiency with Steatorrhea. A new syndrome. Amer. J. Med. 319-326 (1967).
Crabbé, P.A., Nash, D.R., Bazin, H., Eyssen, H., Heremans, J.F.: Antibodies of the IgA type in intestinal plasma cells of germfree mice after oral or parenteral immunisation with ferritin. J. exp. Med. 130, 723-744 (1969).
Davidson, G.P., Bishop, R.F., Townley, R.R.W., Holmes, I.H., Ruck, B.J.: Importance of a new virus in sporadic enteritis in children. Lancet 1975 I, 242-245.
de Sousa, M.: Kinetics of the distribution of thymus and marrow cells in the peripheral lymphoid organs of the mouse; ecotaxis. Clin. Exp. Immunol. 9, 371-380 (1971).
Doe, W.F., Booth, C.C., Brown, D.L.: Evidence for complexes in adult coeliac disease, Crohn's disease and ulcerative colitis. Lancet 1973 I, 404-403.
Douglas, A.P., Crabbé, P.A., Hobbs, S.R.: Immunochemical studies of the serum, intestinal secretions and intestinal mucosa in patients with adult coeliac disease and other forms of the coeliac syndrome. Gastroenterology 59, 414-425 (1970).
Drummond, M.B., Montgomery, R.D.: Acute sprue in Britain. BMJ 2, 340-341 (1970).
Du Pont, A.L., Formal, S.B., Hornick, R.B., Snyder. M.J., Libonati, J.P., Sheahan, D.G., La Brec, E.H., Kalas, J.P.: Pathogenesis of Escherichia coli diarrhoea. New Engl. J. Med. 285, 1-9 (1971).
Eden, A., Bianco, C., Nussenzweig, V.: Mechanisms of binding of soluble immune complexes to lymphocytes. Cell Immunol. 7, 459-473 (1973).
Ferguson, A.: Immunological role of the gastrointestinal tract. Scottish Med. Journal. 17, 111-118 (1972).
Ferguson, A., Parrot, D.M.V.: Growth and development of "antigen-free" grafts of foetal mouse intestine. J. Path. 106, 95-102 (1972).
Ferguson, A., Jarrett, E.E.E.: Hypersensitivity reactions in the small intestine I. Thymus dependence of experimental "partial villous atrophy". Gut 16, 114-117 (1975).

Ferguson, A., MacDonald, T.T., McLure, J.P., Helden, R.J.: Cell mediated immunity to gliadin within the small intestinal mucosa in coeliac disease. Lancet 1975 I, 895-897.

Ferguson, A., Murray, D.: Quantitation of intra-epithelial lymphocytes in human jejunum. Gut 12, 988-994 (1971).

Ferguson, R., Asquith, P., Cooke, O.T.: The jejunal cellular infiltrate in coeliac disease complicated by lymphoma. Gut 15, 458-461 (1974).

Fichtelius, K.E.: The gut epithelium – a first level lymphoid organ. Exp. Cell Res. 49, 87-104 (1968a).

Fichtelius, K.E., Yunis, J.E., Good, R.A.: Occurrence of lymphocytes within the gut epithelium of normal and neonatally thymectomised mice. Proc. Soc. exp. Biol. 128, 185-188 (1968b).

Fisher, J.M., MacKay, I.R., Taylor, K.B., Ungar, B.: An immunological study of categories of gastritis. Lancet 1967 I, 176-180.

Fisher, J.M., Rees, C., Taylor, K.B.: Intrinsic factor antibodies in gastric juice of pernicious anaemia patients. Lancet 1966 II, 88-89.

Fletcher, J., Hinton, J.M.: Tuberculin sensitivity in Crohn's disease. Lancet 1967 II, 753-754.

Franklin, E.C., Lowenstein, J., Bigelow, B., Meltzer, M.: Heavy chain disease, a new disorder of serum γ globulins. Report of the first case. Amer. J. Med. 37, 323-350 (1964).

Fresh, J.W., Versage, P.M., Reyes, V.: Intestinal morphology in human and experimental cholera. Arch. Path. 77, 529-537 (1964).

Fry, L., Kier, P., McMinn, R.M.H., Cowan, J.D., Hoffbrand, A.L.: Small intestinal structure and function and haematological changes in dermatitis and herpetiformis. Lancet 1967 II, 729-733.

Fry, L., Seah, P.P., McMinn, R.M.H., Hoffbrand, A.V.: Lymphocytic infiltration of epithelium in diagnosis of gluten sensitive enteropathy. BMJ 3, 371-374 (1972).

Gatti, R.A., Good, R.A.: Occurence of malignancy in immunodeficiency diseases. Cancer 28, 89-98 (1971).

Gatti, R.A., Stutman, O., Good, R.A.: The lymphoid system. In: Annual Review of Physiology (ed. *V.E. Hall*), pp. 529-546 (1970).

Gelzayd, E.A., Kraft, S.C., Fitch, F.W., Kirsner, J.B.: Distribution of immunoglobulins in human rectal mucosa. "Ulcerative colitis and abnormal mucosal control subjects". Gastroenterology 54, 341-347 (1968).

Gemski, P., Takeuchi, A., Washington, O., Formal, S.B.: Shigellosis due to Shigella dysenteriae 1. Relative importance of mucosal invasion versus toxin production in pathogenesis. J. Infectious disease 126, 523-530 (1972).

Good, R.A.: Experiments of nature in immunobiology. New Engl. J. Med. 279, 1344-1345 (1968).

Gowans, J.L., Knight, E.J.: The route of recirculation of lymphocytes in the rat. Proc. roy. Soc. B 159, 257-282 (1964).

Green, F.H.Y., Fox, H.: The distribution of mucosal antibodies in the bowel of patients with Crohn's disease. Gut 16, 125-131 (1975).

Hall, J.G.: Observations on the migration and localisation of lymphoid cells. In: Progress in Immunology, Vol. 3 (eds. *Brent* and *Holborrow*), pp. 15-24, 1974.

Hall, J.G., Parry, D.M., Smith, M.E.: The distribution and differentiation of lymph borne immunoblasts after intravenous injection on syngeneic recipients. Cell Tissue Kinetics 5, 267-287 (1971).

Hall, J.G., Smith, M.E.: Homing of lymph borne immunoblasts to the gut. Nature 226, 262-263 (1970).

Halstead, T.E., Hall, J.G.: The homing of lymph borne immunoblasts to the small gut of neonatal rats. Transplantation 14, 339-346

Harrison, W.: Autoantibodies against intestinal and gastric mucous cells in ulcerative colitis. Lancet 1965 I, 1346-1350.

Heenan, P.J., Mason, D.Y., Skinner, J.M., Taylor, C.R.: Waldenstroms disease in the jejunum Beiträge zur Pathologie (in press).

Hennig, A. von: Inhalt einer aus Papillen oder Zotten gebildeten Fläche. Mikroskopie 11, 206-213 (1956).

Heremans, J.F., Crabbé, P.A.: IgA deficiency: General considerations and relation to human disease. In: Immunodeficiency Disease of Man (ed. *Good* et al.), pp. 298-307. National Foundation – March of Dimes, 1968.

Hermans, P.E., Huizenga, K.A., Hoffman, H.N., Brown, A.L., Markowitz, H.: Dysgammaglobulinaemia associated with nodular lymphoid hyperplasia of the small intestine. Amer. J. Med. 40, 78-89 (1966).

Herskovic, T., Katz, J., Gryboski, J.D., Spiro, H.M.: Coproantibodies to gluten in coeliac disease. JAMA 203, 887-888 (1968).

Hinz, C.F., Perlmann, P., Hammarström, S.: Reactivity in vitro of lymphocytes from patients with ulcerative colitis. J. Lab. clin. Med. 70, 752-759 (1967).

Hobbs, J.R., Hepner, G.W.: Deficiency of γM globulin in coeliac disease. Lancet 1968 I, 217-220.

Holmes, G.K.T., Asquith, P., Stokes, P.L., Cooke, W.T.: Cellular infiltrate of jejunal biopsies in adult coeliac disease in relation to gluten withdrawal. Gut 15, 278-283 (1974).

Irvine, W.J.: Immunologic aspects of pernicious anaemia. New Engl. J. Med. 273, 432-438 (1965).

Jarnum, S., Jeejeebhoy, K.N., Singh, B.: Dysgammaglobulinaemia in Tropical Sprue. BMJ 4, 416-417 (1968).

Jewell, D.J., MacLennan, I.C.M.: Circulating immune complexes in inflammatory bowel disease. Clin. Exp. Immunol. 14, 219-226 (1973).

Kenrik, K.G., Walker-Smith, J.A.: Immunoglobulins and dietary protein antibodies in childhood coeliac disease. Gut 11, 635-640 (1970).

Kirsner, J.B.: Ulcerative colitis 1970 – recent developments. Scand. J. Gastroent. Suppl. 6, 63-91 (1970).

Kraft, S.C., Kirsner, J.B.: Immunological apparatus of the gut, and inflammatory bowel disease. Gastroenterology 60, 922-951 (1971).

Kraft, S.C., Rimpilla, J.J., Fitch, F.W., Kirsner, J.B.: Immunohistochemical studies of the colon in ulcerative colitis. Arch. Path. 82, 369-378 (1966).

Kyriazis, A.A., Esterly, J.R.: Development of lymphoid tissues in the human embryo and early foetus. Arch. Path. 90, 348-353 (1970).

Kyriazis, A.A., Esterly, J.R.: Foetal and neonatal development of lymphoid tissues. Arch. Path. 91, 444-451 (1971).

Lagercrantz, R., Hammarstrom, S., Pearlmann, P., Gustaffsson, B.E.: Immunological studies in ulcerative colitis. J. exp. Med. 128, 1339-1352 (1968).

Lancet Editorial 1974. Vol. II, p. 31-32.

Lancet Editorial 1975. Rotaviruses of man and animals, p. 257-259.

Maizel, H., Ruffin, J.M., Dobbins, W.O.: Whipples disease. A review of 19 patients from one hospital and a review of the literature since 1950. Medicine 49, 175-205 (1970).

Manousos, O.N., Economidou, J.C., Georgiadon, D.E., Pratsika-Ougourloglou, K.G., Hadziyannis, S.J., Menkas, G.E., Henry, K., Doe, W.F.: Alpha chain disease with clinical, immunological and histological recovery, BMJ 1, 409-412 (1974).

Marcussen, H., Nerup, J.: Fluorescent anti colon and organ specific antibodies in ulcerative colitis. Scand. J. Gastroent. 8, 9-15 (1973).

Mawhinney, H., Tomkin, G.H.: Gluten enteropathy associated with selective IgA deficiency. Lancet 1971 II, 121-123.

Menninger: Report on the transport and catabolism of immunoglobulins. In: Progress in Immunology II, vol 1 (eds. *Brent* and *Holborrow*). North Holland Publishing Co. 1974.

Mitchell, D.N., Cannon, P., Dyer, N.H., Hinton, K.F.W., Willoughby, J.M.T.: Further observations on Kveim test in Crohn's disease. Lancet 1970 II, 496-498.

Nairn, R.C.: Fluorescent antibody tracing 3rd Ed. Edinburgh: Livingston 1969.

Nakane, P.K., Pierce, G.B.: Enzyme labelled antibodies: preparation and application for the localisation of antigens. Histochem. Cytochem. 14, 929-931 (1966).

Nossal, G.V.J., Ada, G.L.: The functional anatomy of the lymphoid system. In: Antigens, Lymphoid Cells and the Immune Response, pp. 61-84. New York: Academic Press 1971.

Ochs, H.D., Ament, M.E., Davis, S.D.: Giardiasis with malabsorption in X linked agammaglobulinaemia. New Engl. J. Med. 287, 341-342 (1972).

Odgers, R.J., Wange, A.G.: Abnormalities in IgA containing mononuclear cells in the gastric lesion of pernicious anaemia. Lancet 1968 II, 846-849.

Parrot, D.M.V., Ferguson, A.: Selective migration of lymphocytes within mouse small intestine. Immunology 26, 571-588 (1974).

Perey, D.Y.E., Good, R.A.: Experimental arrest and induction of lymphoid development in intestinal lymphoepithelial tissues of rabbits. Lab. Invest. 18, 15-26 (1968).

Pierce, N.F., Curlin, G.T., Carpenter, C.C.J.: Possible role of secretory antibodies in cholera. In: The Secretory Immunologic System (ed. *Tomasi*), pp. 287-292. Washinton: Government Printing Office 1971.

Rambaud, J.C., Bognel, C., Prost, A., Bernier, J.J., Le Quintec, Y., Lambling, A., Danon, R., Hurez, D., Seligmann, M.: Clinico-pathological study of a patient with "Mediterranean type of abdominal lymphoma and a new type of IgA abnormality". Digestion 1, 321-336 (1968).

Ramot, B., Shanin, N., Babis, J.J.: Malabsorption syndrome in lymphoma of small intestine: A study of 13 cases. Israel J. Med. Sci. 1, 221-226 (1965).

Rose, M.S., Chanarin, I.: Studies on intrinsic factor antibodies. Brit. Haemat. 15, 325-326 Abstract (1968).

Rose, M.S., Chanarin, I.: Association of intrinsic factor from its antibody: Application to study of pernicious anaemia gastric juice specimens. Brit. med. J. 1969 I, 468-470.

Rubin, C.E., Brandborg, A.L., Flick, A.L., Phelps, P., Parmentier, C., Van Niel, S.: Studies of coeliac sprue: The effect of repeated wheat instillation into the proximal ileum of patients on a gluten free diet. Gastroenterology 43, 621-641 (1962).

Savilahti, E.: Intestinal immunoglobulins in children with coeliac disease. Gut 13, 958-964 (1972).

Schade, S.G., Feick, P., Muckerheide, M., Schilling, R.F.: Occurrence in gastric juice of antibody to a complex of intrinsic factor and vitamin B_{12}. New Engl. J. Med. 275, 528-531 (1966).

Seah, P.P., Fry, L., Rossiter, M.A., Hoffbrand, A.V., Holborrow, E.J.: Anti-reticulin antibodies in childhood coeliac disease. Lancet 1971 II, 681-682.

Seligmann, M., Danon, F., Hurez, D., Mihaeosco, E., Prend'Homme, J.L.: Alpha chain disease: a new immunoglobulin abnormality. Science 162, 1396-1397 (1968).

Shorter, R.G., Spencer, R.J., Huizenga, K.A., Hallenback, G.A.: Inhibition of in vitro cytotoxicity of lymphocytes from patients with ulcerative colitis and granulomatous colitis for allogeneic colonic epithelial cells using horse anti-human thymus serum. Gastroenterology 54, 227-231 (1968).

Siltzbach, L.E., Vieira, L.O.B.D., Topilsky, M., Janowitz, H.D.: Is there Kveim responsiveness in Crohn's disease? Lancet 1971 II, 634-636.
Skinner, J.M., Economidou, J.C., Manousos, O.N.: Lymphoma of the intestine in α chain disease. Clin. Exp. Immunol. In press (1976).
Skinner, J.M., Whitehead, R., Piris, J.: Argentaffin cells in ulcerative colitis. Gut 12, 636-638 (1971).
Skinner, J.M., Whitehead, R.: The plasma cells in inflammatory disease of the colon: A quantitative study. J. clin. Path. 27, 643-646 (1974).
Soltoft, J.: Immunoglobulin containing cells in normal jejunal mucosa and in ulcerative colitis and regional enteritis. Scand. J. Gastroent. A 353-360 (1969).
Soltoft, J.: Intestinal immunoglobulins in pernicious anaemia. Amer. J. dig. Dis. 19, 623-625 (1974).
Soltoft, J., Binder, V., Gudmand-Hoyer, E.: Intestinal immunoglobulins in ulcerative colitis. Scand. J. Gastroent. 8, 293-300 (1973).
Soltoft, J., Soeberg, B.: Immunoglobulin containing cells in the small intestine during acute enteritis. Gut 13, 535-538 (1972a).
Soltoft, J., Soeberg, B.: Immunoglobulin containing cells in the small intestine in viral hepatitis. Acta path. microbiol. scand. B 80, 379-387 (1972b).
Spector, W.G., Heesom, N.: The production of granulomata by antigen-antibody complexes. J. Path. 98, 31-39 (1969).
Sprent, J., Miller, J.F.A.P.: Interaction of thymus lymphocytes with histocompatible cells II recirculating lymphocytes derived from antigen activated thymus cells. Cell Immunol. 3, 385-404 (1972).
Sprintz, A., Sribhibhadh, R., Gangarosa, E.J., Benyajati, C., Kundel, D., Halstead, S.: Biopsy of small bowel of Thai people. Amer. J. clin. Path. 28, 42-51 (1962).
St Marie, G.: A paraffin embedding technique for studies employing immunofluoresceine. J. Histochem. Cytochem. 10, 250-256 (1962).
Stefani, S., Fink, S.: The ulcerative colitis lymphocyte reactions to E. coli 014 and colon antigens. Scand. J. Gastroent. 2, 333-336 (1967).
Strober, W., Flachuk, Z.M., Nelson, D.L., Gebhard, R.M.: The pathogenesis of gluten sensitive enteropathy. In: Progress in Immunology II, vol. 4 (eds. *Brent* and *Holborrow*), pp. 221-229. North Holland Publishing Co. 1974.
Swanson, V.L., Munsey, S.W., Bayless, T.M.: Morphologic effects of folic acid and vitamin B_{12} on the jejunal lesion of Tropical Sprue. Amer. J. Path. 49, 167-185 (1966).
Swanson, V.L., Thomassen, R.W.: Pathology of the jejunal mucosa in tropical sprue. Amer. J. Path. 46, 511-537 (1965).
Taylor, C.R.: The nature of Reed-Sternberg cells and other malignant "reticulin" cells. Lancet 1974 II, 802-807.
Taylor, C.R., Burns, J.: The demonstration of plasma cells and other immunoglobulin containing cells in formalin fixed paraffin embedded tissues using peroxidase labelled antibody. J. clin. Path. 27, 14-20 (1974).
Taylor, K.B., Truelove, S.C.: Circulating antibodies to milk proteins in ulcerative colitis. BMJ 2, 924-929 (1961).
Thayer, W.R.: Crohn's disease (regional enteritis). Scand. J. Gastroent. Suppl. 6, 165-185 (1970).
Thayer, W.R., Brown, M., Sangree, M.H., Katz, J., Hersh, T.: Escherichia coli 014 and colon haemagglutinating antibodies in inflammatory bowel disease. Gastroenterology 57, 311-318 (1969).
Tomasi, T.B.: Secretory immunoglobulins. New Engl. J. Med. 287, 500-506 (1972).

Tomkin, G.H., Mawhinney, A., Nevin, N.C.: Isolated absence of IgA with autosomal dominant inheritance. Lancet 1971 I, 124-125.

Verrier-Jones, J., Housley, J., Ashurst, P.M., Hawkins, C.F.: Development of delayed hypersensitivity to dinitro chlorobenzene in patients with Crohn's disease. Gut 10, 52-56 (1969).

Walker, N.A., Isselbacher, K.J., Block, K.J.: Intestinal uptake of macromolecules: effect or normal immunisation. Science 177, 608-610 (1972).

Watson, D.W.: Immune responses and the gut. Gastroenterology 56, 944-969 (1969).

Watson, D.W., Quigley, A., Bolt, R.S.: Effect of lymphocytes from patients with ulcerative colitis in human colon epithelial cells. Gastroenterology 51, 985-993 (1966).

Warren, K.S., Domingo, E.O., Cowan, R.B.: Granuloma formation around scluotosome eggs as a manifestation of delayed hypersensitivity. Amer. J. Path. 51, 735-756 (1966).

Warshaw, A.L., Walker, A., Cornell, R., Isselbackerk, J.: Small intestinal permeability to macromolecules. Lab. Invest. 25, 675-684 (1971).

Weetman, A.P., Haggith, J., Douglas, A.P.: Enteric loss of lymphocytes in coeliac disease and in Crohn's disease. Gut 15, 923 (1974).

Weibel, E.R.: Principles and methods for the morphometric study of the lung and other organs. Lab. Invest. 12, 131-155 (1963).

Werner, H.-J., Lefevr, H., Raettig, H.: Biphasic occurrence of IgM forming cells in the intestine after oral immunisation. Nature 232, 119-120

Whitehead, R.: Primary lymphadenopathy complicating idiopathic steatorrhoea. Gut 9, 569-575 (1968).

Whitehead, R.: The interruption and significance of morphological abnormalities in jejunal biopsies. J. Clin. Path. 24, Suppl. (Roy Coll. Path.) 5, 108-124 (1971).

Williams, R.C., Gibbons, R.J.: Inhibition of bacterial adherence by secretory immunoglobulin A: A mechanism of antigen disposal. Science 177, 697-699 (1972).

Wright, R., Alp, M.: Autoantibodies to reticulin in patients with various gastrointestinal diseases and their relationship to immunoglobulins and dietry antibodies. Gut 12, 858-859 (1971).

Wright, R., Truelove, S.C.: Circulating antibodies to dietary proteins in ulcerative colitis. BMJ 2, 142-144 (1965).

Wright, R., Truelove, S.C.: Autoimmune reactions in ulcerative colitis. Gut 7, 32-40 (1966).

Wright, R., Whitehead, R., Wangel, A.G., Salem, S.N., Schiller, K.F.R.: Autoantibodies and microscopic appearance of gastric mucosa. Lancet 1966 I, 618-621.

Zipursky, A., Brown, E., Bienenstock, J.: Lack of opsonization potential of 11S human secretory IgA. Proc. Soc. exp. Biol. 142, 181-184 (1973).

Oncofetal and Other Tumor-Associated Antigens of the Human Digestive System *

D.M. GOLDENBERG

* Some of the author's investigations discussed in this paper were supported by U.S. Public Health Service Grants CA-15799 and CA-17742 from the National Cancer Institute.

I. Introduction

Immunology, in all its facets of immunochemistry, humoral immunity, cellular immunity, immunodiagnosis, and immunotherapy, is currently the most rapidly advancing discipline of clinical and experimental oncology. But as in most developing subjects, it is continually beset with problems of methodology and nomenclature, both of which are often intertwined. Indicative of this problem are our circular definitions of antigen and antibody. Another frequent problem is the use of the words "specific" and "associated" when characterizing reactions to tumors or the antigenic properties of neoplasms. When applied to cancer, these terms are obviously very dependent upon the methods used to demonstrate these qualities. Indeed, the very diverse nature and multitude of types of cancer preclude our making generalizations or categorical statements regarding tumor "specificity." Similar problems arise when one considers that many antigens found in malignant tumors share certain properties with embryonic or fetal tissues. First, these observations emphasize a lack of true tumor specificity, for which reason the category of oncofetal antigens has been established. Second, whether or not such antigens are truly oncofetal depends upon the method of detection used, and it has been found that here too specificity decreases as the antigen assay increases in sensitivity. Thus, whether substances can be truly oncofetal in nature still remains a matter of debate, and such terms must therefore be used in an operational sense. The words of *Aldous Huxley* (1924) during his travels "Along the Road" appropriately express these relationships:

> "Most of our mistakes are fundamentally grammatical. We create our own difficulties by employing an inadequate language to describe facts. Thus, to take one example, we are constantly giving the same name to more than one thing, and more than one name to the same thing. The results, when we come to argue, are deplorable. For we are using a language which does not adequately describe the things about which we are arguing."

The purpose of this review is certainly not to offer any solution to this problem, but to focus on possible practical and conceptual meanings that the identification of substances classified as oncofetal may have. It is my objective to summarize the class of antigens associated with digestive tract cancers which have been termed oncofetal because of their supposedly electively sharing immunoreactivity with certain embryonic and/or fetal tissues. It is appropriate to consider such substances in gastrointestinal neoplasia because it is particularly in this system that immunodiagnostic tests for cancer prevail. Further, where other antigens of digestive organs have been described, these have also been included, regardless of whether or not they can be detected during ontogenesis.

II. Background

Antigens associated or supposedly specific for tumors have been demonstrated repeatedly in experimental animals (see reviews by *Haddow*, 1965; *Old* and *Boyse*, 1964) since the pioneering work of *Gross* (1943) and of *Foley* (1953). These are commonly referred to as tumor-specific transplantation antigens, or TSTA, because they were determined by transplantation-rejection techniques in syngeneic hosts. Obviously, ethical considerations preclude similar studies in man, so that the elucidation of antigens distinct for human cancers is limited to demonstrating tumor-distinctive reactions by means of humoral or cellular immune reactions in cancer patients, or by the production of putative tumor-specific antibodies after immunization of xenogeneic animals. These approaches have provided for an accumulation of evidence supporting the antigenic distinctiveness of certain human malignant tumors, such as melanoma (*Morton* et al., 1968), ovarian cancer (*Levi* et al., 1969), bladder carcinoma (*Bubenik* et al., 1970), bronchogenic carcinoma (*Yachi* et al., 1968), sarcomas (*Morton* et al., 1969), neuroblastoma (*Hellström* et al., 1968), leukemias (*Harris* et al., 1971; *Halterman* et al., 1972), and lymphomas (*Buffe* et al., 1970; *Klein* et al., 1969; *Order* et al., 1971), just to mention a few. Publications claiming the existence of antigens specific for various digestive tract neoplasms have been particularly abundant, and will be discussed below. Some of these tumor antigens can be subdivided on the basis of whether or not they are similar to components present in the embryo or fetus but not expressed, or expressed in decreased quantity, in normal adult tissues. For this reason they have been termed oncofetal antigens (*Alexander*, 1972), carcinofetal antigens (*Constanza* and *Nathanson*, 1974), carcinoembryonic antigens (*Gold*, 1971), and variations thereof. The elective occurrence of these substances, including a number of enzymes (*Schapira*, 1971; *Uriel*, 1975), in embryonic or fetal and malignant tissues has resulted in the speculation that these molecules owe their origin to genes which are active during ontogenesis but not expressed during normal adult life except when a "derepression" occurs, thus permitting these genes to be reactivated by some as yet unknown mechanism. Such an explanation would be plausible if there were indeed a truly qualitative difference between embryonic (or fetal) and adult tissues, or between normal adult and malignant tissues of any particular organ or site, and not a mere *quantitative* difference between the amount of antigen present in these various tissues. As we shall see, the evidence in support of truly cancer-distinct or cancer-specific substances or of embryonic- or fetal-specific antigens, in qualitative terms, is still inconclusive for most, if not all, so-called oncofetal antigens, although this field of inquiry has been pursued from as far back as at least 1932, when *Hirszfeld* and coworkers postulated the presence of embryo-specific substances in human tumors. More recently, *Stonehill* and *Bendich* (1970) emphasized this phenomenon in various tumors of the mouse, rat, and hamster induced by physical, viral, and chemical agents, as well as in those occurring spontaneously. These authors proposed that this was a universal phenomenon in tumors which they termed "retrogenetic expression."

At the present time, two oncofetal antigens of the digestive system are receiving the most attention, alpha-fetoprotein (AFP) and carcinoembryonic antigen (CEA). Very sensitive assays to detect these substances have been developed and currently are in clinical use, so that they will be discussed in particular detail. A number of other oncofetal antigens of the gastrointestinal system have also been described in recent years, and likewise will be considered, but less extensively.

III. Alpha-Fetoprotein (AFP)

Since the discovery of fetuin in fetal calf serum by *Pedersen* in 1944, a variety of fetoproteins have been described in several mammalian species, including man (*Bergstrand* and *Czar*, 1956). These substances are distinguished by their being present in fetal serum and absent in the circulation of corresponding adult animals, and their having the mobility of an alpha$_1$-globulin in immunoelectrophoresis. In 1963, *Abelev* and coworkers produced an antiserum to serum proteins of newborn mice and crossabsorbed this with serum from adult mice. The resulting antiserum was shown to react with the sera of adult mice bearing a transplantable hepatoma. This fetal serum protein could also be detected in the blood of adult mice after partial hepatectomy and of mice carrying two other transplantable hepatomas. Mice with transplantable tumors other than hepatomas did not have this antigen in their sera. It has since been shown that fetal calf serum contains several distinct fetoproteins, one of which is alpha$_1$-globulin and the other fetuin, which are distinct from each other (*Kithier* et al., 1968; *Spiro*, 1960; *Spiro* and *Spiro*, 1962). The hepatoma-related fetoprotein has since been found in 18 mammalian species (*Gitlin* and *Boesman*, 1967) for which reason it has been given the general name of alpha-fetoprotein (*Abelev* et al., 1970). In 1964, *Tatarinov* observed that two patients with primary carcinoma of the liver had an antigen in their blood which crossreacted with monospecific antiserum made against a fetal component. AFP has since been identified as elevated in patients with primary liver carcinoma (*Abelev*, 1971), in patients with teratocarcinomas of the testicle and ovary (*Abelev*, 1971), and in patients following partial hepatectomy (*Matray* et al., 1972). Before considering AFP in these clinical situations, attention will first be focused on its behavior in ontogenesis.

1. Fetal Sources

Human AFP can be detected in the 4-week-old fetus and achieves the highest concentration in fetal serum at about 13 to 15 weeks of gestation, reaching levels of about 3 to 4 mg/ml (*Gitlin* and *Boesman*, 1966; *Seller* et al., 1974; *Seppälä* and *Ruoslahti*, 1973). The serum AFP titer rapidly falls near term and is almost completely absent by 2 to 5 weeks after parturition (*Buffe*, 1973; *Seppälä* et al., 1967). The sites of AFP synthesis in the human fetus are liver, yolk sac, thymus, and gastrointestinal tract, the maximal concentration being reached between the tenth and twentieth weeks of gestation (*Gitlin* and *Boesman*, 1966; *Gitlin*, 1971; *Gitlin* et al., 1972; *Linder* and *Seppälä*, 1968; *Wada* et al., 1973). There appears to be an inverse relationship between AFP and albumin concentration in fetal blood since, with increasing fetal age, AFP levels decline and albumin rises. AFP is no longer demonstrable by the end of the fifth week following birth (*Buffe*, 1973; *Seppälä* et al., 1967), unless very sensitive assays are used to show small amounts (between 2 and 25 ng/ml) of AFP persistent in normal adult serum (*Chayvialle* and *Ganguli*, 1973; *Ishiguro* and *Nishimura*, 1973; *Ruoslahti* and *Seppälä*, 1971b; *Ruoslahti* et al., 1973). Small amount of AFP can also be detected in the amniotic fluid (*Field* et al., 1973; *Seppälä* and *Ruoslahti*, 1973). Maternal serum levels of AFP seem to rise during pregnancy, and fall sharply before term (*Ishiguro* and *Nishimura*, 1973). Since very increased levels occur before and after fetal death, it has been proposed that elevated levels of AFP in maternal blood are indications of fetal distress (*Purves* and *Purves*, 1972; *Purves* et al., 1973a; *Seppälä* and *Ruoslahti*, 1972a, b, 1973a, b, c).

2. Physicochemical Properties

Some of the physicochemical properties of AFP deserve brief mention. Human fetal as well as hepatoma AFP is a glycoprotein composed of 96% protein and 4% carbohydrate (*Ruoslahti* et al., 1971a). Its molecular weight ranges between 61,000 and 71,000 (*Hirai* et al., 1973; *Masopust* et al., 1971; *Ruoslahti* and *Seppälä*, 1971a; *Ruoslahti* et al., 1971), it has a sedimentation coefficient between 4.5 and 5.5S (*Gitlin* and *Boesman*, 1966; *Masopust* et al., 1971; *Nishi* and *Hirai*, 1971; *Nishi*, 1970), and, as has already been mentioned, it has a alpha$_1$-globulin mobility in immunoelectrophoresis. Some polydispersity in mobility of AFP is probably due to the presence of small quantities of sialic acid, since treatment with neuraminidase seems to make AFP monodisperse (*Alpert* et al., 1972, 1973; *Purves* et al., 1970b).

3. Clinical Role of AFP

Numerous methods have been employed to detect AFP in various tissues and body fluids, and these are both qualitative and quantitative in nature. Gel diffusion methods (e.g., immunoelectrophoresis, counterelectrophoresis, Ouchterlony two-dimensional diffusion, electroimmunodiffusion, etc.) have been used most frequently. More sensitive techniques, such as radioimmunoassay, are now being utilized increasingly for detecting AFP at very low concentrations, such as in the ng/ml range. Until the development of an AFP radioimmunoassay in 1971 (*Ruoslahti* and *Seppälä*, 1971b), most studies to detect AFP in serum were conducted by means of immunodiffusion tests. Although being less sensitive, the immunodiffusion assays did indicate a great degree of specificity of elevated AFP in hepatocellular cancer and teratocarcinomas of the ovary and testis (*Abelev*, 1971). Nonhepatic primary cancers usually only gave a raised serum AFP once they metastasized to the liver. This was particularly true in cases of pancreatic, gastric, and prostatic carcinomas (*Akai* and *Kato*, 1973; *Alpert* et al., 1971; *Bernades*, 1971; *Bierfield* et al., 1973; *Boureille* et al., 1970; *Geffroy* et al., 1970; *Ishii*, 1973; *Kozower* et al., 1971; *Masseyeff* et al., 1971; *Mehlman* et al., 1971; *Montplaisir* et al., 1973; *Nishi* and *Hirai*, 1973; *Ruoslahti* et al., 1972; *Sauger* et al., 1971). In South Africa, AFP positivity in hepatoma ranged from ca. 75 to 82% (*Purves* et al., 1968a, b, 1970a; *Abelev*, 1971; *Geddes* and *Falkson*, 1970), in the Far East from about 59 to 65 (*Smith* and *Todd*, 1968; *Smith*, 1970), in East Africa and in the United States it was reported at about a 50% rate of positivity (*Abelev*, 1971; *Alpert* et al., 1971a). The highest incidence has been observed in the hepatoma cases of the Bantu population of South Africa (*Abelev*, 1971; *Geddes* and *Falkson*, 1970). Since Africans tend to develop hepatocellular carcinoma two to three decades earlier than Caucasians do elsewhere in the world, this might explain the increased occurrence of elevated AFP levels in the serum of Africans as compared to Caucasians, because the proportion of cases with positive AFP levels in both hepatocellular carcinoma and teratocarcinomas decreases inversely with the age of the patients (*Abelev*, 1971; *Masseyeff*, 1972; *Mawas* et al., 1970). It is also of interest that women with hepatic cancer tend to have lower incidences of AFP positivity than men (*Alpert* et al., 1971a; *Hull* et al., 1970; *O'Conor* et al., 1970). AFP has also been detected in patients with non-neoplastic liver diseases, such as viral hepatitis (*Abelev*, 1971), congenital tyrosinemia (*Buffe* and *Rimbaut*, 1973), Indian juvenile cirrhosis (*Nayak* et al., 1972). These observations could be made with relatively insensitive diffusion methods. Gel diffusion methods also showed that tumor remission or recurrence could be reflected by changes in serum AFP (*Abelev*, 1971; *Elgort* et al., 1973).

The institution of more sensitive assays for serum AFP, such as radioimmunoassay, which can detect AFP in over four logarithmic scales, has indicated that AFP is only quantitatively increased in certain disease states, since it can be found in the sera of healthy adults in a range between 1 and 20 ng/ml (*Chayvialle* and *Ganguli*, 1973; *Ishiguro* and *Nishimura*, 1973; *Purves* et al., 1973a; *Ruoslahti* and *Seppälä*, 1971b). It should be emphasized, however, that even with the most sensitive methods of detecting circulating AFP, abôut 5 to 10% of cases with hepatocellular carcinoma have AFP values lying within the normal range.

The presence of increased levels of AFP in the sera of patients with other common, nonmalignant diseases deserves further attention. Temporary and minimal increases in serum AFP have been found in acute viral hepatitis (*Akeyama* et al., 1972; *Florin-Christian* and *Arana*, 1973; *Geffroy* et al., 1970; *Karvountzis* and *Redeker*, 1974; *Kew* et al., 1973; *Lehmann* et al., 1972; *Nishi* and *Hirai*, 1973; *Ruoslahti* et al., 1973; *Silver* et al., 1974; *Smith*, 1971), in drug or other forms of chronic hepatitis (*Abelev* et al., 1971; *Lehmann* et al., 1972; *Ishii*, 1973), in biliary (*Lehmann*, 1972) and other kinds of liver cirrhosis (*Abelev*, 1971; *Hirai* et al., 1973; *Lehmann* et al., 1972; *Nishi* and *Hirai*, 1973; *Nishioka* et al., 1973), and occasionally in bile duct lesions and obstructive jaundice (*Bloomer* et al., 1975), hemochromatosis (*Geffroy* et al., 1971; *Sarrazin* et al., 1973), ataxia telangectasia (*Waldmann* and *McIntire*, 1972), and in a case of Down's syndrome (*Adinolfi* et al., 1967). In hepatitis, a positive correlation could be found between the detection of AFP in the serum and the severity of the disease (*Karvountzis* and *Redeker*, 1974; *Silver* et al., 1974). In severe hepatitis, a positive level of AFP in the serum is interpreted as an expression of intensive liver cell regeneration, while the absence of AFP in a fulminant hepatitis is considered a poor prognostic sign. It seems, therefore, that the development of radioimmunoassays for AFP has resulted in an increasing number of so-called "false-positive" sera for hepatocellular carcinoma or teratocarcinoma detection. However, the regular use of these methods for AFP may overcome this problem and may provide a means for evaluating more subtle changes in AFP during the management of those patients with malignant tumors having increased circulating AFP titers.

No significant relationship could be found between serum AFP titer and clinical signs or biochemical data in hepatocellular carcinoma patients (*Alpert* et al., 1971a; *Purves* et al., 1970a). However, a degree of correspondence could be demonstrated between AFP serum level and the serum titers of cholesterol, hemoglobin, and protein; these increased together with AFP, while mucoproteins, alpha$_2$-globulin, and CRP fall (*Purves* et al., 1970a; *Purves* et al., 1973a). Several authors have claimed a correlation between AFP content in the tumors and the extent of dedifferentiation (*Alpert* et al., 1971a, c; *Purves* et al., 1970a; *Sasaki* et al., 1973; *Shikata* and *Sakakibara*, 1973; *Sugahara* et al., 1973; *Takahashi* et al., 1971), the more anaplastic tumors showing the highest tumor content of AFP (*Purves* et al., 1970a; *Sakurai* and *Miyaji*, 1973; *Sasaki* et al., 1973; *Takahashi* et al., 1971, 1973). It has also been reported, to confuse the issue, that very well differentiated and highly anaplastic hepatocellular carcinomas have very little or no AFP (*Shikada* and *Sakakibara*, 1973). A correlation has been claimed between the content of AFP in tumors and circulating AFP (*Lehmann* 1972; *Lehmann* et al., 1972), but not between AFP titer in the serum and tumor size, growth rate, stage, severity of the disease, or grade of malignancy (*Abelev*, 1971; *Endo* et al., 1973; *Masseyeff*, 1973; *Nishioka* et al., 1973; *Purves et al., 1968a, b, 1970a, 1973a; Ruoslahti* et al., 1972; *Sakurai* and *Miyaji*, 1973; *Takahashi* et al., 1973; *Uriel* and *de Néchaud*, 1972). However, reports have indicated an increasing occurrence of elevated AFP in the serum with increasing tumor weight, whereby 100 % of the cases were positive when the tumors weighed more than 5 kg (*Alpert* et al., 1971a). However, others have disputed this relationship (*Masseyeff* et al., 1971; *Purves* et al., 1970a). In such studies, one must be cautious in scrutinizing whether these claims were made for the initial level of AFP or during the course of the disease. In studying precisely this point, one investigation reported that the initial level of AFP in the serum had no correlation with tumor size and probably had little, if any, relationship with prognosis (*McIntire* et al., 1972). These problems are further accentuated when we consider that even small tumors can be present when AFP titers in the serum exceed 10 μg/ml (*Lehmann* and *Lehmann*, 1972), while large tumors can have very low AFP titers in the patient's serum (*Sasaki* et al., 1973) or no AFP detectable (*Takahashi* et al., 1973). Further, there has not been a correlation between level of AFP in the serum and survival time after diagnosis of hepatocellular carcinoma (*Vogel* et al., 1974). Therefore, the incidence and level of AFP positivity in circulating blood should not be accepted as a measure of histopathology or biology of the hepatic tumor in question.

Nevertheless, evidence from the production of hepatomas in monkeys (*Hull* et al., 1969) and in rodents (*Kroes* et al., 1972; *Becker* and *Sell*, 1974) indicates that AFP serum levels may be elevated before the tumors are identifiable by other means. This may also be the case in humans in certain situations (*Masseyeff*, 1972). Indeed, in one case it has been reported that the patient with cirrhosis originally had a normal AFP level which then rose to positive titers by gel diffusion seven to twelve months before a hepatic tumor was discovered (*Khasanov* et al., 1971). When considering AFP serum determinations in reference to other measures of diagnosis, it appears that the use of the AFP test is as reliable as, and certainly safer than, percutaneous liver biopsy (*Houstek* et al., 1968).

These results indicate that elevated serum AFP, as detected by radioimmunoassay, does not seem to be pathognomic for cancer in a screening sense. However, persistently high or increasing levels of serum AFP are very strong indications of primary liver cancer or teratocarcinomas of the ovary or testis. Furthermore, serial determinations of AFP are of interest in monitoring the therapeutic effects of various modalities or as a prognostic sign in diseases where the appearance of elevated values of serum AFP is of a transient character, such as in hepatitis and acute liver atrophy. A drop in serum AFP to normal values is an indication of complete tumor resection when AFP was elevated prior to surgery. A rise of a decreased or even normal AFP titer, which was elevated in a patient with hepatocellular carcinoma prior to therapy, is a sign of recurrence. No response in AFP serum titer or just a small response after therapy is indicative of incomplete removal of tumor or the presence of metastasis.

From the clinical standpoint, it is important to appreciate that elevated AFP values in the serum have been found in association with liver metastasis from the following primary tumors: gastric carcinoma (*Akai* and *Kato*, 1973; *Alpert* et al., 1971b; *Bernades*, 1971; *Bierfield* et al., 1973; *Boureille* et al., 1970; *Elgort* et al., 1973; *Geffroy* et al., 1970, 1971; *Kozower* et al., 1971; *Mehlman* et al., 1971; *Montplaisir* et al., 1973; *Ruoslahti* et al., 1972; *Sauger* et al., 1971; *Zawadski* and *Kraj*, 1974), esophageal carcinoma (*Spragins* et al., 1972), bronchogenic carcinoma (*Ishii*, 1973), colonic carcinoma (*Bernades* et al., 1971), pancreatic carcinoma (*Mehlman* et al., 1971), and cholangiocarcinoma (*Ishii*, 1973; *Ruoslahti* et al., 1974). Some other malignancies which have been reported to have increased serum AFP values, but without evidence of metastasis, are hypernephroma (*Piard* et al., 1973), Hodgkin's disease (*Ruoslahti* et al., 1972), and malignant reticulosis (*Ruoslahti* and *Seppälä*, 1972), and other blood disorders (*Abelev* et al., 1971), as well as occasionally in patients with hydatidiform mole (*Ishiguro* and *Nishimura*, 1973; *Seppälä* et al., 1972).

A recent study has shown that the production of AFP is more influenced by the site of tumor origin than by hepatic involvement, since some patients with gastric cancer and elevated AFP serum levels did not have any apparent hepatic metastases (*McIntire* et al., 1974b). This is consistent with an earlier finding that AFP was present in both the primary tumor and the hepatic metastasis of a patient with gastric cancer (*Montplaisir* et al., 1973). Further, in a study of patients with inflammatory bowel diseases, 9 and 5% of patients with ulcerative colitis and regional enteritis, respectively, were seropositive for AFP (*Thompson* et al., 1974). This is not surprising in view of the observation that human fetal gut is capable of a low level of AFP synthesis (*Gitlin*, 1971). These data are of course anecdotal and in need of confirmation and extension. Nevertheless, they caution that liver cancer can be mistakenly identified instead of a carcinoma secondary to the liver. When using very sensitive assays, such as passive hemagglutination, the AFP serum test can be positive in tumors other than those of hepatic or gonadal origin in more than 38% of the cases (*Lehmann* and *Lehmann*, 1973).

These considerations support the view that serum AFP has a definite role in the diagnosis of cancer, but in combination with other diagnostic measures. Serum values in excess of 1 μg/ml are strongly suggestive of the presence of primary hepatocellular carcinoma or of gonadal teratocarcinoma. In the range of 10 to 1,000 ng/ml, several nonmalignant hepatic diseases, such as viral hepatitis, chronic active hepatitis, and cirrhosis, can be associated with elevated serum AFP levels. Also, 25 to 40% of all hepatic tumors and teratocarcinomas, as well as a small percentage of other malignancies, especially gastric cancer, have these lower serum AFP levels.

As already mentioned, the specificity of the tests for hepatic cancer and gonadal teratocarcinoma decreases as the sensitivity of the serum AFP test increases. We may therefore question whether it is perhaps more useful in a clinical setting to use the more qualitative gel diffusion methods which can detect from 50 to 80% of hepatic cancers, but not the benign hepatic diseases also associated with increased AFP production and beyond the sensitivity range of most gel diffusion methods. Unfortunately, about 50% of patients with hepatocellular carcinoma in North America would be negative for AFP in their sera by these methods. Also, since AFP levels in the sera of patients with hepatic cancer can reflect tumor response to therapy on a quantitative basis, this is an important application of the more sensitive assays for serum AFP.

4. Site of AFP in Tumors

The increase in serum AFP seen in patients with partial hepatectomy or with liver damage suggests that increased synthesis and secretion of AFP is associated with reparative hyperplasia following liver injury. Indeed, liver regeneration usually accompanies tumor development and may even occur with metastasis to the liver. However, the evidence is fairly decisive that the tumor cells themselves can synthesize and release AFP, as is supported by tissue culture studies (*Rioche* et al., 1970; *van Furth* and *Adinolfi*, 1969). The cellular localization of AFP has received considerable attention. Immunocytochemical studies have revealed that AFP is present in human liver parenchymal cells of the fetus and newborn, and in hepatocellular carcinoma cells (*Smith* et al., 1971). A correlation between extent of fluorescence in the tumor cells and histological grade of differentiation has been claimed (*Takahashi* et al., 1973). AFP has been observed in fetal hepatocytes and in hepatoma cells to be localized diffusely in the cytoplasm (*Engelhardt* et al., 1971; *Linder* and *Seppälä*, 1968; *Nishioka* et al., 1972, 1973; *Purtilo* and *Yunis*, 1971), as well as also on the cell membrane and in the perinuclear zone of hepatoma cells (*Nishioka* et al., 1972). It has been postulated that AFP is a secretory product, since ultrastructural studies using peroxidase-labeled antibodies to AFP showed antigen to be present mainly in the rough endoplasmic reticulum at the surface, as well as in the free reticulum of a rat hepatoma (*Shikata* and *Sakakibara*, 1973). On the other hand, a binding of tritiated-estrogen to AFP in human hepatocellular carcinoma and in rat hepatoma cells showed by autoradiography that AFP was neither present in the normal nor in the malignant cells, but in the so-called transitional cells participating in normal liver cell regeneration (*Uriel* et al., 1972, 1973, 1974).

5. Biological Function

The biological function of AFP is still obscure. It has already been mentioned that AFP concentration in fetal serum appears to be the inverse of that found for serum albumin during gestation. It is not clear, therefore, whether AFP functions as a "fetal albumin" or as a protein involved in transport functions. AFP can bind estrogen, but not testosterone (*Nunez* et al., 1971; *Uriel* et al., 1972, 1973). This can be explained in terms of a possible protective function for the fetus against maternal estrogen. One could then speculate that if the AFP protective function is deficient, then an increased estrogen stimulation of the liver, as, for example, during the use of oral contraceptives, could be the mechanisms by which an increased occurrence of hepatomas occurs, as has indeed been discussed elsewhere (*Hooglie*, 1974). In laboratory animals, neutralization of AFP by administration of anti-AFP antiserum to pregnant animals resulted in an increased rate of fetal mortality and deformities (*Slade*, 1973), for which reason AFP might be considered to play an important protective role in organogenesis. The question of the role of AFP in oncogenesis in the liver and the gonads has provided much stimulation for conjecture. *Abelev* (1968) and *Lacassagne* (1968) postulate that the genetic information controlling AFP synthesis is due to the persistence of special hepatoblasts, in the case of hepatoma, or of yolk sac entoderm-like cells, in the case of teratocarcinomas. According to *Uriel* (1969), AFP synthesis in hepatomas is due to a retrodifferentiation of hepatocytes. *Pierce* (1970) argues that the increased synthesis of AFP in hepatomas is due to a persistence of undifferentiated stem cells. As was mentioned at the outset, the neosynthesis of a fetal antigen can be explained as a derepression of a repressed gene coding for the synthesis and/or expression of AFP, which is, however, expressed as a normal function in fetal life. The occurrence of AFP in inflammatory conditions of the liver could then be explained in terms of liver cell regeneration (*Abelev*, 1971; *Uriel* and *de Néchaud*, 1973). In the latter case, it is believed that a reversible genetic alteration occurs, whereas the alteration is presumably irreversible during hepatocellular carcinogenesis. Such considerations are obviously intriguing to entertain, but have not resulted in any direct experimental evidence either to elucidate the role and function of this putative oncofetal antigen or the relationships of gene activation or repression to fetal antigen expression or to oncogenesis.

6. Host Reactivity to AFP

Another matter requiring resolution is whether the host synthesizing increased amounts of AFP is capable of eliciting an immunological response to this antigen. No antibodies to AFP have usually been demonstrated in the serum of pregnant women or of patients with cancer (*Alpert* and *Zuckerman*, 1970; *Purves* et al., 1973b; *Ruoslahti* and *Seppälä*, 1972; *Seppälä* and *Ruoslahti*, 1973a). It has been postulated, however, that maternal isoimmunization against AFP could be responsible for congenital abnormalities and spontaneous abortions in humans, because injection of anti-AFP antiserum to pregnant rabbits and rats has such effects (*Slade*, 1973; *Smith*, 1972). However, the nature of the antibodies produced in xenogeneic hosts would be expected to be different from that presumably circulating in an isogeneic situation. It should also be mentioned, in this context, that AFP has been found to be immunosuppressive on antibody synthesis when administered in vivo (*Ogra* et al., 1974), and is a non-cytotoxic suppressor of both the primary and secondary response to sheep erythrocytes in vitro (*Murgita* and *Tomasi*, 1975a). AFP has been found to suppress certain T-cell-dependent functions in mice, such as allogeneic and mitogen-induced lymphocyte transformation (*Murgita* and *Tomasi*, 1975b). Finally, it has been reported that AFP binds to a fraction (about one-third) of murine T-cells (*Dattwyler* et al., 1975), thus suggesting that a subclass of T-cells may be involved in the immunosuppressive effect of AFP. However, it remains to be shown that the levels of AFP found in pregnant or tumor-bearing organisms are immunosuppressive in vitro or in vivo.

IV. Carcinoembryonic Antigen (CEA)

CEA was originally described as a tumor- and organ system-specific antigen of entodermally derived tissues of the gastrointestinal tract (*Gold* and *Freedman*, 1965a). It was also demonstrated in embryonic and fetal digestive tissues of the first two trimesters of gestation (*Gold* and *Freedman*, 1965b), for which reasons it was named the carcinoembryonic antigen of the human digestive system. The original work was performed with adenocarcinoma of the human colon, because this appeared to be a suitable specimen for also obtaining adjacent normal control tissue from the same donor when the tumor-containing segment of the gut was resected. By this means, *Gold* and *Freedman* hoped to distinguish tumor-specific from individual-specific antigenic differences presumably to be found between tumor and normal tissues of the same organ site. Rabbits were then injected with pooled saline extracts of the adenocarcinomas, and the resulting antisera were thought to be made tumor-specific, either by absorption with an excess of corresponding normal colon tissue extract or by using rabbits which previously were made immunologically tolerant to normal colonic mucosa. The antisera prepared by both these procedures were then also absorbed with human plasma, fibrin, and killed gut bacteria. The crossabsorbed antisera, when reacted with tumor extracts, gave a precipitin band in gel diffusion against colonic cancer, but not against extracts of normal mucosa (*Gold* and *Freedman*, 1965a).

These studies showed that all of the colonic adenocarcinomas examined by these authors contained an identical, qualitatively tumor-distinct antigen which was absent from the corresponding normal colonic tissue obtained from the same individuals. It was demonstrated that all human adenocarcinomas arising from the entodermally-derived digestive system epithelium – esophagus, stomach, small intestine, colon, rectum, pancreas, and liver – contain the same tumor-specific constituents. Although this substance could not be detected by gel diffusion in any other normal, diseased, or neoplastic tissues, it was found in embryonic and fetal gut, pancreas, and liver, thus apparently justifying its place as an oncofetal antigen.

These observations resulted in a surge of interest and research on CEA, in particular, and in tumor immunology, in general. In terms of CEA, the efforts principally have been in immunochemical analysis of CEA determinants, structural and biochemical studies, immunodiagnostic tests, and clinical applicability. I will restrict myself here to those salient aspects which I believe are of interest to the subject of gastrointestinal cancer, although mention of the relationship of CEA in other tumors and tissues will be made in an attempt to evaluate the current state and meaning of CEA.

1. Chemical and Physical Properties

Much effort has been expended to purify and analyze the chemical and physical properties of CEA (see reviews by *Terry* et al., 1974; *Fuks* et al., 1975). Suffice it to state that CEA derived from human metastatic colorectal carcinomas is a glycoprotein soluble in perchloric acid and strong salt solutions. It has a sedimentation coefficient of 6.8 S (*Coligan* et al., 1972) and a molecular weight of about 200,000 (*Krupey* et al., 1968). The electrophoretic mobility of CEA at pH 7–8.5 is that of a serum beta-globulin (*Krupey* et al., 1967), although this can vary with different preparations (*Pusztaszeri* and *Mach*, 1973). Isoelectric focusing has revealed that it is heterogeneous in its electrically charged groupings (*Coligan* et al.,1973). The differences in CEA found by isoelectric focusing seen in different specimens would appear to depend upon the tissue source of the antigen, pretreatment with perchloric acid, and individual tumor-CEA variations (*Terry* et al., 1974). Indeed, a similar heterogeneity of CEA fractions following isoelectric focusing of tumor, fetal, and normal colon tissue extracts of CEA has also been reported (*Rule* and *Goleski-Reilly*, 1973). The isoelectric point of CEA has been determined to be 4.8 (*Rosai* et al., 1972). The carbohydrate content of CEA usually varies between 42 and 77% (*Terry* et al., 1974), and its protein content lies at about 25% (*Banjo* et al., 1972). Although the amino acid and monosaccharide compositions vary, the molecule is characterized by a high *N*-acetyl-glucosamine content, whereas *N*-acetyl-galactosamine is low (*Mach* and *Pusztaszeri*, 1972; *Coligan* et al., 1973) or absent (*Krupey* et al., 1968; *Banjo* et al., 1972, 1974a, b). A variable amount of sialic acid is probably responsible for the charge heterogeneity of CEA molecules from different tumor specimens. The amino acids glutamine, asparagine, serine, and threonine account for 40% of the protein content of the molecule. Despite some variation in amino acid composition in different preparations of CEA, the amino acid sequence analysis has revealed a constant sequence for the first 24 amino terminal residues (*Terry* et al., 1972, 1974). It appears that sialic acid and fucose comprise the end position of the polysaccharide chain (*Terry* et al., 1974). Different investigators have shown that the *N*-terminal amino acid of CEA from colonic cancer is lysine (*Terry* et al., 1972; *Turberville* et al., 1973). Amino acid sequencing of five different CEA preparations from colonic cancers showed identical sequences of the first 20 to 30 amino acid residues (*Terry* et al., 1972). A similar sequence was obtained when the CEA synthesized by a human colon carcinoma serially propagated in hamsters (*Goldenberg* et al., 1966) was analyzed (*Terry* et al., 1974). On the other hand, there is wider variation in the values reported for the monosaccharides of CEA preparations (*Westwood* et al., 1974). Studies of the glycopeptides obtained from CEA have provided indirect evidence for the involvement of *N*-acetyl-glucosamine in the carbohydrate-protein linkage (*Banjo* et al., 1974a). Asparagine-*N*-acetyl-glucosamine showed weak inhibitory activity in the CEA radioimmunoassay (*Banjo* et al., 1974a). However, the chemical identity of the CEA determinant(s) is still a subject of investigation. Removal of sialic acid by neuraminidase treatment was not found to alter CEA activity (*Coligan* et al., 1973; *Banjo* et al., 1974b). Similarly, fucose did not appear to be important for immunological activity on the basis of controlled periodate treatment not affecting CEA activity (*Coligan* et al., 1974; *Egan* et al., 1974). After treating CEA by neuraminidase and then by nagase, a proteolytic enzyme made from *B. subtilis,* the fractions that were active were reported to contain *N*-acetyl-glucosamine (*Banjo* et al., 1972), but one or another lacked fucose, galactose, or mannose. Thus, it was suggested that *N*-acetyl-glucosamine is perhaps essential for CEA immunoreactivity (*Banjo* et al., 1974a). Recent evidence of reduction and alkylation of the CEA molecule diminishing binding activity to anti-CEA antibody suggests that the protein conformation is of importance to CEA immunoreactivity (*Thomas* et al., 1974; *Hammarström* et al., 1975). *Westwood* et al. (1974) showed that treatment of CEA with alkali, even under mild conditions, destroyed the antigenic activity, which was attributed to damage of the protein chain and consequent destruction of the tertiary structure. Also, treatment of CEA with weak acid cleaved the protein chain and reduced CEA activity. This reduction in activity could also be accomplished by treatment with pepsin. Thus, *Westwood* and coworkers (1974) concluded that the integrity of the protein chain of CEA is critical for its immunoreactivity. *Morris* et al. (1975) have also indicated that the protein portion of CEA is responsible for a major part of its antigenicity. However, we must be aware that it is extremely difficult to affect the protein portion of the molecule without concomitantly altering adjacent carbohydrate groups which may indeed be important for CEA's antigenicity.

Among the reactive groups that are known to be associated with CEA, but which are not necessarily an integral part of the molecule, are blood-group determinants (*Gold* et al., 1972; *Turner* et al., 1972; *Gold* and *Gold*, 1973). Also, determinants associated with CEA bind some lectins (*Terry* et al., 1974). The blood group activity of certain CEA preparations has been found generally to be related to the blood group of the patient from whom the CEA was obtained (*Holburn* et al., 1974), and could not be separated from CEA during extraction and isolation. Immunochemical studies have indicated that the CEA and blood group determinants are on the same molecule, but they are distinct from one another (*Gold* and *Gold*, 1973; *Holburn* et al., 1974). Distinct chemical differences have been found between CEA and blood group substances (*Terry* et al., 1974). Blood group substances have been found to be relatively inefficient in inhibiting CEA in the radioimmunoassay (*Terry* et al., 1974), and, as already mentioned, the CEA blood group activity correlated well with the blood group of the donor. Additional evidence supporting a distinction between CEA and blood group substances include the following: Monospecific anti-CEA antibody does not agglutinate blood group A erythrocytes, and blood-group A and B do not inhibit CEA-anti-CEA binding (*Gold* et al., 1972); *N*-acetyl-D-galactosamine, the immunodominant sugar of A antigen, is conspicuously absent or very negligible in most CEA preparations (*Gold* et al., 1973); treating CEA with anti-CEA and anti-i immunoabsorbents causes no reduction in its CEA activity (*Cooper* et al., 1974), and although the blood group precursors I and i can be found in extracts of colonic cancers, they can be separated from CEA by gel filtration (*Feizi* et al., 1975). These findings thus suggest that the blood group substances associated with CEA are extracted and purified along with CEA as non-covalently-linked molecules. In support of this contention, a recent report has shown a clearly different localization of CEA and blood group antigens on the surface of colonic tumor cells in culture by means of fluorescent microscopy (*Rosenthal* et al., 1975).

2. Clinical Role

In 1969, *Thomson* and coworkers in Montreal reported the development and application of a radioimmunoassay for CEA, based upon the Farr technique, which could detect nanogram quantities of CEA in the sera of cancer patients (*Thomson* et al., 1969). It was reported that all except 1 of 36 patients with colonic or rectal cancer had elevated serum CEA titers which became undetectable after successful resection. Only 1 of 30 cases with cancer of other parts of the digestive tract (a disseminated pancreatic carcinoma) had a high CEA level. Non-digestive tract cancers and non-neoplastic diseases gave negative results for circulating CEA. It was concluded that the CEA test was diagnostic of digestive tract cancer, and that this test was sufficiently specific and with such a high degree of positivity that it would be suitable for screening purposes. Unfortunately, subsequent research has revealed that this was a wrong projection, and the original results could not be confirmed by other groups or by these investigators themselves, either with the Farr radioimmunoassay method or other assays developed for CEA. Subsequent studies of circulating and tissue CEA have clearly shown that this antigen is neither tissue- nor cancer-specific, so that the CEA blood test could neither be used as a diagnostic screen for cancer nor as a test for digestive tract cancers.

However, it should be appreciated that an important advance in the clinical applicability of the CEA blood test was accomplished by the development of a rapid and more suitable radioimmunoassay for routine laboratory use by *Hansen* and his collaborators (1971) at Hoffmann-La Roche, Nutley, New Jersey. This assay, which has a sensitivity of 0.5 ng/ml of plasma, can be completed within 24 h, and is now in widespread clinical use throughout the USA and a number of other countries. Although a number of excellent studies using the Hansen assay for CEA have been reported since the original paper by *Lo Gerfo* et al. (1971), perhaps the most elaborate documentation of the clinical application of this assay is the Hoffmann-La Roche collaborative study (*Hansen* et al., 1974). Approximately 10,000 patients ranging in age from less than 1 year to over 80 years in more than 100 institutions in the US, Canada, and Great Britain were involved. The same biological reagents and standardized materials were used by all participants. Plasma CEA values were determined in a controlled group of 2,677 apparently healthy subjects. A second group of 2,039 patients with histologically-confirmed cancers of diverse origins was included, and every effort was made to obtain a pre-therapy and at least 2 post-therapy plasma samples. A third group consisted of 2,010 patients with previously proven metastatic or non-metastatic malignant disease, in which plasma samples were requested every 30 days. A total of 3,340 patients with a variety of non-malignant conditions constituted a fourth group, from which at least 1 plasma sample was obtained. The "normal" range of plasma CEA was reported as 0–2.5 ng/ml. The results among the group of apparently healthy individuals indicated that their smoking history affected the plasma CEA titer. Whereas 97% of healthy nonsmokers had CEA titers below 2.6 ng/ml (3% were between 2.6 and 5.0 ng/ml), 19% of cigarette smokers had CEA levels above 2.5 ng/ml in their plasma. An analysis of CEA levels in the plasma of women in all stages of pregnancy revealed that in 97% the levels were in the normal range (i.e., below 2.6 ng/ml).

In the group in which CEA titers were determined in patients suspected of having malignant disease, later to be confirmed, where true, histologically, abnormal CEA titers were obtained in 73% of the patients with colorectal cancer, in 76% of those with pulmonary cancer, in 91% of patients with pancreatic cancer, and in 61% of those with gastric cancer. As already mentioned, all these entodermally-derived digestive tract cancers were histologically confirmed, as was the case in all other cancer patients that were diagnosed as such. It is important to note that a significant number of these patients had CEA levels of 5.0 ng/ml or greater. Over 50% were between 5 and 10 ng/ml, and approximately 30% were above 10 ng/ml. In other kinds of cancer, it was found that abnormal CEA titers were present in 47% of patients with breast cancer (13% were in the 5.1–10.0 ng/ml range, while 14 % were above 10.0 ng/ml), and in about 50% of patients with other kinds of cancer (prostate, head and neck, ovary, cervix). In patients with lymphoreticular neoplasia, 37% had elevated CEA titers in acute and chronic leukemia, and 35% in a group of assorted malignant lymphomas. Elevated CEA titers in patients with leukemia and Hodgkin's disease were associated with disease activity, so that the CEA level was generally below 2.6 ng/ml when the disease was in remission. Finally, in patients with sarcoma, 31% had elevated CEA titers. In general, it is noteworthy that patients with carcinomas had a higher percentage of CEA levels above 5.0 or above 10.0 ng/ml than those with malignancies of the lymphoreticular or connective tissues.

In the part of the study in which CEA levels were determined in patients with known metastatic and non-metastatic malignant diesease, it was learned that the percentage of elevated titers rises as the condition of the patient deteriorates. Also, the percentage of elevated titers in patients with metastatic disease is greater regardless of whether the patient had a significant response to therapy, was afforded relief but not cured, or had no response to treatment, than for those with non-metastatic malignant disease.

A very significant portion of this extensive clinical investigation was the analysis of CEA titers in patients with non-malignant diseases. Although 34% of 3,340 patients had titers of 2.6 ng/ml or higher, less than 10% of all except those with gastrointestinal inflammation had titers above 5.0 ng/ml and less than 1% were above 10.0 ng/ml. In almost all cases the titer elevations occurred while the disease was in a clinically active state, and when remission occurred or the inflammatory disease was no longer present, the titer usually fell to the normal range. It is further important to note that 57% of patients with pulmonary emphysema, 70% with alcoholic cirrhosis, 47% with granulomatous colitis, 45% with gastric ulcer, 53% with pancreatitis, 56% of kidney transplant patients, 65% who were alcohol addicts, and 46% of patients with pneumonia had abnormally elevated CEA titers. This list is just an example of some of the diseases in which a marked percentage of individuals had elevated CEA levels. However, the majority of the titers were in the mildly elevated zone of 2.6–5.0 ng/ml, with an extremely small percentage with titers above 10.0 ng/ml. For example, in pulmonary emphysema only 16% were in the range of 5.1 to 10.0 ng/ml and 4% above

Table 1. Circulating CEA levels in various conditions [a]

Clinical Status	% Elevated CEA
Normal	
Healthy, unselected	11
Healthy, nonsmokers	3
Healthy, smokers	19
Healthy, pregnant	3
Nonmalignant diseases	
Alcoholic cirrhosis of liver	70
Alcohol addiction	65
Pulmonary emphysema	57
Kidney transplant	56
Pancreatitis	53
Granulomatous colitis	47
Pneumonia	46
Gastric ulcer	45
Ulcerative colitis	31
Malignant diseases	
Colorectum, all stages	72–81
Dukes' A	38–44
Dukes' B	60–76
Dukes' C	60–75
Metastasized	80–89
Stomach	61
Pancreas	91
Breast	47
Lung	76
Prostate	40
Bladder	42
Gynecologic	65
Lymphomas	35
Acute and chronic leukemias	37

[a] Compiled from results in *Hansen* et al. (1974), *Reynoso* et al. (1972), *Laurence* et al. (1972), *LoGerfo* et al. (1971), *Hall* et al. (1973), *Laurence* and *Neville* (1972), *Khoo* (1974), and *Martin* et al. (1976).

10.0 ng/ml; 24% of patients with alcoholic cirrhosis were in the 5.1 to 10.0 ng/ml range, while 2% were over 10.0 ng/ml; 8% of patients with ulcerative colitis were in the 5.1–10.0 ng/ml range, while 5% were above 10.0 ng/ml; 15% in granulomatous colitis were in the 5.1 to 10.0 ng/ml group, while 2% had titers above 10.0 ng/ml, etc. Except for patients with alcohol addiction (12% above 10.0 ng/ml CEA), patients with these non-malignant diseases rarely constituted more than 5% with plasma CEA above 10.0 ng/ml. Thus, almost all the healthy non-smoking and smoking subjects and patients with clinically active non-malignant disease who had elevated CEA titers showed levels in the range of 2.6 to 5.0 ng/ml. However, it should be emphasized that CEA titers below 2.6 ng/ml are not proof of the absence of malignant diesease, particularly when other positive clinical findings are available. A summary of the percentage of cases with elevated blood CEA titers is presented in Table 1.

Most of the benign conditions that produce elevations in circulating CEA rarely exceed 10 ng/ml CEA, and most of these are between 2.5 and 5.0 ng/ml (i.e., polyps, ulcerative colitis, regional enteritis, chronic lung disease, heavy smoking, pancreatitis). Hence, when evaluating patients for cancer, levels exceeding 10 ng/ml are very suggestive of a cancer being present. In this context, serial determinations are being recommended widely, particularly when other tests are not conclusive. Indeed, serial determinations showing a rising CEA titer are often the only early indicator of recurrent cancer. For example, cases have been reported in which the patients were asymptomatic but the CEA levels were increasing, and where recurrent cancer was finally demonstrated (*Zamcheck*, 1975).

In one particular study, 47% of 81 patients with non-specific gastrointestinal problems and positive CEA assays were found to evidence gastrointestinal cancers during extended evaluation with repeated radiological and/or endoscopic investigations over a two-year period (*Gold* et al., 1973). *McCartney* and *Hoffer* (1974) have reported evidence suggesting that combining the CEA assay and barium enema results in a higher detection rate of colon cancer than either test alone.

The highest percentage of elevated titers was in carcinomas of entodermal origin (colorectal, pulmonary, pancreatic, gastric) (Table 1), and this group also yielded the greatest number of titers above 5.0 ng/ml. About 50% with non-entodermally derived carcinomas (e.g., breast, head and neck) had CEA titer elevations. But except when metastatic disease was present, the values were not as high as in the sites already listed. The results of this study thus suggest that CEA plasma titers could play an important role in the management of patients with neoplastic disease, especially when the values are obtained from serial specimens and show a consistently increasing or decreasing trend. Indeed, rising CEA levels may preceed clinical recurrence of cancer (*Holyoke* et al., 1975; *Sorokin* et al., 1974). The duration between rise in CEA titer and appearance of clinical or other laboratory evidence of tumor recurrence has varied from two weeks to ten months (*Holyoke et al.*, 1972, 1975; *Mach* et al., 1974; *Khoo* and *Mackay*, 1973, 1974; *Sorokin* et al., 1974). Likewise, it is clear from the data obtained in patients with diseases other than neoplasia that the CEA plasma test cannot be used as a screening test to detect cancer in the general population. Whether or not it will prove of significant value in patients with an increased risk for certain kinds of cancer needs more intensive investigation before answering.

The relationship of CEA plasma levels to inflammatory bowel disease is an intriguing question, since these diseases, particularly ulcerative colitis, are known to have a high proclivity for malignant change. Whether the persistently elevated CEA titers in such patients have any prognostic significance with regard to the possible transition into cancer certainly merits further investigation. In 15 of 17 sera from patients with ulcerative colitis, the CEA activity could be removed by extraction with perchloric acid (*Khoo* et al., 1973). This would suggest that the inhibitory component(s) in the CEA radioimmunoassay in the unextracted sera was probably not the same CEA measured after PCA-extraction, thus emphasizing the heterogeneity of glycoproteins indicating CEA activity in the radioimmunoassay.

At the present time, the principal application of the CEA blood test is to monitor tumor response to therapy in those cases where previously increased CEA titers fell to normal values after total resection of colorectal, pancreatic, and other cancers (*Booth* et al., 1973; *Dhar* et al., 1972; *Gold* et al., 1973; *Laurence* et al., 1972; *LoGerfo* et al., 1972; *Mach* et al., 1974; *Meeker* et al., 1973; *Moore* et al., 1971; *Reynoso* et al., 1972; *Sorokin* et al., 1974; *Thomson* et al., 1969) or during chemotherapy (*Mulcare* and *LoGerfo*, 1972; *Skarin* et al., 1974; *Martin* et al., 1976). Partial or failure of a drop in elevated titers has been observed in incomplete resection or in cases of metastasis or recurrence, particularly during the symptom-free interval (*Booth* et al., 1973; *Holyoke* et al., 1972; *Laurence* et al., 1972; *Mach* et al., 1974; *Sorokin* et al., 1974). In such cases a generally increased or elevated CEA titer falls to normal within 1 to 4 weeks after total tumor resection in cases without metastasis (*Booth* et al., 1973; *Dhar* et al., 1972; *Laurence* et al., 1972; *LoGerfo* et al., 1972; *Mach* et al., 1974; *Reynoso* et al., 1972; *Sorokin* et al., 1974; *Thomson* et al., 1969). This observation agrees with the metabolism of human CEA when it is injected into dogs or hamsters, where the majority of the injected material clears from the circulation within an hour, most of it accumulating in the liver (*Shuster* et al., 1973; *Primus* et al., 1974). It is interesting, however, that there is a delayed clearance observable in hamsters bearing CEA-producing human tumors (*Primus* et al., 1974).

To a certain extent, there is a correlation between the degree of CEA elevation and the stage of disease; e.g., in colonic cancers classified according to Dukes' Classification (*Dukes*, 1932), as was shown in Table 1. In the early stage (Dukes' A) when colonic cancer is still highly curable, more than half of the cases have normal circulating CEA values. No direct relationship between blood CEA titer and grade of tumor differentiation has been reported (*Laurence* et al., 1972; *Meeker* et al., 1973), as well as a lack of correlation with age (*Miller*, 1972) of the cancer patients. However, a correlation between CEA elevation and stage of the disease, duration of the disease, age of the patient, and response to therapy was found in cases with inflammatory bowel diseases (*Rule* et al., 1973).

Whether or not the CEA being measured in the plasma of patients with various kinds of cancer is the same as that found in the blood of patients with digestive tract carcinomas is a question of continual concern, and points to one of the major problems of this area of research; namely, the lack of a standard and highly purified preparation of CEA with known chemical composition and physical structure. Without such a standard, the CEA's found in many studies cannot be compared except in their capacity to react with certain antibody preparations in a number of immunological tests. This problem is exacerbated when radioimmunoassays are obtained in different laboratories using different reagents or different tests, and even different means of extracting CEA from blood. On the basis of physicochemical and immunochemical criteria, however, we have been able to show the identity of CEA circulating in the blood of patients with ovarian, cervical, bronchogenic, and other cancers with a preparation of colonic carcinoma CEA (*Goldenberg* et al., 1976c; *Pletsch* and *Goldenberg*, 1974). These results are certainly not unexpected when one reacts CEA's from various tumors, including colonic cancer, with anti-CEA antibody prepared against colonic cancer CEA in gel diffusion (Fig. 1). A complete precipitin line of identity is obtained, thus indicating the immunological identity of the CEA's in these different kinds of cancer. Although this finding is in contradiction to the results originally reported by *Gold* and *Freedman* (1965a) using similar immunodiffusion methods, it may well be that the antiserum they initially used was qualitatively different or quantitatively less potent than the anti-CEA antisera now more commonly available.

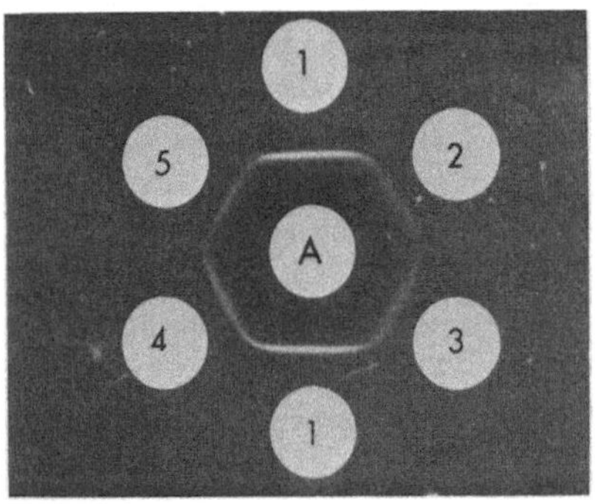

Fig. 1. Gel diffusion plate showing identical precipitin bands in reactions of goat anti-CEA antibody (A) against CEA in colonic cancer (1, 3), GW-39 human colonic cancer transplant system (2), cervical cancer (4), and ovarian cancer (5)

The combined role of CEA and AFP in tumor detection and diagnosis has received only limited attention. A comparison of circulating CEA and AFP in gastric and colorectal cancer has shown that both antigens measured simultaneously significantly increased the incidence of positive diagnosis in patients with gastric cancer but not in colorectal cancer (*McIntire* et al., 1974a). This study further showed that a single tumor could produce both these oncofetal antigens, and that the production of AFP is more influenced by the site of tumor origin than by hepatic involvement, since some patients with gastric cancer and elevated AFP serum levels did not have any evidence of hepatic metastasis. However, as was to be expected, elevations of both AFP and CEA were more frequent among patients with liver metastasis than those without (*McIntire* et al., 1974a). In a comparison of circulating CEA and AFP in a series of patients with colorectal cancer with hepatic metastases, of cases with bronchogenic or mammary carcinoma, of miscellaneous chronic liver disease (cirrhosis, ethanol abuse, chronic hepatitis, obstructive jaundice), and cases with miscellaneous tumors, it was found that measurement of CEA is, by itself, a more reliable index of disease activity than measurement of plasma AFP (*Grigor* et al., 1975).

In a study of CEA and AFP in patients with ulcerative colitis or regional enteritis, no serum was positive for both CEA and AFP (*Thompson* et al., 1974). It is not surprising, however, to find 9 and 5% of patients with ulcerative colitis and regional enteritis, respectively, to be seropositive for AFP (*Thompson* et al., 1974) in view of the observation that human fetal gut is capable of a low level of AFP synthesis (*Gitlin*, 1971).

As was the case for AFP, CEA has been detected in minute quantities in normal plasma since the advent of a radioimmunoassay for its determination (*Chu* et al., 1972; *LoGerfo* et al., 1971; *Thomson* et al., 1969). CEA was also detected in the urine of healthy individuals (*Guinan* et al., 1974; *Hall* et al., 1972). Other body fluids containing CEA include amniotic fluid (*Goldenberg* et al., 1972b) and lavages of the bronchial tree (*Blair* and *Goldenberg*, 1974) or the intestinal tract (*Go* et al., 1975). The presence of CEA in amniotic fluid and meconium stimulated the proposal that increased levels of CEA in amniotic fluid obtained at amniocentesis could reflect meconium content and, in turn, perhaps serve as a quantitative measure of fetal distress (*Goldenberg* et al., 1972b). CEA could also be detected in stool (*Freed* and *Taylor*, 1972). However, because it is present in the stool of 27% of adults with gastrointestinal cancer, in 18% of patients with extra-gastrointestinal cancers, in individuals without cancer, and in pregnant women, it does not appear that the detection of CEA in the stool of patients with cancer will be of any diagnostic value (*Freed* and *Taylor*, 1972; *Hirsch-Marie* et al., 1973). Mention should be made that CEA has been extracted from normal colonic mucosa (*Dyce* and *Haverback*, 1974; *Khoo* et al., 1973; *LoGerfo* et al., 1972; *Martin* and *Martin*, 1970, 1972; *Rosai* et al., 1972), normal and cirrhotic liver (*Dyce* and *Haverback*, 1974; *Khoo* et al., 1973; *Kupchik* and *Zamcheck*, 1972), normal lung (*Dyce* and *Haverback*, 1974; *Khoo* et al., 1973; *LoGerfo* et al., 1972; *Pusztaszeri* and *Mach*, 1973; *Tillack* et al., 1974), lactating breast (*Pusztaszeri* and *Mach*, 1973), and from the erythrocyte membranes of normal individuals and of patients with hemorrhoids and hemochromatosis (*Nery* et al., 1973). An interesting observation was made by *Taylor* and *Freed* (1976) that human erythrocytes contain a "sticky" substance which can bind to CEA. This probably explains the CEA-like substance which was extracted from erythrocyte stromata by *Nery* et al. (1973), as well as the apparently higher CEA levels found in plasma stored in contact with its cells than the same specimen when fresh (*Laurence* et al., 1972). One must again caution that we are dealing here with substances which are "immunoreactive" with anti-CEA antibody in the radioimmunoassay, and not necessarily the same molecule as that found to be the major immunodeterminant for CEA in colonic and other carcinomas. Indeed, if the anti-CEA antibody still contains immunoreactivity for the cross-reacting antigens of CEA, such as NCA and its associated molecules (*vide infra*), then so-called CEA will be detectable in many different tissues and cells.

3. Localization

Immunofluorescent (*Bordes* et al., 1973; *Burtin* et al., 1973b; *Denk* et al., 1972; *Gold* et al., 1968; *von Kleist* and *Burtin*, 1969; *Tappeiner* et al., 1973) and electron-microscopic (*Gold* et al., 1970; *Huitric*, 1973) studies have revealed that CEA is localized on the surface of the cells which lies along the lumen of the acini of gastrointestinal adenocarcinoma, preferentially in the glycocalyx of "fuzzy coat" intimately associated with the plasma membrane. Due to this localization and because CEA is seen in the glandular lumen, it has been suggested that it is more a secretory product than a structural component of the cell (*Denk* et al., 1972; *Huitric* et al., 1976; *Rogalsky*, 1975). On the other hand, the studies of others (*Gold* et al., 1970; *Rosai* et al., 1972) indicate that CEA is a cellular structural glycoprotein. Recently, CEA was shown to be present both intracellularly and in or near the cell membrane of colonic carcinoma as well as putatively normal colonic mucosal cells by means of immunoperoxidase electron microscopy (*Huitric* et al., 1976), which could be interpreted as support of CEA being a secretory product of the cell. However, it is not convincing that the reaction seen was truly CEA and no other crossreactive substances, such as NCA. Indeed, at a recent meeting where these results were presented and discussed, a retraction was made for the intracellular localization of CEA in either normal or malignant colon cells (*Huitric* and *Burtin*, 24th Meeting of Protides of the Biological Fluids, Brugge, April, 1976). Further, recent evidence showing a so-called fluorescence capping or redistribution of CEA when anti-CEA antiserum was reacted with colonic tumor cells in culture (*Rosenthal* et al., 1975) would support the view that CEA is a peripheral membrane component similar to certain antigenic determinants on lymphocytes. Nevertheless, CEA has been shown to be produced and released by numerous malignant cell types grown in culture (*Breborowicz* et al., 1973; *Burtin* et al., 1970; *Egan* and *Todd*, 1972; *Goldenberg* et al., 1972a; *Tomkins* et al., 1974; *Tom* et al., 1976), where it is released into the medium. Such observations emphasize that CEA is indigenous to the tumor cells, which is also supported by the finding that human colonic carcinoma cells serially passaged in unconditioned golden hamsters continue to produce and release CEA into the animal host (*Goldenberg* and *Hansen*, 1972a, b), and are even capable of evoking anti-CEA IgM antibodies (*Primus* et al., 1976). However, the release of CEA in culture medium does not unequivocally prove that active release is occurring, since dead or dying tumor cells may account for the values obtained in the medium. More quantitative data, using radiolabeled precursors, are therefore needed to resolve this question.

The immunocytochemical demonstration of CEA in extra-gastrointestinal tract cancers and in other tissue specimens has been the subject of a number of studies, some of which have produced conflicting results. Whereas one group reported that squamous cell carcinoma of the bronchus and cystadenocarcinoma of the ovary, as well as mammary carcinoma and a few other tumors, were all negative for CEA by immunofluorescence (*Denk* et al., 1972), another study claimed positive immunofluorescence for CEA in lung, mammary, renal, and laryngeal cancers, and no stainable CEA in pharyngeal, anal, and ovarian carcinomas (*Bordes* et al., 1973). Moreover, immunofluorescent staining of CEA has been shown in colonic adenomas (*Burtin* et al., 1972; *Tappeiner* et al., 1973), in normal juvenile mucosa, normal mucosa surrounding or somewhat distant from colonic cancer (*Bordes* et al., 1973; *Burtin* et al., 1972a,b; *Tappeiner* et al., 1973; *von Kleist* and *Burtin*, 1969), and in ulcerative colitis mucosa and inflamed colonic mucosa (*Bordes* et al., 1973; *Burtin* et al., 1972). These differences are probably more attributable to differences in techniques and antibody specificities (perhaps containing crossreactive antibodies to NCA and similar substances [*vide infra*]) than to actual differences in CEA content between such specimens.

In order to investigate the presence and localization of CEA in tissue specimens, particularly in a surgical pathology setting, we undertook the further development and application of a triple-bridge, indirect, peroxidase-antiperoxidase method for demonstrating CEA in frozen, ethanol-fixed or formalin-fixed, paraffin-embedded specimens, as we described elsewhere (*Primus* et al., 1975). Up to the present time, we have examined 511 tissue specimens, including 328 malignant tumors, 71 benign tumors, 56 non-neoplastic, diseased tissues, and 56 normal specimens. CEA could be demonstrated fairly consistently, frequently, and almost exclusively in a group of cancers, including carcinomas of the stomach, colon, rectum, pancreas, lung, and cervix. Malignant tumors of the breast, prostate, kidney, larynx, brain, lymphoreticular and connective tissues were devoid of CEA demonstrable by this technique (Table 2). As can be seen in this table, the cancers with the highest frequency of staining

Table 2. Immunoperoxidase-CEA results in malignant tumors

Organ/Histopathology	No. Pos./Total	% Pos.
Esophagus/Squamous cell ca.	0/5	0
Esophago-gastric/Adenoca.	2/4	50
Stomach/Adenoca.	5/12	42
Colon/Adenoca.	35/45	78
Rectum/Adenoca.	5/10	50
Pancreas/Adenoca.	2/8	25
Liver/Hepatocellular ca.	0/9	0
Liver/Cholangioca.	1/1	100
Larynx/Squamous cell ca.	0/7	0
Parotid/Squamous cell ca.	0/1	0
Kidney/Renal cell ca.	0/6	0
Lung/Squamous cell ca.	9/35	26
Lung/Adenoca.	1/11	9
Breast/Scirrhous ca.	0/11	0
Breast/Medullary ca.	0/1	0
Breast/Adenoca.	0/16	0
Brain/Various type	0/16	0
Urinary bladder/Transitional cell ca.	1/10	10
Urinary bladder/Squamous cell ca.	0/3	0
Prostate/Adenoca.	0/11	0
Ovary/Mucinous cystadenoca.	1/12	8
Ovary/Serous cystadenoca.	0/7	0
Ovary/Adenoca. and miscellaneous	0/5	0
Endometrium/Adenoca.	0/10	0
Uterine cervix/Squamous cell ca.	10/28	36
Uterine cervix/Ca. in situ	0/17	0
Lymphoreticular tissue/Lymphosarcoma, reticulum cell ca., Hodgkin's disease	0/7	0
Skin/Basal cell ca.	0/9	0
Skin/Squamous cell ca.	0/5	0
Skin/Melanoma	0/3	0

Table 3. Immunoperoxidase-CEA results in benign tumors

Organ/Histopathology	No. Pos./Total	% Pos.
Stomach/Leiomyoma	0/1	0
Colon/Villous adenoma [a]	2/4	50
Colon/Polypoid adenoma	7/26	27
Colon/Juvenile polyp	4/5	80
Rectum/Villous adenoma	1/3	33
Ovary/Cystic teratoma	0/5	0
Ovary/Mucinous cystadenoma	0/3	0
Ovary/Serous cystadenoma	1/5	20

[a] Not included in this group were 2 mixed villous-adenomatous polyps. These were positive and included in group of polypoid adenoma.

for CEA were adenocarcinoma of the colon, adenocarcinoma of the rectum, squamous cell carcinoma of the uterine cervix, adenocarcinoma of the stomach, squamous cell carcinoma of the lung, and pancreatic adenocarcinoma, thus confirming and extending our initial study with this method (*Goldenberg* et al., 1976d). The staining reaction for CEA in such tumor specimens can be appreciated best by comparing it with an adjacent tissue section from the same specimen which, however, was instead reacted with a CEA-neutralized, control antiserum, as is shown in Figure 2 for a colonic adenocarcinoma fixed in formalin and embedded in paraffin. The test reaction shown in Figure 3 demonstrates specific staining for CEA at the glandular border of the tumor acini and in some intraglandular deposits. Benign colonic tumors were positive for CEA in 27% of the cases examined, while a single serous cystadenoma of the ovary also showed CEA staining by immunoperoxidase (Table 3). The immunoperoxidase test and control reactions for CEA in a polypoid adenoma of the colon are shown in Figures 4 and 5, respectively. Of the non-neoplastic, diseased tissues studied, only inflammatory conditions of the bowel showed a CEA-staining reaction (Table 4). The results for normal tissues tested by this technique are summarized in Table 5. It appears that normal tissues were devoid of stainable CEA, except for a weak cytoplasmic reaction in 2 colonic

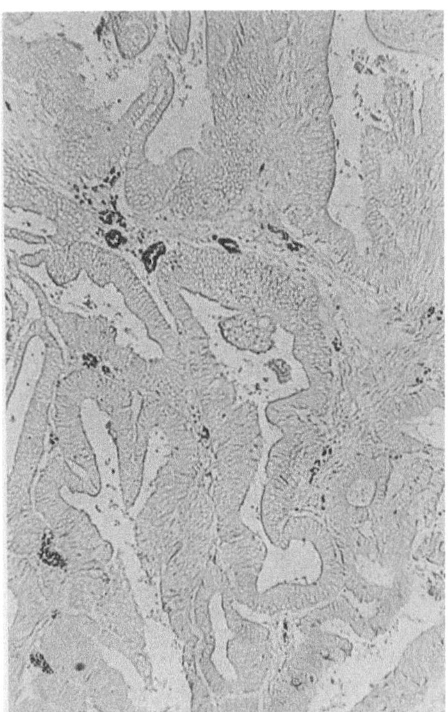

Fig. 2

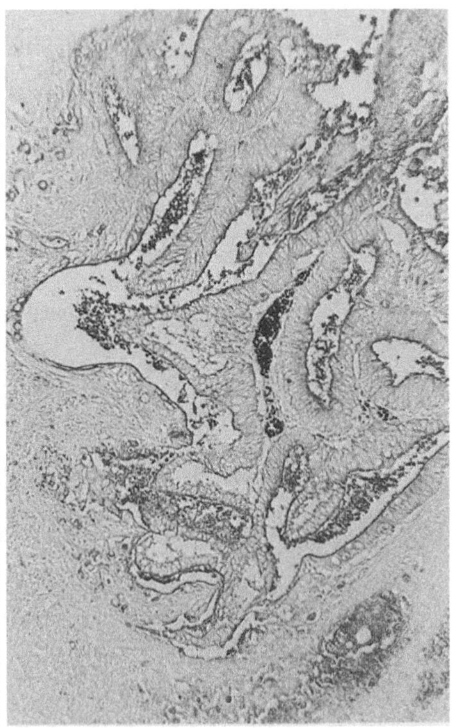

Fig. 3

Fig. 2. Control immunoperoxidase reaction for CEA in colonic carcinoma specimen fixed in formalin and embedded in paraffin. Orig. x 100

Fig. 3. Immunoperoxidase reaction for CEA in specimen of Fig. 2, showing staining of the surface of the malignant glands bordering the lumen and of material within the lumen. Orig. x 100 mucosa specimens from the resection margins of colonic carcinomas which were fixed in ethanol (Fig. 6). However, the same sections proved to be negative for CEA after formalin-paraffin processing, thus indicating that the CEA present was very close to the threshold quantity demonstrable by immunoperoxidase testing. Measurement of tumor CEA content by radioimmunoassay has revealed that this relative specificity of the immunoperoxidase test for CEA is due to a different concentration of CEA between the various tissue specimens, and because the threshold for CEA staining was usually above the CEA concentration found in non-neoplastic specimens. An analysis of the formalin-paraffin-treated sections showed that CEA positivity by immunoperoxidase reflected tissular CEA levels of about 3.0–5.0 μg/g or more, thus permitting retrospective estimates of minimal tissue CEA concentrations to be made in older histopathology specimens by the immunoperoxidase reaction; indeed, formalin-paraffin sections as old as ten years still had demonstrable CEA (*Goldenberg* et al., 1976d). Whereas tumor CEA concentration correlated well with immunoperoxidase staining for CEA, it was found that plasma CEA titer did not necessarily reflect tumor CEA concentration. A strong correlation was also seen between CEA positivity in primary and in secondary tumors, as well as somewhat with level of tumor differentiation (*Goldenberg* et al., 1976d). This study, which documented that

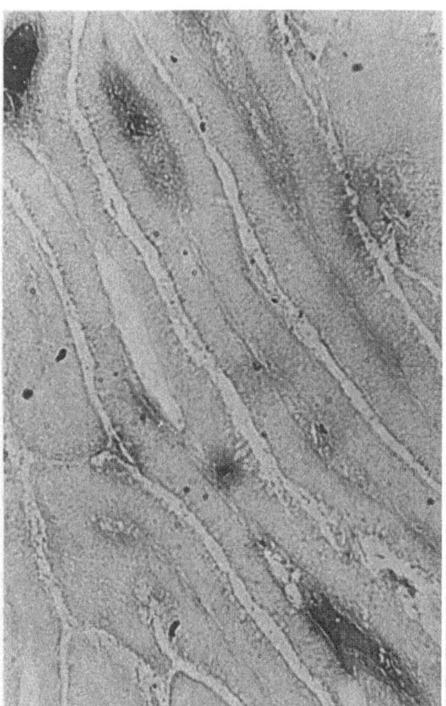

Fig. 4

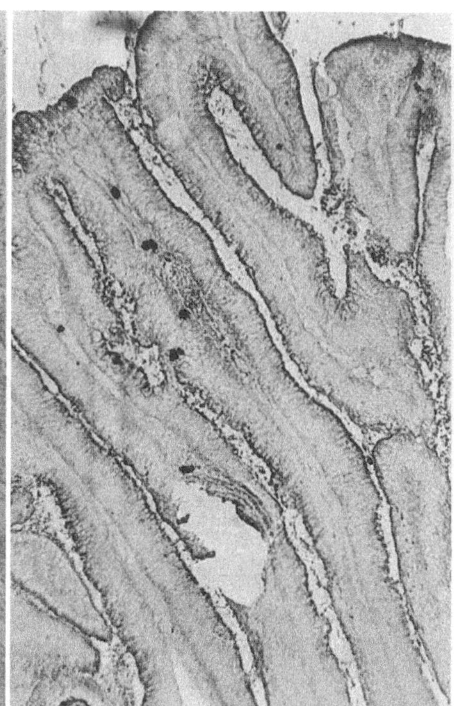

Fig. 5

Fig. 4. Control immunoperoxidase reaction for CEA in a colonic polypoid adenoma. Orig. x 100

Fig. 5. Immunoperoxidase reaction for CEA in specimen of Figure 4, showing an intensive staining reaction. Orig. x 100

Table 4. Immunoperoxidase-CEA results in non-malignant, diseased tissues

Organ/Histopathology	No. Pos./Total	%Pos.
Stomach/Ulcer	0/6	0
Colon/Nonspecific colitis	0/4	0
Colon/Ulcerative colitis	2/15	13
Colon/Granuloma	0/2	0
Colon/Inflam. polyp	1/2	50
Colon/Regional enteritis	0/1	0
Rectum/Pseudomembran. colitis	1/1	100
Liver/Cirrhosis	0/5	0
Liver/Viral hepatitis	0/2	0
Lung/Chron. bronchitis	0/6	0
Lung/Bronchiolectasis	0/1	0
Lung/Pneumonitis	0/1	0
Lung/Pneumonia	0/1	0
Urin. bladder/Cystitis	0/3	0
Endometrium/Hyperplasia	0/1	0
Uterine cervix/Cervicitis	0/5	0
Uterine cervix/Metaplasia	0/2	0
Uterine cervix/Dysplasia	0/2	0

Table 5. Immunoperoxidase-CEA results in normal tissues

Organ	No. Pos./Total	% Pos.
Brain	0/1	0
Thymus	0/4	0
Esophagus	0/4	0
Stomach	0/5	0
Colon	0/9	0
Colon near carcinoma	2/13	15
Lung	0/4	0
Liver	0/3	0
Gall bladder	0/3	0
Kidney	0/1	0
Urinary bladder	0/5	0
Cervix	0/4	0

CEA could be detected in specimens routinely processed for histopathology as paraffin sections, indicates that the evaluation of this immunological marker in malignant tissues is now readily feasible for the histopathologist. It further emphasizes that an oncofetal antigen such as CEA, which is only quantitatively increased in malignant as compared to non-malignant or certain benign tumor specimens, can be exploited by methods less sensitive than radioimmunoassay for demonstrating tumor-specific reactions. Of course, use of such less sensitive tests increases the number of false-negative reactions, so that negative immunocytochemical results only indicate relatively low levels of tissular CEA. What low or high levels of tissular CEA may mean in terms of tumor biology, progression, and patient survival remains to be investigated in restrospective and prospective studies.

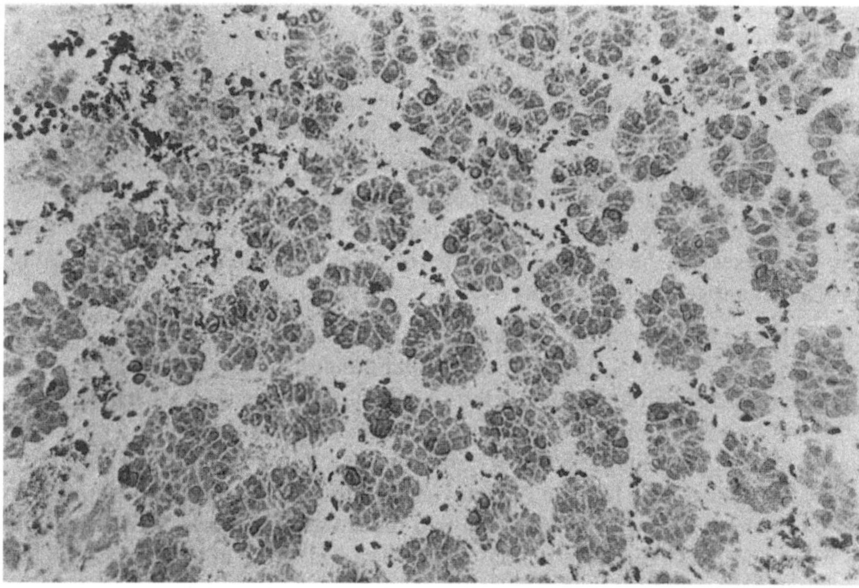

Fig. 6. Immunoperoxidase reaction for CEA in resection margin of a colonic carcinoma specimen, showing staining of normal-appearing glands. Orig. x 100

4. Host Immunity to CEA

As with many issues concerning CEA, the question of whether or not there exists host immunity or reactivity to CEA has been much debated and little resolved. In 1967 (*Gold*, 1967) and later (*Gold* et al., 1972), it was reported that anti-CEA antibodies could be detected in 70% of patients with nonmetastatic gastrointestinal tract cancers and in pregnant and postpartum women. These results were then contested by others (*Collatz* et al., 1971; *LoGerfo* et al., 1972). More recently, *Gold* reported that by means of radioimmunoelectrophoresis, 19% of patients without anti-A antibodies had anti-CEA IgM antibodies, which was also true for 80% of patients with anti-A isoantibodies (*Gold* et al., 1972). Alongside 2 pregnant women, the positive cases included those with disseminated carcinomas of the gastrointestinal tract and of the urinary bladder. Although anti-A antiserum could be absorbed with purified CEA, anti-CEA antiserum could not be absorbed with A-erythrocytes or blood group A and B substances. *Constanza* et al. (1973) recently showed the presence of diffuse granular precipitates of IgG, IgA, IgM, beta$_{1A}$-globulin, and CEA in the kidney glomeruli of patients with colon carcinoma, membranous nephropathy, and nephrotic syndrome. It was suggested that these cases had membranous nephropathy due to CEA-anti-CEA complexes. Evidence in support of such a contention would be stronger had these authors succeeded in extracting antigen-antibody complexes which could be dissociated to show CEA and anti-CEA antibody, since the presence of immunoglobulins alongside with CEA is only presumptive support that CEA-antibody complexes were involved in the nephropathy. Another report of the glomerular deposition of a tumor antigen apparently distinct from CEA in a colonic cancer patient with membranous nephropathy has also appeared (*Couser* et al., 1974). These investigators showed that the patient's serum 1 week post tumor resection could lose its reactivity to an antigen deposited on the glomerular basement membrane when the serum was absorbed with homogenates of the patient's tumor, but not by absorption with normal colon, colonic polyps, liver or spleen. Since the antigen did not react with several antisera to CEA (including that used by *Constanza* et al., 1973), *Couser* and coworkers (1974) concluded that the antigen on the glomerular basement membrane was not CEA. This work emphasizes two major points: (1) The possibility of tumor antigen-antibody complexes being implicated in membranous nephropathy of cancer patients; and (2) such tumor-associated antigen-antibody complexes may be eluted and dissociated for the isolation and characterization of tumor-distinct antigens and antibodies.

Cell-mediated immunity against colonic carcinoma cells has been demonstrated in vitro by *Hellström* et al. (1970, 1971) using colony inhibition or microcytotoxicity methods, and it was claimed that colon carcinomas have a common type-specific cell surface antigen(s) not shared by other tumor types. This was confirmed by *Embleton* (1973), who further showed that papain-solubilized tumor membrane extracts of colon cancer, but not of normal colon or melanoma, inhibited cytotoxicity by sensitized lymphocytes from colon carcinoma patients. The evidence suggested that the antigen(s) responsible for this effect was not CEA, since high concentration of CEA in the extracts did not correlate with lymphocyte inhibitory activity (*Embleton*, 1973). Using a purified preparation of mixed human peripheral blood lymphocytes and monocytes in an inhibition-of-migration assay for cell-mediated immunity to cancer of the colon, *Bull* and colleagues (1973) found that 24 of 27 patients with this disease showed inhibited migration in response to membrane-rich homogenates of colonic adenocarcinomas. The migration pattern of 52 cancer-free controls, including those who were surgically cured of colon cancer, in contrast, were unaffected. No further effort was undertaken, however, to characterize the antigen(s) responsible for the migration inhibition. Other studies supporting the non-identity between CEA and lymphocyte reactive colon carcinoma-associated antigen have been published by *Hollinshead* et al. (1970, 1972) using skin delayed-hypersensitivity reactions in colon carcinoma patients. Pure CEA did not elicit skin reactions, and the skin-reactive antigen(s) was separated from CEA by polyacrylamide gel electrophoresis (*Hollinshead* et al., 1972).

5. Prospects of Tumor Localization with Radioantibodies to CEA

Since CEA is a surface marker which is quantitatively increased in a number of malignant tumors, consideration has been given to using anti-CEA antibodies as carriers of cytotoxic chemicals or radioisotopes, or of gamma-emitting radioisotopes for external tumor localization. A major difficulty in pursuing such studies, however, is the requirement of clinical studies being performed to test suitable antibody preparations for these purposes, since CEA is known to be synthesized only by human tumors. Tissue culture studies could be of some value in this regard, but the obvious problems of host metabolism, degradation, and clearance of these antibody preparations would require investigations in vivo. Many of these difficulties were resolved with the availability of a serially transplantable human colonic carcinoma in hamsters, the GW-39 tumor system (*Goldenberg* et al., 1966), which was found to synthesize and release CEA despite its long-term passage in an unconditioned animal host (*Goldenberg* and *Hansen*, 1972a). The GW-39 tumor grows in various body sites of normal, unconditioned golden hamsters (Fig. 7), and has a predominantly signet-ring tumor cell morphology, with occasional aborted acini being distinguished (Fig. 8). Radioimmunoassay of this tumor has revealed that it contains between 20 and 200 μg CEA per g of tissue, intimately associated with the tumor's abundance of mucoproteins. CEA is

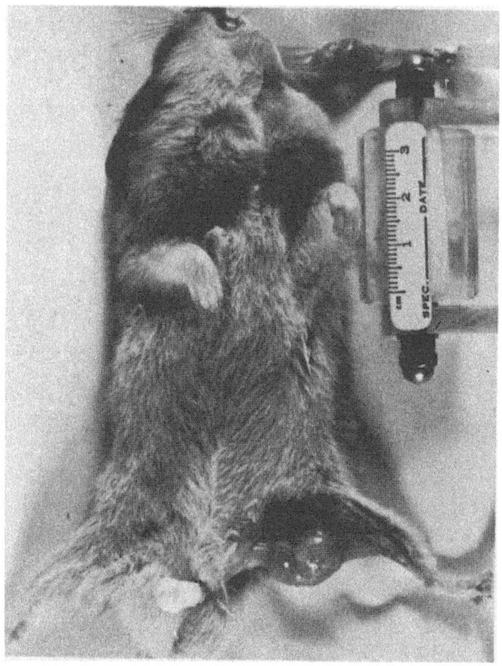

Fig. 7. GW-39 human colonic tumors growing in cheek pouch and hind limb of an unconditioned, normal adult golden hamster for 22 days

released into the circulation when GW-39 tumor is grown intramuscularly or subcutaneously (*Goldenberg* and *Hansen*, 1972b; *Munjal* and *Goldenberg*, 1976), while circulating IgM antibodies to CEA could also be demonstrated in tumor-bearing hamsters (*Primus* et al., 1976). Further, surgical resection of i.m. GW-39 tumors results in a rapid drop of circulating CEA titers (*Munjal* and *Goldenberg*, 1976). These conditions thus appear to reflect the clinical situation for CEA-producing human tumors in many ways. We therefore undertook a program of developing radioantibodies to CEA which could be used to localize GW-39 tumors in hamsters by photoscanning techniques, and which will be summarized briefly at this time. Our initial studies have already appeared in detail elsewhere (*Primus* et al., 1973; *Goldenberg* et al., 1974).

Goats were immunized with purified CEA, from which the IgG was separated and radioiodinated with either ^{125}I or ^{131}I by the procedure of *Greenwood* et al. (1953), as modified by *McConahey* and *Dixon* (1969). The specific activity of the labeled IgG preparations was 4 to 8 μCi/μg. The radioactivity injected per hamster ranged from 10 to 50 μCi. Prior to injection, each radiolabeled IgG preparation was counted in a well-type gamma-scintillation counter, so that in each animal the organ radioactivity measured in cpm at the termination of the experiment could be compared to the total dose injected. Blood and tissue levels of radioactivity were determined by exsanguinating the anesthetized animals by cardiac puncture and counting 1.0 ml aliquots of unclotted blood and the removed intact organs in a well-type scintillation counter. The organs were weighed and the organ radioactivity was computed on a gram basis. Thereafter, the amount of radioactivity in cpm/g was calculated as a percentage of the injected dose of radioactivity, this then corresponding to the proportion of radioactivity recovered per g of tissue examined. Six days after transplanting GW-39 tumors to hamster cheek pouches, the radiolabeled IgG was injected intracardially

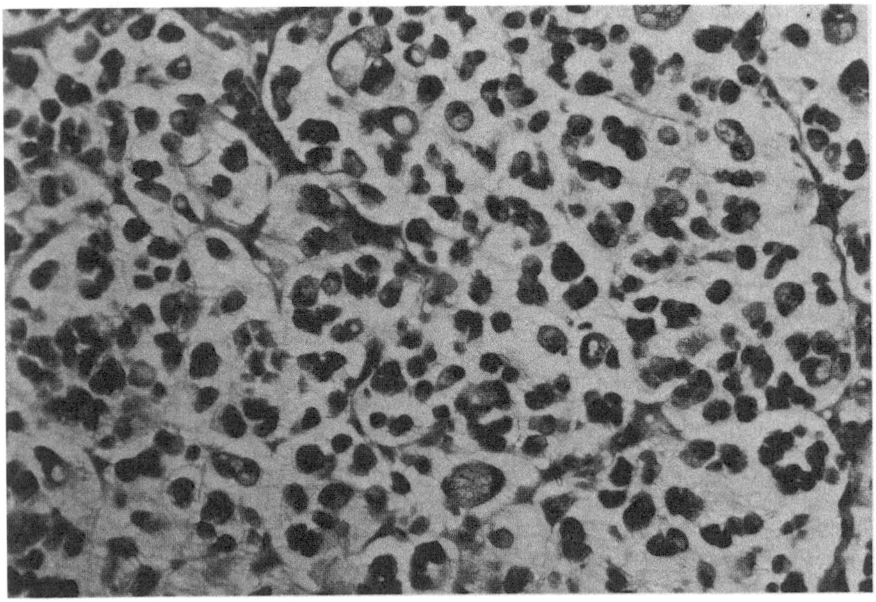

Fig. 8. Microscopic morphology of GW-39 human colonic carcinoma cells growing in the hamster cheek pouch. H & E, orig. x 250

in a volume of 0.1 to 0.3 ml. All hamsters received KI solution in their drinking water during the entire experimentation period in order to block uptake of free iodine by the thyroid. Hamsters bearing GW-39 cheek pouch tumors received either anti-CEA radiolabeled IgG or radiolabeled control goat IgG, whereas a group of normal hamsters received either one of these two preparations. Thereafter, total-body scans of the anesthetized hamsters were performed with a Picker rectilinear scanner equipped with a 7.5-cm diameter crystal, as well as a special low energy 73-hole, medium resolution, collimator with a 6.3-cm focal length. Each scan took about 30 min, during which time the hamsters were immobilized on their backs.

Our photoscanning experiments demonstrated a preferential tumor localization of anti-CEA IgG in hamsters bearing GW-39 cheek pouch tumors (*Goldenberg* et al., 1974). Indeed, cheek pouch tumors weighing as little as 70 mg were visualized after injecting 10 μCi of ^{125}I-labeled anti-CEA IgG (Fig. 9). The tumor vs. organ counts of radioactivity at the termination of this experiment support a preferential localization of this radioantibody preparation in the tumor (legend to Figure 9). In addition to radioactivity being seen over the tumor in the cheek pouch, some activity was seen in the region of the lungs, heart and upper part of the liver and also over the urinary bladder. The poor localization seen in the control tumor-bearing group receiving normal goat radiolabeled IgG, as well as the lack of specific uptake seen in control, normal hamsters receiving either the specific radioantibody or the control preparation, further confirmed the specific localizing ability of our anti-CEA radioantibody.

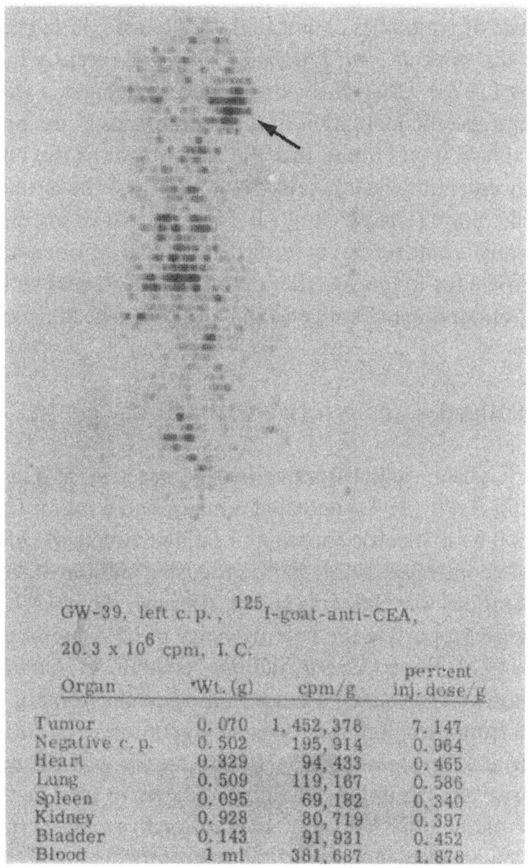

GW-39, left c.p., ^{125}I-goat-anti-CEA, 20.3 x 10^6 cpm, I.C.

Organ	*Wt. (g)	cpm/g	percent inj. dose/g
Tumor	0.070	1,452,378	7.147
Negative c.p.	0.502	195,914	0.964
Heart	0.329	94,433	0.465
Lung	0.509	119,167	0.586
Spleen	0.095	69,182	0.340
Kidney	0.928	80,719	0.397
Bladder	0.143	91,931	0.452
Blood	1 ml	381,687	1.878

Fig. 9. Total-body photoscan of a hamster bearing a 70 mg GW-39 tumor in its left cheek pouch (arrow). This scan was made 6 days after injection of 10 μCi ^{125}I-labeled anti-CEA IgG intracardially (having an initial activity of 20.3 x 10^6 cpm). The table records the tissue radioactivity found after sacrificing the animal, indicating the percent of the injected dose (in cpm) per g of tissue

The percentages of radioactivity recovered per g of tissue at 6 days postinjection of 10 μCi radioiodinated anti-CEA IgG into hamsters bearing tumors in their left cheek pouches weighing an average of 90 mg indicate an 8 to 20-fold increased localization in the tumor as compared to other organs of the animals (excluding blood, where 1 ml had only 4.5-fold less activity than 1 g of tumor) (*Goldenberg* et al., 1974). Both our photoscanning and organ radioactivity data thus support our contention that radioantibodies to CEA could be used to localize tumors in the body by means of external scanning techniques. Whether or not this is feasible in patients having variable levels of circulating CEA must eventually be resolved in clinical trials. In the meantime, however, we have been able to grow GW-39 tumor in the cheek pouches of stumptail monkeys (*Macaca speciosa*) for sufficient periods of time as to show tumor localization with anti-CEA radioantibodies (*Goldenberg* et al., manuscript in preparation), which adds further justification for the pursuit of clinical studies with such tumor-localizing radioantibody preparations.

The use of antibodies conjugated with cytotoxic substances has been advocated at least since the work of *Paul Ehrlich* (1906), and recently has been brought into perspective by *Parker* (1973). Using antibodies to CEA conjugated with glucose oxidase, an enzyme which permits specific iodination of cell membranes in the presence of glucose, iodide, and lactoperoxidase, it was found that the attachment of this enzyme to the antibody produced an enhancement of the inherent cytotoxicity of the antibody to colon tumor cells propagated in cell culture (*Shearer* et al., 1974). Whether or not similar mechanisms can function in vivo must await further investigation, but the principle of using tumor-specific antibodies as carriers for toxins or other cytotoxic substances will become increasingly important as truly tumor-distinct antigens and antibodies become known and available.

V. Antigens Crossreactive with CEA

CEA has been viewed from various perspectives as a heterogeneous substance. *Rule* and *Goleski-Reilly* (1973) detected 6 major and 6 minor CEA reactive peaks between pH 2.0 and 9.0 by isoelectric focusing of saline extracts of colonic tumors. *Coligan* et al. (1973) also demonstrated by isoelectric focusing and ion-exchange chromatography that their CEA preparations were heterogeneous, although these were immunochemically similar. Other evidence supporting the heterogeneity of CEA preparations has also been reported (*Eveleigh*, 1974; *Rogers, Searle* and *Bagshawe*, 1974; *Ichiki* et al., 1976). Recently, *Edgington* and coworkers isolated a single homogeneous isomeric species of CEA, termed CEA-S, purified from perchloric acid-soluble glycoprotein of colonic cancer metastatic to the liver (*Plow* and *Edgington*, 1975). Clincal studies of CEA-S have revealed that it is at least as sensitive as CEA in the detection of digestive tract cancer (80.4%), while yielding much fewer elevated CEA-S values in nondigestive cancers (primarily of the lung and breast) and in non-neoplastic diseases of the gastrointestinal tract and the kidney (*Edgington* et al., 1975). Since gastrointestinal cancers usually have the highest circulating titers of CEA, just raising the "normal" cutoff level of CEA-S could by itself be responsible for the apparent increased gastrointestinal cancer specificity of patients with advanced cancer (and thus having elevated CEA levels) which were evaluated. Hence these questions will have to be resolved before any improved clinical value can be ascribed to CEA-S. Nevertheless, this work will prove to be an encouragement of further efforts to re-examine and possibly refine the immunological determinant(s) of CEA.

A number of other antigens which have some crossreactivity with CEA have been identified and more extensively characterized. *Von Kleist* et al. (1972) described a "nonspecific cross reacting antigen" (NCA) because of its reactivity with CEA and its lack of tissue and cancer specificity. NCA was found in perchloric acid extracts of gastrointestinal tumors and in reduced amounts in extracts of normal gastrointestinal mucosa, lung and spleen. The apparently same antigen has been described by others under different names, such as normal glycoprotein, NGP (*Mach* and *Pusztaszeri*, 1972), CCEA-2 (*Turberville* et al., 1973), and colon carcinoma antigen-III, CCA-III (*Newman* et al., 1974). NCA is a glycoprotein of beta-globulin mobility in electrophoresis, and has a molecular weight of about 50,000 and a sedimentation constant of 3.5 S. It contains 25% carbohydrate and is similar to CEA in its location on the cell surface. *Burtin* and colleagues (1975) have subsequently shown that NCA is present in the cytoplasm and on the surface of human neutrophils and monocytes, and in the cytoplasm of macrophages.

A second NCA, NCA-2, has also been reported by *Burtin* et al. (1973a), but its relationship to NCA, CEA, and other tissue antigens is still under investigation. Since these crossreactive antigens with CEA were not appreciated in the earlier literature on CEA, it is not clear which studies used anti-CEA antibodies free of NCA immunoreactivity, particularly with immunocytochemical techniques.

VI. Other Tumor-associated Antigens

The early literature on human tumor antigens has been critically reviewed by *Day* (1965), thus not requiring repetition at this time except for a few interesting observations on gastrointestinal cancers. Already in 1930, *Witebsky* claimed to obtain antibodies apparently specific against an alcohol-soluble antigen of rectal cancer. Antigastric cancer serum was found by *Hirszfeld* et al. (1929) to react with stomach free of cancer and in increased frequency with stomachs of cancer patients. *Hirszfeld* and coworkers (1929) were able to demonstrate a gastric cancer-specific antigen after crossabsorbing his antibody preparation with normal stomach tissue. It is interesting to note that other so-called "normal" organs of cancer patients had an increased frequency of tumor antigen positivity than the same organs from individuals free of cancer. In more recent studies, *Zilber* (1962) showed that water extracts of gastric cancer, when used to immunize rabbits, resulted in antisera with both normal gastric tissue- and gastric cancer-specific antibodies, as demonstrated by immunodiffusion. Interestingly, *Zilber* was able to show reactivity of purified antiserum to human spleen against one of the antigens of gastric cancer, whereas antiserum against gastric cancer did not react with antigens of the spleen. In retrospect, it is tempting to speculate that *Zilber* was dealing with an NCA immunoreactivity in his anti-spleen antibody preparation which was apparently absent or less active in the antibody to gastric cancer. Thus, claims for the existence of tumor-specific antigens of gastrointestinal cancers will soon approach a half-century in longevity, and will most likely be "rediscovered" in more recent studies, although it remains to be seen whether true tumor-specificity or even organ-specificity will be demonstrated. A number of putatively tumor-associated or tumor-specific antigens of gastrointestinal tissues have been described in recent years, and the more prominent of these will be reviewed.

1. Fetal Sulfoglycoprotein (FSA)

Häkkinen and coworkers (1968a, b) have described 3 sulfoglycoproteins as appearing in the human fetal gastrointestinal tract at about the seventh or eighth week of gestation. They were localized in fetal gut mucosa and in gastric cancer juice. Only one of the three, FSA, was restricted to the digestive tract (*Häkkinen*, 1972). It is interesting, however, that absorption of the anti-FSA antiserum with normal colon, colonic cancer, or gastric cancer, as well as with acid glycoproteins of cancerous gastric juice, totally inhibited the specific reaction of anti-FSA antibody against CEA in immunodiffusion. It was also found that FSA of gastric origin and CEA of colonic cancer crossreact. Using antibody to CEA, a precipitin line can be obtained against FSA, and this precipitin line could be inhibited by absorbing the anti-CEA antiserum with FSA of cancerous gastric juice. On the other hand, the precipitin line between anti-CEA antibody and CEA is not inhibited by absorbing the antibody with FSA. Absorption of anti-FSA antibody with CEA also inhibited the formation of precipitin lines of anti-FSA reacted against FSA and anti-FSA reacted against CEA. On the basis of these results, it has been suggested that the CEA molecule has a second determinant which is identical with FSA (*Häkkinen*, 1972, 1974). Certainly, these data are at present inadequate to clarify the apparent relationship between FSA and CEA, but clearly indicate that there is a degree of crossreactivity. Nevertheless, some of the clinical findings with FSA deserve mention.

In a survey of 14,000 Finnish people, FSA was found in the gastric juice in about 3% of the industrial and in 5 to 7% of the rural population. Three histologically verified cases and 1 suspected case of gastric cancer, all clinically symptom-free, were found among the FSA-positive group during a 4-year follow-up (*Häkkinen*, 1974). *Häkkinen* (1974) suggested that there is a class of FSA secretors within the population, and this group may have a predilection for the development of gastric cancer. However, it is not clear why 14% of subjects with peptic ulcer have FSA detectable in their gastric juice, unless these cases have a high proclivity for malignant change in spite of this percentage exceeding the expected incidence of malignant transformation in patients with peptic ulcer. Whether these relationships are unique to the Finnish population remains to be determined. Unfortunately, many questions about the specificity and diagnostic accuracy of FSA remain unresolved, as is likewise the relationship of FSA to other gastrointestinal tract antigens.

2. Fetal Gut Antigen (FGA)

A fetal gut antigen, FGA, has also been described by *Smith* and *O'Neill* (1971) after immunizing rabbits with human fetal gut extracts (from the entire GI tract) and obtaining an antiserum which reacted in immunodiffusion with 87% of gut extracts from human fetuses, 31.7% of extracts of human gastrointestinal carcinomas, and 8.7% of normal adult gut tissue extracts, as well as with an extract of ulcerative colitis tissue and with the mucosa overlying a carcinoma of the rectum. FGA was reported to have the electrophoretic mobility of a beta-globulin, but could not be detected in the serum of patients with gastrointestinal cancers. It is interesting, however, that a Wilms' tumor also contained FGA. This antigen may be similar to that described by *Burtin* et al. (1967), using antiserum prepared against human fetal intestine. However, FGA was not found in human fetal serum, whereas the antigen of

Burtin et al. was. By means of immunofluorescent techniques, *Norland* et al. (1969) described a colon tumor antigen which also migrated as a beta-globulin in electrophoresis, and also occurred in the colon of a patient with ulcerative colitis. Although *Smith* and *O'Neill* (1971) argued that FGA is not CEA, they did not provide any evidence for this in their publication. Indeed, it would be of interest to determine whether FGA has any determinants in common with CEA or its related crossreactive antigens.

3. Pancreas Oncofetal Antigen

Banwo and coworkers (1974) described an oncofetal antigen complex specific to the pancreas after raising antisera to whole human fetal pancreas and crossabsorbing the antisera with normal adult pancreas and albumin. The antisera reacted with sera from 36 of 37 patients with carcinoma of the pancreas, with extracts of fetal pancreas and pancreatic carcinoma, but not with sera from 38 other patients (including 8 positive for CEA and 2 positive for AFP, and 17 with acute or chronic pancreatitis) by gel diffusion and by immunoelectrophoresis. Other fetal tissues tested, such as colon and liver, proved devoid of this antigen. Because of the difficulty in diagnosing carcinoma of the pancreas, particularly in the tail or body of the pancreas, the development of a test for early diagnosis of this tumor type based upon a pancreatic cancer-distinct antigen is urgently needed, and one must hope that the encouraging observations of *Banwo* et al. are confirmed and extended.

4. Beta-Oncofetal Antigen (BOFA)

Fritsch and *Mach* (1975) have also claimed to have identified a new oncofetal antigen associated with several types of human carcinomas, which they termed BOFA, or beta-oncofetal antigen, because of its beta-mobility in immunoelectrophoresis. The antigen was identified by rabbit antisera raised against semipurified fractions of colon carcinoma extracts, and then found to be present in carcinomas of the colon, lung, breast, liver, pancreas, and melanomas. In addition, it was present in fetal intestine, lung, liver, and kidney. BOFA was present in only low levels in normal adult tissues, but was in relatively high concentration in placenta and in cord serum at the end of gestation, and even persisted in normal adult serum, but at very low levels. Since elevated serum levels of BOFA did not seem to be limited to a particular type of cancer despite the fact that the original immunogen was made from a colon cancer extract, BOFA would appear to be a general oncofetal antigen very similar in its distribution and specificity to CEA, since both can be detected in minute quan-size (1.5 x 10^7 daltons) and is extracted by phenol-water and then precipitated in ethanol, similar to our own procedure for isolating CSA's (*vide infra*). An antigenic determinant of CMA has recently been reported as specific for colon cancer as compared to normal colon (*Gold* and *Miller*, 1975), although no results supporting the restriction of this determinant to colonic as compared to other cancer types were presented in this publication.

6. Zinc Glycinate Marker (ZGM)

A more gentle method for extracting tumor antigens has been described recently by *Pusztaszeri* et al. (1976), who claim to have identified a new component of colon cancer after immunizing rabbits made tolerant to normal human tissue antigens. ZGM has an alpha$_2$-mobility in immunoelectrophoresis and a molecular weight of about 2 million. This substance apparently differs from AFP, CEA, NCA, ferritin-like molecules, and blood group substances A, B, H, and Lewis a and b, and was not detected by immunodiffusion in normal tissues. A little less than half of a small series of extracts of colon carcinomas, however, was found to contain ZGM. Since only gel diffusion methods were used to study ZGM, we must await the development of more sensitive assays for detecting this substance before its role in tumor diagnosis can be evaluated.

7. Colon-specific Antigen-p (CSAp)

In the course of isolating and studying glycoprotein antigens other than CEA which are associated with normal and neoplastic colon tissues (*Goldenberg* et al., 1975, 1976a), we discovered immunoreactivity in our antisera which was more directed to a protein-rich antigen in colon cancer (*Goldenberg* et al., 1976b), and which was later found to be quantitatively increased in fetal and neoplastic colon tissues (*Goldenberg* and *Pant*, 1976a, b). Since the antisera raised in hamsters to this antigen had immunoreactivity to the other CSA's we have identified (*vide infra*), we chose to name this component CSAp. At present, immunodiffusion and hemagglutination-inhibition methods have indicated that CSAp is restricted to gastrointestinal polyps and cancers, to fetal gut, and is present in reduced quantities in normal adult colon. Thus, it appears to be an oncofetal antigen truly restricted to gastrointestinal tissues and quantitatively increased in neoplasia. In contrast to the cell-surface localization usually ascribed to other antigens. CSAp is predominantly a cytoplasmic component, as based upon immunofluorescent studies (*Goldenberg* et al., 1976b). Since we are engaged in purifying CSAp and, ultimately, developing a very sensitive assay, it is still premature to predict if it will eventually serve any useful role in gastrointestinal cancer immunodiagnosis.

VII. Organ- or Tissue-associated Antigens

Most investigators' approach to cancer immunology is to identify distinct or so-called "neoantigens" of tumors, as compared to the normal adult tissue counterparts. The question of what organ- or tissue-distinct, or differentiation, antigens are retained and expressed in certain malignant tumors has rarely received serious and consistent consideration, although numerous studies have called attention to the capacity of certain tumors and tumor cell lines maintained in vitro to possess biochemical and other markers of their histogenetic origins. Certainly, the retention or loss of these properties during oncogenesis and the progression of tumors to more advanced states of malignancy would appear to be as revealing, from the conceptual standpoint, as the discovery of inappropriate molecules produced by the malignant lesion. Unfortunately, few truly organ- or tissue-specific substances are known for normal tissues, no less for those that have become malignant.

The problem of defining and demonstrating organ- or tissue-specific antigens was appreciated by *Witebsky* and his coworkers a little less than half a century ago (*Witebsky,* 1930; see also *Witebsky* et al., 1956). At this time, *Witebsky* (1930) reported the existence of an organ-specific antigen of the intestine, while *Hirszfeld* et al. (1929) described an antigen which was organ-specific for the stomach by preparing antisera against gastric cancer. Subsequently, a number of reports have claimed to demonstrate antigens either specific or associated with various tissues of the gastrointestinal system (*Baur* et al., 1965; *Broberger* et al., 1959; *Gibbs* and *French*, 1971; *Gold* and *Miller*, 1974; *Goldenberg* et al., 1975, 1976a, b; *Henry* et al., 1967; *Karitzky* and *Burtin*, 1967; *Kobayashi*, 1956a, b; *Murray* and *Thal*, 1960; *Nairn* et al., 1962a, b; *Norland* et al., 1969; *Rapp* et al., 1964; *Sannela,* 1957; *Tappeiner* et al., 1973; *Zweibaum* et al., 1975). Embryonic antigens present in adult human stomach and intestine were demonstrated by *Remacle-Bonnet* and *Depieds* (1974) by means of immunofluorescence. These studies on colon-associated antigens were reviewed recently elsewhere (*Goldenberg* et al., 1976a).

Most of the earlier work did not always consider the crossreactivity between different organs and tissues, while the relatively low sensitivity of the assays usually employed further conflicted with any true tissue- or organ-specificity. Nevertheless, the morphological and functional differentiation of adult tissues suggest that organ- or tissue-distinct antigens should indeed exist. If so, then a malignant tumor still expressing some features of its histogenetic origin likewise should possess organ-specific antigens to a certain degree, as was indeed claimed by *Hirszfeld* in 1929 when antibodies were prepared to gastric carcinoma and then found to be immunoreactive with normal gastric tissue. Similarly, we have recently extracted a family of glycoproteins from our serially transplantable colon carcinoma, GW-39, one of which, "HMW/CSA" (high molecular weight/colon-specific antigen), appears to be truly distinct in immunodiffusion for human gastrointestinal tissues, increasing in concentration from the esophagus to the rectum (*Goldenberg* et al., 1976a). With antisera to this antigen, we have been able to confirm the intestinal, epithelial origin of certain human tumor cell lines propagated in vitro (*Goldenberg* et al., 1976a; *Tom* et al., 1976).

On the other hand, a loss of organ-specificity has been more generally ascribed as a feature of malignancy (*Nairn* et al., 1966; *Weiler*, 1956). Indeed, in colon cancer, the loss of such organ antigens has been reported (*Burtin* et al., 1971; *Nairn* et al., 1962b). A mucous epithelial antigen of the stomach found in adults and fetal specimens was reported by *Lynranen* and *de Boer* (1969). A similar antigen of the intestines was reported by *Nairn* et al. (1962a) by means of immunofluorescence. Upon examining gastric mucosa for both antigens, it was found that the intestinal component disappears soon after birth and re-emerges in senescence and in metaplasia and neoplasia, while the gastric antigen, which normally persists in adult life, is depleted in these conditions (*deBoer, Forsyth* and *Nairn*, 1969). Similar observations were made by *Häkkinen* et al. (1968). It is apparent that some of this earlier work needs to be re-evaluated for the possible implication of CEA. Clearly, there may well be different classes of antigens present in any organ or tissue, and these would be expected to segregate differentially during oncogenesis, depending, perhaps, on which cell populations are emerging as the dominant parties of the neoplasm, and to what extent cell selection and loss, and even such processes as gene amplification and so-called derepression, are occurring. Basic to all such considerations, However, is an understanding of the antigenic composition and character of the tissues and organs from which neoplasms develop, and which supposedly give rise to the developmental gene products termed oncofetal antigens. Unfortunately, this has remained a relatively unexplored area of immunology.

VIII. Concluding Remarks

Do Qualitatively Distinct Oncofetal Antigens Exist?

A number of other embryonic or fetal antigens associated with tumors have been described in human material, but, for the most part, these are even less tissue-specific than those already reviewed. These include the gamma-fetoprotein of *Edynak* (*Edynak* et al., 1972), the universal carcinoplacental antigen of *Tal* (*Tal*, 1964, 1970), the carcinoplacental Regan isoenzyme of alkaline phosphatase (*Fishman* et al., 1968; *Nathanson* and *Fishman*, 1971), alpha$_2$-H ferroglobulin (*Buffe* et al., 1972), leukemia-associated antigen (*Harris* et al., 1971), the universal carcinofetal antigen of *Klavins* et al. (1971), a glioblastoma-associated antigen (*Trouillas*, 1971), beta-S-fetoprotein (*Takahashi* et al., 1967), a Hodgkin's disease antigen (*Chism* et al., 1973), and perhaps several sarcoma-related antigens (*Buttle* et al., 1962; *Mukherji* and *Hirschaut*, 1973). Although this list is not intended to be complete, it does demonstrate that there is certainly no paucity of claims of oncofetal antigens in humans. However, as was witnessed for AFP, CEA, and the others reviewed, most appear to represent quantitatively increased levels in neoplastic and fetal tissues as compared to normal adult tissues and body fluids. Under these circumstances, one may pose the question raised at the beginning of this section, since can a substance be considered as oncofetal if it is found in adult tissues in minute amounts? In my own view, although there may be substances truly specific for tissues at various stages of development, a tumor product having crossreactivity or even identity with a similar substance found in fetal or embryonic tissues should not necessarily be restricted to neoplastic and gestational tissues if this molecule is synthesized in the tumor because of a so-called retrogenetic expression. If the neoplasm evolved from primitive cells that did not undergo tissue differentiation prior to birth, then one would expect an oncofetal substance which is not detectable in normal adult tissues. This could be so for embryonal tumors or teratoblastomas if one were to isolate antigens from these types of neoplasia. Further support for this view would be gained if specific antibodies to fetal or embryonic tissues were produced and shown to be exclusively present in neoplastic, and not normal tissues of the adult. In other words, there may well be truly embryonic or fetal antigens in neoplasms, but antigens isolated directly from tumors which are not dysontogenetic may not have qualitatively distinct embryonic or fetal characteristics. Indeed, if the tumors in question evolve from mature, differentiated cells by a series of developmental steps, then uniquely oncofetal antigens should not be expected. On the other hand, the quantitative increase in tumors of certain substances likewise increased in fetal or embryonic tissues suggests that the proliferative character of the neoplasm has come to resemble that of ontogenetic tissues, including many of the biochemical, immunological, and other gene products prevalent during this developmental phase of the organism.

Whether these observations and realizations pertaining to oncofetal substances and the processes termed genetic derepression, retrogenetic differentiation, etc., have as much meaning and significance for oncology as has been contended in much of the literature on this subject remains to be decided by the historian. Nevertheless, I venture to say that for the immediate future, the major contribution of oncofetal antigens is as aids for monitoring the course of certain cancers, and the group of malignant tumors that eppears to have been influenced most by the exploration of this subject is that of the human digestive system.

References

Abelev, G.I.: Production of embryonal serum α-globulin by hepatomas: Review of experimental and clinical data. Cancer Res. 28, 1344-1350 (1968).

Abelev, G.I.: Alpha-fetoprotein in ontogenesis and its association with malignant tumors. Advanc. Cancer Res. 14, 295-358 (1971).

Abelev, G.I.: Alpha-fetoprotein production by normal liver and liver tumors. In: Protides of the Biological Fluids (ed. *H. Peeters*), pp. 203-209. Oxford: Pergamon Press 1971.

Abelev, G.I., Alpert, E., Hull, E.W., Masseyeff, R., De Nechaud, B., Tatarinov, Y., Uriel, J.: Les protéines sériques foeto-spécifiques. Recommandations en vue d'une normalisation de la terminologie. Bull. Org. mond. Santé 43, 311-312 (1970).

Abelev, G.I., Perova, S.D., Khramkova, N.I., Postnikova, Z.A., Irlin, I.S.: Production of embryonal alpha-globulin by transplantable mouse hepatomas. Transplantation 1, 174-180 (1963).

Abelev, G.I., Tsvetkov, V.S., Biryulina, T.I., Él'gort, D.A., Olovnikov, A.M., Gusev, A.I., Yazova, A.K., Perova, S.D., Rubtsov, I.V., Shaborina, S.V., Kantorovich, B.A., Tur, V.M., Khazanov, A.I., Levina, D.M.: Value of highly sensitive methods of α-fetoprotein determination for the diagnosis of hepatocellular cancer and teratoblastoma (in Russian). Bull. exp. Biol. Med. 4, 75-81 (1971).

Adinolfi, M., Gardner, B., Martin, W.: Fetal proteins and immunoglobulins in Down's syndrome. Atti. Assoc. Genet. ital. 12, 133-143 (1967).

Akai, S., Kato, K.: Serum alpha-fetoprotein-positive stomach cancer. Gann Monogr. on Cancer Res. 14, 149-154 (1973).

Akeyama, T., Koyama, T., Kamada, T.: Alpha-fetoprotein in acute viral hepatitis. New Engl. J. Med. 287, 989 (1972).

Alexander, P.: Foetal "antigens" in cancer. Nature (Lond.) 235, 137-140 (1972).

Alpert, E., Drysdale, J.W., Isselbacher, K.J.: Isoelectric focusing of human α-fetoprotein: An aid in purification and characterization of microheterogeneity. Ann. N.Y. Acad. Sci. 209, 387-396 (1973).

Alpert, E., Drysdale, J.W., Isselbacher, K.J., Schur, P.H.: Human α-fetoprotein. Isolation, characterization, and demonstration of microheterogeneity. J. biol. Chem. 247, 3792-3798 (1972).

Alpert, E., Hershberg, R., Schur, P.H., Isselbacher, K.J.: α-Fetoprotein in human hepatoma: Improved detection in serum and quantitative studies using a new sensitive technique. Gastroenterology 61, 137-143 (1971a).

Alpert, E., Pinn, V.W., Isselbacher, K.J.: Alpha-fetoprotein in a patient with gastric carcinoma metastatic to the liver. New Engl. J. Med. 285, 1058-1059 (1971b).

Alpert, E., Starzl, T.E., Schur, P.H., Isselbacher, K.J.: Serum alpha-fetoprotein in hepatoma patients after liver transplantation. Gastroenterology 61, 144-148 (1971c).

Alpert, E., Zuckerman, J.: Absence of alpha-1-fetoprotein antigen or antibody in maternal sera. Lancet 1970 II, 465.

Banjo, C., Gold, P., Freedman, S.O., Krupey, J.: Immunologically active heterosaccharides of carcinoembryonic antigen of human digestive system. Nature New Biol. (Lond.) 238, 183-185 (1972).

Banjo, C., Gold, P., Gehrke, C.W., Freedman, S.O., Krupey, J.: Preparation and isolation of immunologically active glycopeptides from carcinoembryonic antigen (CEA). Int. J. Cancer 13, 151-163 (1974a).

Banjo, C., Shuster, J., Gold, P.: Intermolecular heterogeneity of the carcinoembryonic antigen. Cancer Res. 34, 2114-2121 (1974b).

Banwo, O., Versey, J., Hobbs, J.R.: New oncofetal antigen from human pancreas. Lancet 1974 I, 643-645.

Baur, S., Roitt, I.M., Doniach, D.: Characterization of the human gastric parietal cell auto-antigen. Immunology 8, 62-68 (1965).

Becker, F.F., Sell, S.: Early elevation of alpha$_1$-fetoprotein in N-2-fluorenylacetamide hepatocarcinogenesis. Cancer Res. 53, 289-291 (1974).

Bergstrand, C.G., Czar, B.: Demonstration of a new protein fraction in serum from human fetus. Scand. J. clin. Lab. Invest. 8, 174 (1956).

Bernades, P.: Alpha-1-foeto-protéine et cancers digestifs primitifs en dehors de l'hépatome. Ann. Gastroent. Hépatol. 7, 565-570 (1971).

Bernades, P., Smadja, M., Rueff, B., Bonnefond, A., Tursz, T., Martin, E., Bognel, C., Barge, J., Uriel, J.: Présence de l'alpha-foeto-protéine sérique dans quartre cas de cancers digestifs primitifs autres que l'hépatome. Presse méd. 79, 1585-1587 (1971).

Bierfield, J.L., Scheiner, M.I., Schultz, D.R., Moral, M.D., Rogers, A.I.: Alpha-fetoprotein and carcinoembryonic antigen in a case of gastric carcinoma metastatic to the liver. Amer. J. dig. Dis. 18, 517-520 (1973).

Bivins, B.A., Meeker, W.R., jr., Griffen, W.O., jr.: Carcinoembryonic antigen levels and tumor histology in colon cancer. J. Surg. Res. 18, 257-261 (1975).

Blair, O.M., Goldenberg, D.M.: A correlative study of bronchial cytology, bronchial washing carcinoembryonic antigen, and plasma carcinoembryonic antigen in the diagnosis of bronchogenic cancer. Acta cytologica 18, 510-514 (1974).

Bloomer, J.R., Waldmann, T.A., McIntire, K.R., Klatskin, G.: Relationship of serum α-fetoprotein to the severity and duration of illness in patients with viral hepatitis. Gastroenterology 68, 342-350 (1975).

Booth, S.N., King, J.P.G., Leonard, J.C., Dykes, P.W.: Serum carcinoembryonic antigen in clinical disorders. Gut 14, 794-799 (1973).

Bordes, M., Michiels, R., Martin, F.: Detection by immunofluorescence of carcinoembryonic antigen in colonic carcinoma, other malignant or benign tumors, and non-cancerous tissues. Digestion 9, 106-115 (1973).

Boureille, J., Metayer, P., Sauger, F., Matray, F., Fondimare, A.: Existence d'alpha-foetoprotéine au cours d'un cancer secondaire du foie d'origine gastrique. Presse méd. 78, 1277-1278 (1970).

Breborowicz, J., Easty, G.C., Neville, A.M.: In-vitro production of carcinoembryonic antigen by normal and neoplastic colon. Lancet 1973 II, 1393.

Broberger, O., Perlmann, P.: Autoantibodies in human ulcerative colitis. J. exp. Med. 110, 657-674 (1959).

Bubenik, J., Perlmann, P., Helmstein, K., Moberger, G.: Immune response to urinary bladder tumors in man. Int. J. Cancer 5, 39-46 (1970).

Buffe, D.: Fetoproteins and children's tumours. Gann Monogr. on Cancer Res. 14, 117-128 (1973).

Buffe, D., Rimbaut, C.: L'α_1-foetoprotéine dans les atteintes hépatiques et les maladies métaboliques de l'enfant. Biomed. 19, 172-176 (1973).

Buffe, D., Rimbaut, C., Fuccaro, C., Burtin, P.: Isolement et caractérisation d'une ferroprotéine tissulaire l'α_2 H-globuline. Ann. Inst. Pasteur 123, 129-142 (1972).

Buffe, D., Rimbaut, C., Lemerle, J., Schweisguth, O., Burtin, P.: Présence d'une ferroprotéine d'origine tissulaire, l'α_2 H, dans le sérum des enfants porteurs de tumeurs. Int. J. Cancer 5, 85-87 (1970).

Bull, L.M., Leibach, J.R., Williams, M.A., Helms, R.A.: Immunity to colon cancer assessed by antigen-induced inhibition of mixed mononuclear cell migration. Science 181, 957-959 (1973).

Burtin, P., Buffe, D., von Kleist, S., Wolff, E., Wolff, Et.: Mise en évidence de l'antigène carcinoembryonnaire spécifique des cancers digestifs dans les tumeurs humaines entretenues en culture organotypique. Int. J. Cancer 5, 88-95 (1970).

Burtin, P., Chavanel, G., Hirsch-Marie, H.: Characterization of a second normal antigen that cross-reacts with CEA. J. Immunol. 111, 1926-1928 (1973a).

Burtin, P., von Kleist, S., Buffe, D.: Étude sur les antigènes foetaux humaines. I. Étude immunoélectrophorétique des antigènes du sérum foetal humaine absents de sérum adulte. Bull. Soc. Chim. biol. (Paris) 49, 1389-1398 (1967).

Burtin, P., von Kleist, S., Sabine, M.C.: Loss of a normal colonic membrane antigen in human cancers of the colon. Cancer Res. 31, 1038-1041 (1971).

Burtin, P., von Kleist, S., Sabine, M.C., King, M.: Immunohistological localization of carcinoembryonic antigen and nonspecific crossreacting antigen in gastrointestinal normal and tumoral tissues. Cancer Res. 33, 3299-3305 (1973b).

Burtin, P., Martin, E., Sabine, M.C., von Kleist, S.: Immunological study of polyps of the colon. J. nat. Cancer Inst. 48, 25-32 (1972a).

Burtin, P., Quan, P.C., Sabine, M.C.: Nonspecific cross reacting antigen as a marker for human polymorphs, macrophages and monocytes. Nature (Lond.) 255, 714-716 (1975).

Burtin, P., Sabine, M.C., Chavanel, G.: Presence of carcinoembryonic antigen in children's colonic mucosa. Int. J. Cancer 10, 72-76 (1972b).

Buttle, G.A.H., Eperon, J.L., Kovacs, E.: An antigen in malignant and in embryonic tissues. Nature (Lond.) 194, 780 (1962).

Chayvialle, J.A., Ganguli, P.C.: Radioimmunoassay of alpha-fetoprotein in human plasma. Lancet 1973 I, 1355-1357.

Chism, S.E., Order, S.E., Hellman, S.: Tumor-fetal antigens in Hodgkin's disease and immunoelectrophoresis analysis. Amer. J. Roentgenol. 117, 5-11 (1973).

Chu, T.M., Reynoso, G., Hansen, H.J.: Demonstration of carcinoembryonic antigen in normal human plasma. Nature (Lond.) 238, 152-153 (1972).

Coligan, J.E., Henkart, P.A., Todd, C.W., Terry, W.D.: Heterogeneity of the carcinoembryonic antigen. Immunochemistry 10, 591-600 (1973).

Coligan, J.E., Lautenschleger, J.T., Egan, M.L., Todd, C.W.: Isolation and characterization of carcinoembryonic antigen. Immunochemistry 9, 377-386 (1972).

Coligan, J.E., Todd, C.W.: Structural studies on carcinoembryonic antigen. Periodate oxidation. Biochem. 14, 805-810 (1975).

Collatz, E., von Kleist, S., Burtin, P.: Further investigations of circulating antibodies in colon cancer patients: On the autoantigenicity of carcinoembryonic antigen. Int. J. Cancer 8, 298-303 (1971).

Constanza, M.E., Nathanson, L.: Carcinofetal antigens. Progr. Clin. Immunol. 2, 191-224 (1974).

Constanza, M.E., Pinn, V., Schwartz, R.S., Nathanson, L.: Carcinoembryonic antigen-antibody complexes in a patient with carcinoma and nephrotic syndrome. New Engl. J. Med. 289, 520-522 (1973).

Cooper, A.G., Brown, M.C., Kirch, M.E., Rule, A.H.: Relationship of carcinoembryonic antigen to blood substances A and i: Evidence that the antigenic sites are on different molecules. J. Immunol. 113, 1246-1251 (1974).

Couser, W.G., Wagonfeld, J.B., Spargo, B.H., Lewis, E.J.: Glomerular deposition of tumor antigen in membranous nephropathy associated with colonic carcinoma. Amer. J.Med. 57, 962-970 (1974).

Darcy, D.A., Turberville, C., James, R.: Immunological study of carcinoembryonic antigen (CEA) and a related glycoprotein. Brit. J. Cancer 28, 147-160 (1973).

Dattwyler, R.J., Murgita, R.A., Tomasi, T.B.: Binding of α-fetoprotein to murine T cells. Nature (Lond.) 256, 656-657 (1975).

Day, E.D.: The Immunochemistry of Cancer. Springfield, Ill.:Charles C Thomas 1965.

DeBoer, W.G.R.M., Forsyth, A., Nairn, R.C.: Gastric antigens in health and disease: Behaviour in early development, senescence, metaplasia and cancer. Brit. med. J. 1969 III, 93-94.

Denk, R., Tappeiner, G., Eckerstorfer, R., Holzner, J.H.: Carcinoembryonic antigen (CEA) in gastrointestinal and extragastrointestinal tumors and its relationship to tumor-cell differentiation. Int. J. Cancer 10, 262-272 (1972).

Deutsch, E., Apffel, C.A., Mori, H., Walker, J.E.: A tumor-associated antigen in gastric cancer secretions. Cancer Res. 33, 112-116 (1973).

Dhar, P., Moore, T., Zamcheck, N., Kupchik, H.Z.: Carcinoembryonic antigen in colonic cancer. Use in preoperative diagnosis and prognosis. J. Amer. med. Ass. 221, 31-35 (1972).

Dukes, C.E.: The classification of cancer of the rectum. J. Path. Bact. 35, 323-332 (1932).

Dyce, B.J., Haverback, B.J.: Free and bound carcinoembryonic antigen in neoplasms and in normal adult and fetal tissue. Immunochemistry 11, 423-430 (1974).

Edgington, T.S., Astarita, R.W., Plow, E.F.: Association of an isomeric species of carcinoembryonic antigen with neoplasia of the gastrointestinal tract. New Engl. J. Med. 293, 103-107 (1975).

Edynak, E.M., Old, L.J., Vrana, M., Lardis, M.P.: A fetal antigen associated with human neoplasia. New Engl. J. Med. 286, 1178-1183 (1972).

Egan, M.L., Coligan, J.E., Todd, C.W.: Radioimmune assay for the diagnosis of human cancer. Cancer 34, 1504-1509 (1974).

Egan, M.L., Todd, C.W.: Carcinoembryonic antigen: Synthesis by a continuous line of adenocarcinoma cells. J. nat. Cancer Inst. 48, 887-889 (1972).

Ehrlich, P.: Collected Studies on Immunity, translated by *C. Boldman*, pp. 441-442. New York: Wiley & Sons 1906.

Elgort, D.A., Abelev, G.I., Levina, D.M., Marienbach, E.V., Martochkina, G.A., Laskina, A.V., Solovjeva, E.A.: Immunoradioautography test for alpha-fetoprotein in the differential diagnosis of germinogenic tumors of the testis and in the evaluation of effectiveness of their treatment. Int. J. Cancer 11, 586-594 (1973).

Embleton, M.J.: Significance of tumor associated antigens on human colonic carcinomata. Brit. J. Cancer 28 (Suppl. I), 142-152 (1973).
Endo, Y., Kanai, K., Iino, S., Oda, T.: Clinical significance of alpha-fetoprotein with special reference to primary cancer of the liver. Gann Monogr. on Cancer Res. 14, 67-78 (1973).
Engelhardt, N.V., Goussev, A.I., Shipova, L.Ja., Abelev, G.I.: Immunofluorescent study of alpha-fetoprotein (αfp) in liver and liver tumors. I. Technique of αfp localization in tissue sections. Int. J. Cancer 7, 198-206 (1971).
Eveleigh, J.W.: Heterogeneity of carcinoembryonic antigen. Cancer Res. 34, 2122-2124 (1974).
Feizi, T., Turberville, C., Westwood, J.H.: Blood-group precursors and cancer-related antigens. Lancet 1975 II, 391-393.
Feldman, J.M., Plonk, J.W.: Carcinoembryonic antigen and carcinoid tumors. Ann. Intern. Med. 83, 82-83 (1975).
Field, B., Mitchell, G., Garrett, W., Kerr, C.: Amniotic alpha-fetoprotein levels and anencephaly. Lancet 1973 II, 798.
Fishman, W.H., Inglis, N.R., Green, S., Antiss, C.L., Ghosh, N.K., Reif, A.E., Rustigan, R., Krant, M.J., Stolbach, L.L.: Immunology and biochemistry of Regan isoenzyme of alkaline phosphatase in human cancer. Nature (Lond.) 219, 697-699 (1968).
Florin-Christensen, A., Arana, R.M.: Alpha_1-fetoprotein and anti-alpha_1-fetoprotein in acute viral hepatitis. Brit. med. J. 1973 II, 94-95.
Foley, E.J.: Antigenic properties of methylcholanthrene-induced tumors in mice of the strain of origin. Cancer Res. 13, 835-837 (1953).
Freed, D.L.J., Taylor, G.: Carcinoembryonic antigen in faeces. Brit. med. J. 1972 I, 85-87.
Fritsche, R., Mach, J.P.: Identification of a new oncofoetal antigen associated with several types of human carcinomas. Nature (Lond.) 258, 734-737 (1975).
Fuks, A., Banjo, C., Shuster, J., Freedman, S.O., Gold, P.: Carcinoembryonic antigen (CEA): Molecular biology and clinical significance. Biochim. biophys. Acta (Amst.) 417, 123-152 (1975).
Furth, R. van, Adinolfi, M.: In vitro synthesis of the foetal α_1-globulin in man. Nature (Lond.) 222, 1296-1299 (1969).
Geddes, E.W., Falkson, G.: Malignant hepatoma in the Bantu. Cancer 25, 1271-1278 (1970).
Geffroy, Y., Boureille, J., Denis, P., Colin, R., Metayer, P.: Bilan d'une recherche systématique de l'alpha-1-foetoprotéine dans 224 hépatopathies. Sem. Hôp. Paris 47, 1281-1285 (1971).
Geffroy, Y., Denis, P., Colin, R., Sauger, F., Matray, F., Fondimare, A.: Présence d'alpha-1-foetoprotéine chez l'adulte au cours d'une hépatite virale traitée par corticothérapie. Presse méd. 78, 1107-1108 (1970).
Geffroy, Y., Metayer, P., Denis, P., Phillipe, J., Matray, F., Sauger, F., Laumonier, R., Duval, C.: Alpha-foeto-protéine et cancer secondaire du foie. Presse méd. 78, 1896 (1970).
Gibbs, N.M., French, L.W.: The colon mucus antibody. J. clin. Path. 24, 867-869 (1971).
Gitlin, D.: Sites of α-fetoprotein synthesis. New Engl. J. Med. 285, 1436-1437 (1971).
Gitlin, D., Boesman, M.D.: Serum α-fetoprotein, albumin, and γG-globulin in the human conceptus. J. clin. Invest. 45, 1826-1838 (1966).
Gitlin, D., Boesman, M.D.: Fetus-specific proteins in several mammals and their relation to human α-fetoprotein. Comp. Biochem. Physiol. 21, 327-336 (1967).
Gitlin, D., Perricelli, A., Gitlin, G.:, Synthesis of α-fetoprotein by liver, yolk sac and gastrointestinal tract of the human conceptus. Cancer Res. 32, 979-982 (1972).

Go, V.L.W., Ammon, H.V., Holtermuller, K.H., Krag, E., Phillips, S.F.: Quantification of carcinoembryonic antigen-like activities in normal human gastrointestinal secretions. Cancer 36, 2346-2350 (1975).
Gold, D.V., Miller, F.: Characterization of human colonic mucoprotein antigen. Immunochemistry 11, 369-375 (1974).
Gold, D., Miller, F.: Chemical and immunological differences between normal and tumoural colonic mucoprotein antigen. Nature (Lond.) 255, 85-87 (1975).
Gold, J.M., Banjo, C., Freedman, S.O., Gold, P.: Immunochemical studies of the intramolecular heterogeneity of the carcinoembryonic antigen (CEA) of human digestive system. J. Immunol. 111, 1872-1879 (1973).
Gold, J.M., Freedman, S.O., Gold, P.: Human anti-CEA antibodies detected by radioimmunoelectrophoresis. Nature New Biol. (Lond.) 239, 60-62 (1972).
Gold, J.M., Gold, P.: The blood group A-like site on the carcinoembryonic antigen. Cancer Res. 33, 2821-2824 (1973).
Gold, P.: Circulating antibodies against carcinoembryonic antigens of the human digestive system. Cancer 20, 1663-1667 (1967).
Gold, P.: Antigenic reversion in human cancer. Ann. Rev. Med. 22, 85-94 (1971).
Gold, P., Freedman, S.O.: Demonstration of tumor-specific antigens in human colonic carcinomata by immunological tolerance and absorption techniques. J. exp. Med. 121, 439-462 (1965a).
Gold, P., Freedman, S.O.: Specific carcinoembryonic antigens of the human digestive system. J. exp. Med. 122, 467-481 (1965b).
Gold, P., Gold, M., Freedman, S.O.: Cellular location of carcinoembryonic antigens of the human digestive system. Cancer Res. 28, 1331-1334 (1968).
Gold, P., Krupey, J., Ansari, H.: Position of the carcinoembryonic antigen of the human digestive system in ultrastructure of tumor cell surface. J. nat. Cancer Inst. 45, 219-225 (1970).
Gold, P., Thomson, D.M.P., Freedman, S.O.: Circulating carcinoembryonic antigens. Clin. Res. 17, 476 (1969).
Gold, P., Wilson, T., Romero, R., Shuster, J., Freedman, S.O.: Immunology and colonic cancer: Further evaluation of the radioimmunoassay for carcinoembryonic antigen of the human digestive system as an adjunct in cancer diagnosis. Dis. Colon. Rect. 16, 358-365 (1973).
Goldenberg, D.M., Hansen, H.J.: Carcinoembryonic antigen present in human colonic neoplasms serially propagated in hamsters. Science 175, 1117-1118 (1972a).
Goldenberg, D.M., Hansen, H.J.: GW-39: A human tumor – animal model for carcinoembryonic antigen (CEA). Proc. Amer. Ass. Cancer Res. 13, 80 (1972b).
Goldenberg, D.M., Pant, K.D.: Studies of carcinoembryonic antigen and other markers of a xenografted human colonic carcinoma, GW-39. In: Protides of the Biological Fluids (ed. *H. Peeters*), 24, in press (1976a).
Goldenberg, D.M., Pant, K.D.: Colonic cancer-associated antigens in a heterografted human tumor, GW-39. In: Onco-Developmental Gene Expression (eds. *W.H. Fishman, S. Sell*), in press (1976 b).
Goldenberg, D.M., Pant, K.D., Dahlman, H.L.: Antigens associated with normal and malignant gastrointestinal tissues. Cancer Res. 36, 3455-3463 (1976a).
Goldenberg, D.M., Pant, K.D., Dahlman, H.: A new oncofetal antigen associated with gastrointestinal cancer. Proc. Amer. Ass. Cancer Res. 17, 155 (1976b).
Goldenberg, D.M., Pavia, R.A., Hansen, H.J., Vandevoorde, J.P.: Synthesis of carcinoembryonic antigen in vitro. Nature New Biol. (Lond.) 239, 189-190 (1972).

Goldenberg, D.M., Pegram, C.A., Vazquez, J.J.: Identification of a colon-specific antigen (CSA) in normal and neoplastic tissues. J. Immunol. 114, 1008-1013 (1975).
Goldenberg, D.M., Pletsch, Q.A., Nagell, J.R. van, jr.: Characterization and localization of carcinoembryonic antigen in a squamous cell carcinoma of the cervix. Gynecol. Oncol. in press (1976c).
Goldenberg, D.M., Preston, D.F., Primus, F.J., Hansen, H.J.: Photoscan localization of GW-39 tumors in hamsters using radiolabeled anti-carcinoembryonic antigen immunoglobulin G. Cancer Res. 34, 1-9 (1974).
Goldenberg, D.M., Sharkey, R.M., Primus, F.J.: Carcinoembryonic antigen in histopathology: Immunoperoxidase staining of conventional tissue sections. J. nat. Cancer Inst. 57, 11-22 (1976d).
Goldenberg, D.M., Tchilinguirian, N.G.O., Hansen, H.J., Vandevoorde, J.P.: Carcinoembryonic antigen present in meconium: The basis of a possible new diagnostic test of fetal distress. Amer. J. Obstet. Gynecol. 113, 66-69 (1972b).
Goldenberg, D.M., Witte, S., Elster, K.: GW-39: A new human tumor serially transplantable in the golden hamster. Transplantation 4, 760-763 (1966).
Greenwood, F.C., Hunter, W.M., Coloner, J.S.: The preparation of ^{131}I-labeled human growth hormone of high specific radioactivity. Biochem. J. 89, 114-123 (1963).
Grigor, K.M., Detre, S.I., Laurence, D.J.R., Stevens, U., Neville, A.M.: Comparison of plasma carcinoembryonic antigen and alpha-fetoprotein in various tumours. Lancet 1975 II, 412.
Gross, L.: Intradermal immunization of C3H mice against a sarcoma that originated in an animal of the same line. Cancer Res. 3, 326-333 (1943).
Guinan, P., John, T., Sadoughi, N., Ablin, R.J., Bush, I.: Urinary carcinoembryonic-like antigen levels in patients with bladder carcinoma. J. Urol. (Baltimore) 111, 350-352 (1974).
Haddow, A.: Immunology of the cancer cell: Tumour-specific antigens. Brit. Med. Bull. 21, 133-139 (1965).
Häkkinen, I.P.T.: Immunological relationship of the carcinoembryonic antigen and the fetal sulforglycoprotein antigen. Immunochemistry 9, 1115-1119 (1972).
Häkkinen, I.P.T.: FSA – Foetal sulphoglycoprotein antigen associated with gastric cancer. Transplant. Rev. 20, 61-76 (1974).
Häkkinen, I.P.T., Jarvi, O., Gironroos, J.: Sulphoglycoprotein antigens in the human alimentary canal and gastric cancer. An immunohistochemical study. Int. J. Cancer 3, 572-581 (1968a).
Häkkinen, I.P.T., Korhonen, L.K., Saxen, L.: The time of appearance and distribution of sulphoglycoprotein antigens of the human foetal alimentary canal. Int. J. Cancer 3, 582-592 (1968b).
Hall, R.R., Laurence, D.J.R., Darcy, D., Stevens, U., James, R., Roberts, S., Neville, A.M.: Carcinoembryonic antigen in the urine of patients with urothelial carcinoma. Brit. Med. J. 1972 III, 609-611.
Halterman, R.H., Leventhal, B.G., Mann, D.L.: An acute-leukemia antigen: Correlation with clinical status. New Engl. J. Med. 287, 1272-1274 (1972).
Hammarström, S., Engvall, E., Johansson, B.G., Svensson, S., Sundblad, G., Goldstein, I.J.: Nature of the tumor-associated determinant(s) of carcinoembryonic antigen. Proc. nat. Acad. Sci (Wash.) 72, 1528-1532 (1975).
Hansen, H.J., Lance, K.P., Krupey, J.: Demonstration of an ion sensitive antigenic site on carcinoembryonic antigen using zirconyl phosphate. Clin. Res. 19, 143 (1971).
Hansen, H.J., Snyder, J.J., Miller, E., Vandevoorde, J.V., Miller, O.N., Hines, L.R., Burns, J.J.: Carcinoembryonic antigen (CEA) assay. A laboratory adjunct in the diagnosis and management of cancer. Human Pathol. 4, 139-147 (1974).

Hara, M., Watanabe, S., Kitagawa, M., Yasutomi, M.: Detection of carcinoembryonic antigen in feces for the diagnosis of colonic rectal cancers. Amer. J. Proctol. 25, 67-76 (1974).

Harris, R., Viza, D., Todd, R., Phillips, J., Sugar, R., Jennison, R.F., Marriott, G., Gleeson, M.H.: Detection of human leukaemia associated antigens in leukaemic serum and normal embryos. Nature (Lond.) 233, 556-557 (1971).

Hellström, I., Hellström, K.E., Pierce, G.E., Bill, A.H.: Demonstration of cell-bound and humoral immunity against neuroblastoma cells. Proc. nat. Acad. Sci. (Wash.) 60, 1231-1238 (1968).

Hellström, I., Hellström, K.E., Shepard, T.H.: Cell-mediated immunity against antigens common to human colonic carcinomas and fetal gut epithelium. Int. J. Cancer 6, 346-351 (1970).

Hellström, I., Hellström, K.E., Sjögren, H.O., Warner, G.A.: Demonstration of cell-mediated immunity to human neoplasms of various histological types. Int. J. Cancer 7, 1-16 (1971).

Henry, C., Bernard, D., Depieds, R.: Étude biochimique et immunochimique des antigènes solubles de la muqueuse du gros intestin humain. I. Extraction et fractionnement. Ann. Inst. Pasteur 114, 395-416 (1968).

Hirai, H., Nishi, S., Watabe, H., Tsukada, Y.: Some chemical, experimental, and clinical investigations of α-fetoprotein. Gann Monogr. on Cancer Res. 14, 19-34 (1973).

Hirsch-Marie, H., Chavanel, G., Burtin, P.: Carcinoembryonic antigens (CEA) and non specific cross-reacting antigens in feces. Digestion 9, 193-198 (1973).

Hirszfeld, L., Halber, W., Laskowski, J.: Untersuchungen über die serologischen Eigenschaften der Gewebe. II. Mitteilung. Ueber serologische Eigenschaften der Neubildungen. Z. Immunitätsforsch. 64, 81-113 (1929).

Hirszfeld, L., Halber, W., Rosenblat, J.: Untersuchungen über Verwandtschaftsreaktionen zwischen Embryonal- und Krebsgewebe. II. Vorläufige Mitteilung: Menschenembryo und Menschenkrebs. Z. Immunitätsforsch. 75, 209-216 (1932).

Holburn, A.M., Mach, J.P., MacDonald, D., Newlands, M.: Studies of the association of the A, B and Lewis blood group antigens with carcinoembryonic antigen (CEA). Immunology 26, 831-843 (1974).

Hollinshead, A., Glew, D., Bunnag, B., Gold, P., Herberman, R.: Skin-reactive soluble antigen from intestinal cancer-cell-membranes and relationship to carcinoembryonic antigens. Lancet 1970 I, 1191-1195.

Hollinshead, A.C., McWright, C.G., Alford, T.C., Gold, P., Herberman, R.B.: Separation of skin reactive intestinal cancer antigen from the carcinoembryonic antigen of Gold. Science 177, 887-889 (1972).

Holyoke, E.D., Chu, T.M., Murphy, G.P.: CEA as a monitor of gastrointestinal malignancy. Cancer 35, 830-836 (1975).

Holyoke, D., Reynoso, G., Chu, T.M.: Carcinoembryonic antigen (CEA) in patients with carcinoma of the digestive tract. Ann. Surg. 176, 559-564 (1972).

Hooglie, R.: Benign hepatomas and oral contraceptives. Lancet 1974 I, 630.

Houstek, J., Masopust, J., Kithier, K., Radl, J.: Hepatocellular carcinoma in association with a specific fetal α_1-globulin fetoprotein. J. Pediat. 72, 186-193 (1968).

Huitric, E.: An ultrastructural study of the localization of the carcinoembryonic antigen in adenocarcinomas of the human colon. Ann. Immunol. (Inst. Pasteur) 124C, 603-608 (1973).

Huitric, E., Laumonier, R., Burtin, P., Kleist, S. von, Chavanel, G.: An optical and ultrastructural study of the localization of carcinoembryonic antigen (CEA) in normal and cancerous human rectocolonic mucosa. Lab. Invest. 34, 97-107 (1976).

Hull, E.W., Carbone, P.P., Gitlin, D., O'Gara, R.W., Kelly, M.G.: α-Fetoprotein in monkeys with hepatoma. J. nat. Cancer Inst. 42, 1035-1044 (1969).

Hull, E.W., Carbone, P.P., Moertel, C.G., O'Conor, G.T.: Serum alpha-fetoprotein in the U.S.A. Lancet 1970 I, 779-780.

Huxley, A.: Along the Road. Notes and Essays of a Tourist, p. 139. New York: G.H. Doran Co. 1925.

Ichiki, A.T., Wenzel, K.L., Quirin, Y.P., Lange, R.D., Eveleigh, J.: Immunochemical studies of carcinoembryonic antigen (CEA) variants. Brit. J. Cancer 33, 273-278 (1976).

Ishiguro, T., Nishimura, T.: Radioimmunoassay of maternal serum alpha-fetoprotein associated with pregnancy. Amer. J. Obstet. Gynecol. 116, 27-33 (1973).

Ishii, M.: Radioimmunoassay of α-fetoprotein. Gann Monogr. on Cancer Res. 14, 89-98 (1973).

Karitzky, D., Burtin, P.: Isolement de l'autoantigène, responsable de la formation d'autoanticorps chez les malades atteints de cancer gastrique. Eur. J. Biochem. 1, 411-418 (1967).

Karvountzis, G.G., Redeker, A.G.: Relation of alpha-fetoprotein in acute hepatitis to severity and prognosis. Ann. Intern. Med. 80, 156-160 (1974).

Kew, M.C., Purves, L.R., Bersohn, I.: Serum alpha-fetoprotein levels in acute viral hepatitis. Gut 14, 939-942 (1973).

Khasanov, A.I., Abelev, G.I., Perova, S.D., Polenko, V.K., Ryapsova, U.K., Shirenkova, O.: Vopr. Onkol (1971); cited by *Abelev* (1971).

Khoo, S.K., Mackay, I.R.: Carcinoembryonic antigen in serum in diseases of the liver and pancreas. J. clin. Path. 26, 470-475 (1973).

Khoo, S.K., Warner, N.L., Lie, J.T., Mackay, I.R.: Carcinoembryonic antigenic activity of tissue extracts: A quantitative study of malignant and benign neoplasms, cirrhotic liver, normal adult and fetal organs. Int. J. Cancer 11, 681-687 (1973).

Kithier, K., Masopust, J., Radl, J.: Fetal alpha-globulin of bovine serum differing from fetuin. Biochim. Biophys. Acta 160, 135-137 (1968).

Klavins, J.V., Mesa-Fejada, R., Weiss, M.: Human carcinoma antigens cross-reacting with anti-embryonic antibodies. Nature New Biol. (Lond.) 234, 153-154 (1971).

Klein, G., Clifford, P., Henle, G., Henle, W., Geering, G., Old, L.J.: EBV-associated serological patterns in a Burkitt lymphoma patient during regression and recurrence. Int. J. Cancer 4, 416-421 (1969).

Kleist, S. von, Burtin P.: Localisation cellulaire d'un antigène embryonnaire de tumeurs coliques humaines. Int. J. Cancer 4, 874-879 (1969).

Kleist, S. von, Chavanel, G., Burtin, P.: Identification of an antigen from normal human tissue that cross-reacts with the carcinoembryonic antigen. Proc. nat. Acad. Sci. (Wash.) 69, 2492-2494 (1972).

Kobayashi, K.: Studies on the specific antigens of human gastric cancer. I. Tohoku J. Exp. Med. 63, 185-190 (1956).

Kobayashi, K.: Studies on the specific antigens of human gastric cancer. II. Tohoku J. Exp. Med. 63, 191-202 (1956).

Kozower, M., Gawaz, K.A., Miller, H.M., Kaplan, M.M.: Positive alpha-fetogolubulin in a case of gastric carcinoma. New Engl. J. Med. 285, 1059-1060 (1971).

Kroes, R., Williams, G., Weisburger, J.H.: Early appearance of serum α-fetoprotein during hepatocarcinogenesis as a function of age of rats and extent of treatment with 3'-methyl-4-dimethylamino-azobenzene. Cancer Res. 32, 1526-1532 (1972).

Krupey, J., Gold, P., Freedman, S.O.: Purification and characterisation of carcinoembryonic antigens of the human digestive system. Nature (Lond.) 215, 67-68 (1967).

Krupey, J., Gold, P., Freedman, S.O.: Physicochemical studies of the carcinoembryonic antigens of the human digestive system. J. exp. Med. 128, 387-398 (1968).
Kupchik, H.Z., Zamcheck, N.: Carcinoembryonic antigen(s) in liver disease. II. Isolation from human cirrhotic liver and serum and from normal liver. Gastroenterology 63, 95-101 (1972).
Lacassagne, A.: Sur l'histogenèse des carcinomes hépatiques. A propos des foetoprotéines specifiques. Bull. Cancer 55, 181-204 (1968).
Laurence, D.J.R., Stevens, U., Bettelheim, R., Darcy, D., Lesse, C., Turberville, C., Alexander, P., Johns, E.W., Neville, A.M.: Role of plasma carcinoembryonic antigen in diagnosis of gastrointestinal, mammary, and bronchial carcinoma. Brit. med. J. 1972 III, 605-609.
Lehmann, F.G.: Der Nachweis von α_1-Fetoprotein bei internen Erkrankungen. Aktueller Stand des Problems. Internist 13, 332-339 (1972).
Lehmann, F.G., Lehmann, D.: Neue immunologische Techniken und quantitative Bestimmung von Alpha$_1$-Fetoproteinen in der Tumordiagnostik. Verh. dtsch. Ges. inn. Med. 78, 841-845 (1972).
Lehmann, F.G., Lehmann, D.: Vergleich verschiedener Methoden zum serologischen Nachweis von α_1-Foetoproteinen in der Tumordiagnostik. Verh. dtsch. Ges. inn. Med. (1973).
Lehmann, F.G., Lehmann, D., Martini, G.A.: α_1-Foetoprotein in liver diseases. Digestion 6, 249-250 (1972).
Lejtenyi, M.C., Freedman, S.O., Gold, P.: Response of lymphocytes from patients with gastrointestinal cancer to the carcinoembryonic antigen of the human digestive system. Cancer 28, 115-120 (1971).
Levi, M.M., Keller, S., Maudl, I.: Antigenicity of a papillary serous cystadenocarcinoma tissue homogenate and its fractions. Amer. J. Obstet. Gynecol. 105, 856-861 (1969).
Linder, E., Seppälä, M.: Localization of α-foetoprotein in the human foetus and placenta. Acta path. microbiol. scand. 73, 565-571 (1968).
Livingstone, A.S., Hampson, L.G., Shuster, J., Gold, P., Hinchey, E.J.: Carcinoembryonic antigen in the diagnosis and management of colorectal carcinoma. Current status. Arch. Surg. 109, 259-264 (1974).
LoGerfo, P., Herter, F., Hansen, H.J.: Demonstration of tumor associated antigen in normal colon and lung. J. Surg. Oncol. 4, 1-7 (1972).
LoGerfo, P., Krupey, J., Hansen, H.J.: Demonstration of an antigen common to several varieties of neoplasia. New Engl. J. Med. 285, 138-141 (1971).
Lynraven, G.S., de Boer, W.G.R.M.: A specific antiserum for gastric mucous epithelium. Pathology 1, 57-60 (1969).
Mach, J.P., Jaeger, P., Berthelot, M.M., Ruegsegger, C.H., Loosli, R.M., Pettavel, J.: Detection of recurrence of large-bowel carcinoma by radioimmunoassay of circulating carcinoembryonic antigen (CEA). Lancet 1974 II, 535-540.
Mach, J.P., Pusztaszeri, G.: Carcinoembryonic antigen (CEA): Demonstration of a partial identity between CEA and a normal glycoprotein. Immunochemistry 9, 1031-1034 (1972).
Martin, E.W., jr., Kibbey, W.E., DiVecchia, L., Anderson, G., Catalano, P., Minton, J.P.: Carcinoembryonic antigen. Clinical and historical aspects. Cancer 37, 62-81 (1976).
Martin, F., Martin, M.S.: Demonstration of antigens related to colonic cancer in the human digestive system. Int. J. Cancer 6, 352-360 (1970).
Martin, F., Martin, M.S.: Radioimmunoassay of carcinoembryonic antigen in extracts of human colon and stomach. Int. J. Cancer 9, 641-647 (1972).
Masopust, J., Tomášová, H., Kotál, L.: Some physicochemical characteristics of human α_1-fetoprotein. In: Protides of the Biological Fluids (ed. *H. Peeters*) 18, 37-42 (1971).

Masseyeff, R.: Human alpha-fetoprotein. Path. Biol. 20, 703-725 (1972).
Masseyeff, R.F.: Factors influencing α-fetoprotein biosynthesis in patients with primary liver cancer and other diseases. Gann Monogr. on Cancer Res. 14, 3-18 (1973).
Masseyeff, R., Basteris, B., Leblanc, L.: Use of the alpha-fetoprotein test for the diagnosis of primary liver cancer. In: Protides of the Biological Fluids (ed. *H. Peeters*) 18, 217-220 (1971).
Matray, F., Sauger, F., Borde, J., Mitrofanoff, P., Grosley, M., Bourg, M., Laumonier, R., Hemet, J.: Présence d'alpha-foetoprotéine au cours d'une régénération hépatique après hépatectomie gauche pour hépatomie gauche pour hépatome chez un enfant. Path. Biol. 20, 353-356 (1972).
Mawas, C., Buffe, D., Burtin, P.: Influence of age on alpha-fetoprotein incidence. Lancet 1970 I, 1292.
McCartney, W.H., Hoffer, P.B.: The value of carcinoembryonic antigen (CEA) as an adjunct to the radiological colon examination in the diagnosis of malignancy. Radiology 110, 325-328 (1974).
McConahey, P.J., Dixon, F.J.: A method of trace iodination of proteins for immunologic studies. Arch. Allergy Appl. Immunol. 29, 185-189 (1969).
McIntire, K.R., Vogel, C.L., Princler, G.L., Patel, I.R.: Serum α-fetoprotein as a biochemical marker for hepatocellular carcinoma. Cancer Res. 32, 1941-1946 (1972).
McIntire, K.R., Waldmann, T.A., Go, V.L.W., Moertel, C.G., Ravry, M.: Simultaneous radioimmunoassay for carcinoembryonic antigen (CEA) and alpha-fetoprotein (αFP) in neoplasms of the gastrointestinal tract. Ann. Clin. Lab. Sci. 4, 104-108 (1974a).
McIntire, K.R., Waldmann, T.A., Moertel, C.G., Go, V.L.W.: Serum α-fetoprotein in patients with neoplasms of the gastrointestinal tract. Cancer Res. 35, 991-996 (1974b).
Meeker, W.R., jr., Kashmiri, R., Hunter, L.: Clinical evaluation of carcinoembryonic antigen test. Arch. Surg. 107, 266-274 (1973).
Mehlman, D.J., Bulkley, B.H., Wiernik, P.H.: Serum α-fetoglobulin with gastric and prostatic carcinomas. New Engl. J. Med. 285, 1060-1061 (1971).
Miller, A.B.: A joint National Cancer Institute of Canada/American Cancer Society investigation. A collaborative study of a test for carcinoembryonic antigen (CEA) in the sera of patients with carcinoma of the colon and rectum. Canad. Med. Ass. J. 107, 25-33 (1972).
Montplaisir, S., Rabin, B., Pelletier, M., Rose, N.R., Alpert, E.: Alpha$_1$-fetoprotein content of gastric carcinoma and hepatic metastases. Amer. J. dig. Dis. 18, 416-418 (1973).
Moore, T.L., Kupchik, H.Z., Marcon, N., Zamcheck, N.: Carcinoembryonic antigen assay in cancer of the colon and pancreas and other digestive tract disorders. Amer. J. dig. Dis. 16, 1-8 (1971).
Morris, J.E., Egan, M.L., Todd, C.W.: The binding of carcinoembryonic antigen by antibody and its fragments. Cancer Res. 35, 1804-1808 (1975).
Morton, D.L., Malmgren, R.A., Hall, W.T., Schidlovsky, G.: Immunologic and virus studies with human sarcomas. Surgery 66, 152-161 (1969).
Morton, D.L., Malmgren, R.A., Holmes, E.C., Ketcham, A.S.: Demonstration of antibodies against human malignant melanoma by immunofluorescence. Surgery 64, 233-240 (1968).
Mukherji, B., Hirschaut, Y.: Evidence for fetal antigen in human sarcoma. Science 181, 440-442 (1973).
Mulcare, R., LoGerfo, P.: Tumor associated antigen in the chemotherapy of solid tumors. J. Surg. Oncol. 4, 407-417 (1972).
Munjal, D., Goldenberg, D.M.: Circulating and tumor levels of glucose phosphate isomerase and carcinoembryonic antigen in hamsters xenografted with the GW-39 human colonic tumor. In: Program and Abstracts of Third International Symposium on Detection and Prevention of Cancer, pp. 425-430 (1976).

Murgita, R.A., Tomasi, T.B., jr.: Suppression of the immune response by α-fetoprotein. I. The effect of mouse α-fetoprotein on the primary and secondary antibody response. J. exp. Med. 141, 269-286 (1975a).
Murgita, R.A., Tomasi, T.B., jr.: Suppression of the immune response by α-fetoprotein. II. The effect of mouse α-fetoprotein on mixed lymphocyte reactivity and mitogen-induced lymphocyte transformation. J. exp. Med. 141, 440-452 (1975b).
Murray, M.J., Thal, A.P.: The clinical significance of circulating pancreatic antibodies. Ann. Intern. Med. 53, 548-555 (1960).
Nagell, J.R. van, jr., Pletsch, Q.A., Goldenberg, D.M.: A study of cyst fluid and plasma carcinoembryonic antigen in patients with cystic ovarian neoplasms. Cancer Res. 35, 1433-1437 (1975).
Nairn, R.C., Fothergill, J.E., McEntegart, M.G., Porteus, I.B.: Gastro-intestinal-specific antigen: An immunohistological and serological study. Brit. med. J. 1962a I, 1788-1790.
Nairn, R.C., Fothergill, J.E., McEntegart, M.G., Richmond, H.G.: Loss of gastro-intestinal-specific antigen in neoplasia. Brit. med. J. 1962b I, 1791-1793.
Nairn, R.C., Ghose, T., Tannenberg, A.E.G.: Kidney specific antigen deletion in human renal carcinomas. Brit. J. Cancer 20, 756-759 (1966).
Nathanson, L., Fishman, W.H.: New observations on the Reagen isoenzyme of alkaline phosphatase in cancer patients. Cancer 27, 1388-1397 (1971).
Nayak, N.C., Malaviya, A.N., Chawla, V., Chandra, R.K.: α-Fetoprotein in Indian childhood cirrhosis. Lancet 1972 I, 68-69.
Nery, R., Bullman, H., Barsoum, A.: Carcinoembryonic antigen of erythrocyte membranes. Nature New Biol. (Lond.) 246, 44-46 (1973).
Newman, E.S., Petras, S.E., Georgiadis, A., Hansen, H.J.: Interrelationship of CEA and colon carcinoma antigen-III. Cancer Res. 34, 2125-2130 (1974).
Nishi, S.: Isolation and characterization of a human fetal alpha-globulin from the sera of fetuses and a hepatoma patient. Cancer Res. 30, 2507-2513 (1970).
Nishi, S., Hirai, H.: Purification and chemical characterization of human alpha-fetoprotein. In: Protides of the Biological Fluids (ed. *H. Peeters*). 18, 43-47 (1971).
Nishi, S., Hirai, H.: Radioimmunoassay of α-fetoprotein in hepatoma, other liver diseases, and pregnancy. Gann Monogr. on Cancer Res. 14, 79-87 (1973).
Nishioka, M., Ibata, T., Miyazato, K., Okita, K., Hironaga, K., Fujita, T.: Immunofluorescence studies on α-fetoprotein in hepatoma tissue. Gann Monogr. on Cancer Res. 14, 205-218 (1973).
Nishioka, M., Ibata, T., Okita, K., Harada, T., Fujita, T.: Localization of α-fetoprotein in hepatoma tissues by immunofluorescence. Cancer Res. 32, 162-166 (1972).
Nishioka, M., Okamoto, Y., Shigeta, K., Hironaga, K., Fujita, T.: Further observations on alpha-fetoprotein in the diagnosis of diseases of the digestive tract. Digestion 8, 396-406 (1973).
Norland, C.C., Maass, E.G., Kirsner, J.B.: Identification of colon carcinoma by immunofluorescent staining. Cancer 23, 730-739 (1969).
Nunez, E., Engelmann, F., Benassay, G., Jayle, M.F.: Identification et purification préliminaire de la foetoprotéine liant les oestrogènes dans le sérum de rats nouveau-nés. C.R. Acad. Sci. (Paris) 273, 242-245 (1971).
O'Conor, G.T., Tatarinov, Y.S., Abelev, G.I., Uriel, J.: A collaborative study for the evaluation of a serologic test for primary liver cancer. Cancer 25, 1091-1098 (1970).
Ogra, S.S., Margita, R.A., Tomasi, T.B., jr.: Immunosuppressive activity of mouse amniotic fluid. Immunol. Commun. 3, 497-508 (1974).
Old, L.J., Boyse, E.A.: Immunology of experimental tumors. Ann. Rev. Med. 15, 167-186 (1964).

Ona, F.V., Zamcheck, N., Dhar, P., Moore, T., Kupchik, H.Z.: Carcinoembryonic antigen (CEA) in the diagnosis of pancreatic cancer. Cancer 31, 324-327 (1973).

Opolon, P., Hirsch-Marie, H., Gateau, P., Caroli, J.: Apparition de l'alpha-1-foetoprotéine circulante au cours de l'atrophie aiguë du foie. Ann. Med. Interne 124, 883-888 (1973).

Parker, C.W.: The immunotherapy of cancer. Pharmacol. Rev. 25, 325-342 (1973).

Pedersen, K.O.: Fetuin, a new globulin isolated from serum. Nature (Lond.) 154, 575-576 (1944).

Piard, A., Mabille, J.P., Putelat, R.: Syndrome paranéoplastique à manifestations multiples révélateur d'un hypernéphrome avec présence d'alpha-foetoprotéine. Sem. Hôp. Paris. 49, 341-346 (1973).

Pierce, G.B.: Differentiation of normal and malignant cells. Fed. Proc. 29, 1248-1254 (1970).

Pletsch, Q.A., Goldenberg, D.M.: Molecular size of carcinoembryonic antigen in the plasma of patients with malignant disease. J. nat. Cancer Inst. 53, 1201-1204 (1974).

Plow, E.F., Edgington, T.S.: Isolation and characterization of a homogenous isomeric species of carcinoembryonic antigen: CEA-S. Int. J. Cancer 15, 748-761 (1975).

Primus, F.J., Hansen, H.J., Goldenberg, D.M.: Altered metabolism of carcinoembryonic antigen in hamsters bearing GW-39 tumours. Nature (Lond.) 249, 837-838 (1974).

Primus, F.J., Wang, R.H., Cohen, E., Hansen, H.J., Goldenberg, D.M.: Antibody to carcinoembryonic antigen in hamsters bearing GW-39 human tumors. Cancer Res. 36, 2176-2181 (1976).

Primus, F.J., Wang, R.H., Goldenberg, D.M., Hansen, H.J.: Localization of human GW-39 tumors in hamsters by radiolabeled heterospecific antibody to carcinoembryonic antigen. Cancer Res. 33, 2977-2982 (1973).

Primus, F.J., Wang, R.H., Sharkey, R.M., Goldenberg, D.M.: Detection of carcinoembryonic antigen in tissue sections by immunoperoxidase. J. Immun. Methods 8, 267-276 (1975).

Purtilo, D.T., Yunis, E.J.: α-Fetoprotein. Its immunofluorescent localization in human fetal liver and hepatoma. Lab. Invest. 25, 291-294 (1971).

Purves, L.R., Bersohn, I., Geddes, E.W.: Serum alpha-fetoprotein and primary cancer of the liver in man. Cancer 25, 1261-1270 (1970).

Purves, L.R., Branch, W.R., Geddes, E.W., Manso, C., Portugal, M.: Serum α-fetoprotein. VII. The range of apparent serum values in normal people, pregnant women, and primary liver cancer high risk populations. Cancer 31, 578-587 (1973).

Purves, L.R., Macnab, M., Bersohn, I.: Fetoglobulin and primary liver cancer. Lancet 1968 II, 634.

Purves, L.R., Macnab, M., Geddes, E.W., Bersohn, I.: Serum alpha-fetoprotein and primary hepatic cancer. Lancet 1968 I, 921-922.

Purves, L.R., Manso, C., Torres, F.O.: Serum α-fetoprotein levels in people susceptible to primary cancer in Southern Africa. Gann Monogr. on Cancer Res. 14, 51-66 (1973).

Purves, L.R., Purves, M.: Serum α-fetoprotein. VI. The radioimmunoassay. Evidence for the presence of α-fetoprotein in the serum of normal people and pregnant women. S. Afr. Med. J. 46, 1290-1297 (1972).

Purves, L.R., van der Merwe, E., Bersohn, I.: Variants of α-fetoprotein. Lancet 1970 II, 464-465.

Pusztaszeri, G., Mach, J.P.: Carcinoembryonic antigen (CEA) in non-digestive cancerous and normal tissues. Immunochemistry 10, 197-204 (1973).

Pusztaszeri, G., Saravis, C.A., Zamcheck, N.: The zinc glycinate marker in human colon carcinoma. J. nat. Cancer Inst. 56, 275-278 (1976).

Rapp, W., Aranson, S.B., Burtin, P., Grabar, P.: Constituents and antigens of normal human gastric mucosa as characterized by electrophoresis and immunoelectrophoresis in agar gel. J. Immunol. 92, 579-595 (1964).

Remacle-Bonnet, M., Depieds, R.: Study of the antigenic constituents of human colon connective tissue. Path. Biol. 22, 113-117 (1974).

Reynoso, G., Chu, T.M., Holyoke, D., Cohen, E., Nemoto, T., Wang, J.J., Chuang, J., Guinan, P., Murphy, G.P.: Carcinoembryonic antigen in patients with different cancers. J. Amer. med. Ass. 220, 361-365 (1972).

Rioche, M., Quelin, S., Aeck, I., Jacquesson, M., Basteris, B., Masseyeff, R.: Culture in vitro de cellules de cancer primitif de foie humaine. C.R. Acad. Sci. (Paris) 271, 1148-1151 (1970).

Rogalsky, V.Y.: Variations in carcinoembryonic antigen localization in tumors of the colon. J. nat. Cancer Inst. 54, 1061-1065 (1975).

Rogers, G.T., Searle, F., Bagshawe, K.D.: Heterogeneity of carcinoembryonic antigen and its fractionation by con A affinity chromatography. Nature (Lond.) 251, 519-521 (1974).

Rosai, J., Tillack, T.W., Marchesi, V.T.: Membrane antigens of human colonic carcinoma and non-tumoral colonic mucosa: Results obtained with a new isolation method. Int. J. Cancer, 10, 357-367 (1972).

Rosenthal, L., Palmer, J.L., Harris, J.A., Rawls, W.E., Tompkins, W.A.F.: Antibody-induced redistribution of CEA on the cell surface: Utilization in separation of CEA and isoantigen A. J. Immunol. 115, 1049-1053 (1975).

Rule, A.H., Goleski-Reilly, C.: Carcinoembryonic antigen (CEA): Separation of CEA-reacting molecules from tumor, fetal gut, meconium and normal colon. Immunol. Commun. 2, 213-226 (1973).

Rule, A.H., Goleski-Reilly, C., Sachar, D.B., Vandevoorde, J., Janowitz, H.D.: Circulating carcinoembryonic antigen (CEA): Relationship to clinical status of patients with inflammatory bowel disease. Gut 14, 880-884 (1973).

Ruoslahti, E., Salaspuro, M., Pihko, H., Andersson, L., Seppälä, M.: Serum α-fetoprotein: Diagnostic significance in liver disease. Brit. med. J. 393, 527-529 (1974).

Ruoslahti, E., Seppälä, M.: Studies of carcino-fetal proteins. Physical and chemical properties of human α-fetoprotein. Int. J. Cancer 7, 218-225 (1971).

Ruoslahti, E., Seppälä, M.: Studies of carcino-fetal proteins. III. Development of a radioimmunoassay for α-fetoprotein. Demonstration of α-fetoprotein in serum of healthy human adults. Int. J. Cancer 8, 374-383 (1971).

Ruoslahti, E., Seppälä, M.: Normal and increased α-fetoprotein in neoplastic and non-neoplastic liver disease. Lancet 1972 II, 278-279.

Ruoslahti, E., Seppälä, M., Pihko, H., Vuopio, P.: Studies of carcino-fetal proteins. II. Biochemical comparison of α-fetoprotein from human fetuses and patients with hepatocellular cancer. Int. J. Cancer 8, 283-288 (1971).

Ruoslahti, E., Seppälä, M., Rasanen, J.A., Vuopio, P., Helske, T.: Alpha-fetoprotein and hepatitis B antigen in acute hepatitis and primary cancer of the liver. Scand. J. Gastroent. 8, 197-202 (1973).

Ruoslahti, E., Seppälä, M., Vuopio, P., Saksela, E., Peltokallio, P.: Radioimmunoassay of α-fetoprotein in primary and secondary cancer of the liver. J. nat. Cancer Inst. 49, 623-650 (1972).

Sukarai, M., Miyaji, T.: α-Fetoprotein and the morphology of hepatoma in man. Gann. Monogr. on Cancer Res. 14, 185-198 (1973).

Sannela, J.J.: Antigenic Properties of Normal Human Intestinal Mucosa. Dissertation, University of Buffalo, pp. 1-34 (1957).

Sarrazin, A., Emerit, J., Bousquet, O., Lanoe, J.: Hémochromatose avec alpha-foetoprotéine positive, un nouveau cas. Nouv. Presse méd. 2, 2602 (1973).

Sasaki, K., Miyakawa, A., Mito, M., Kasai, Y.: Histology of hepatoma in man with regard to α-fetoprotein. Gann Monogr. on Cancer Res. 14, 199-203 (1973).

Sauger, F., Duval, C., Fondimare, A., Matray, F., Buffe, D.: Systematic analysis of alpha-fetoprotein in 5000 sera. Rev. Europ. Etud. Clin. Biol. 16, 471-473 (1971).

Schapira, F.: Foetal enzyme patterns in cancer tissues. Rev. Europ. Etud. Clin. Biol. 16, 205-208 (1971).

Seller, M., Singer, J.D., Coltart, T.M., Campbell, S.: Maternal serum alpha-fetoprotein levels and prenatal diagnosis of neural tube defects. Lancet 1974 I, 428-429.

Seppälä, M., Bagshawe, K.D., Ruoslahti, E.: Radioimmunoassay of alpha-fetoprotein: A contribution ot the diagnosis of choriocarcinoma and hydatidiform mole. Int. J. Cancer 10, 478-481 (1972).

Seppälä, M., Ruoslahti, E.: Alpha-fetoprotein in abortion. Brit. med. J. 1972a III, 769-771.

Seppälä, M., Ruoslahti, E.: Radioimmunoassay of maternal serum alpha-fetoprotein during pregnacy and delivery. Amer. J. Obstet. Gynec. 112, 208-212 (1972b).

Seppälä, M., Ruoslahti, E.: Alpha-fetoprotein in Rh-immunized pregnancies. Obstet. Gynec. 42, 701-706 (1973a).

Seppälä, M., Ruoslahti, E.: Alpha-fetoprotein: Physiology and pathology during pregnancy and application to antenatal diagnosis. J. Perinat. Med. 1, 104-113 (1973b).

Seppälä, M., Ruoslahti, E.: Alpha-fetoprotein in maternal serum: A new marker for detection of fetal distress and intrauterine death. Amer. J. Obstet. Gynec. 115, 48-52 (1973c).

Seppälä, M., Tallberg, T., Ehnholm, C.: Studies on embryo-specific proteins. Physiological characteristics of embryo-specific alpha-globulins. Ann. Med. Exp. Fenn. 45, 16-19 (1967).

Shearer, W.T., Turnbaugh, T.R., Coleman, W.E., Aach, R.D., Philpott, G.W., Parker, C.W.: Cytotoxicity with antibody-glucose oxidase conjugates specific for a human colonic cancer and carcinoembryonic antigen. Int. J. Cancer 14, 539-547 (1974).

Shikata, T., Sakakibara, K.: Relationship between α-fetoprotein and histological patterns of hepatoma, and localization of α-fetoprotein in hepatoma cells using the peroxidase antibody technique. Gann Monogr. on Cancer Res. 14, 269-277 (1973).

Shuster, J., Silverman, M., Gold, P.: Metabolism of human carcinoembryonic antigen in xenogeneic animals. Cancer Res. 33, 65-68 (1973).

Silver, H.K., Deneault, J., Gold, P., Thompson, W.G., Shuster, J., Freedman, S.O.: The dectection of α_1-fetoprotein in patients with viral hepatitis. Cancer Res. 34, 244-247 (1974)

Skarin, A.T., Delwiche, R., Zamcheck, N., Lokich, J.J., Frei, E., III: Carcinoembryonic antigen: Clinical correlation with chemotherapy for metastatic gastrointestinal cancer. Cancer 33, 1239-1245 (1974).

Slade, B.: Antibodies to alpha-fetoprotein cause foetal mortality in rabbits. Nature (Lond.) 246, 493 (1973).

Smith, J.A.: Alpha-fetoprotein: A possible factor necessary for normal development of the embryo. Lancet 1972 I, 851.

Smith, J.A., Francis, T.I., Edington, G.M., Williams, A.O.: Immunofluorescent localization of human alpha-fetoprotein in fetal and neonatal livers and cultured cells from hepatocellular carcinoma. Brit. J. Cancer 25, 343-349 (1971).

Smith, J.B.: Occurrence of alpha-fetoprotein in acute viral hepatitis. Int. J. Cancer 8, 421-424 (1971).

Smith, J.B.: Alpha-fetoprotein: Occurrence in certain malignant diseases and review of clinical applications. Med. Clin. N. Amer. 54, 797-803 (1970).

Smith, J.B., O'Neill, R.T.: Fetal gut antigen: A substance in fetal gut and its relationship to gut carcinoma. Res. Commun. Chem. Path. Pharmacol. 2, 1-15 (1971).

Smith, J.B., Todd, D.: Foetoglobulin and primary liver cancer. Lancet 1968 II, 833.

Sorokin, J.J., Sugarbaker, P.H., Zamcheck, N., Pisick, M., Kupchik, H.Z., Moore, F.D.: Serial carcinoembryonic antigen assays. Use in detection of cancer recurrence. J. Amer. Med. Ass. 228, 49-53 (1974).

Spiro, M.J., Spiro, R.G.: Composition of the peptide portion of fetuin. J. biol. Chem. 237, 1507-1510 (1962).

Spiro, R.G.: Studies of fetuin, a glycoprotein of fetal serum. I. Isolation, chemical composition, and physicochemical properties. J. biol. Chem. 235, 2860-2869 (1960).

Spragins, J., Hall, W.H., White, H.J.: Fetoprotein from esophageal squamous cell carcinoma. Ann. Int. Med. 77, 322-323 (1972).

Stonehill, E.H., Bendich, A.: Retrogenetic expression: The reappearance of embryonal antigens in cancer cells. Nature (Lond.) 228, 370-372 (1970).

Sugahara, K., Kashii, A., Kogure, H.: Serum alpha-fetoprotein and resection of primary hepatic cancer. Arch. Surg. 105, 63-65 (1973).

Takahashi, M., Kawaguchi, A., Kawamata, K., Yasuma, T.: α-Fetoprotein by the immunofluorescent antibody technique in primary liver carcinoma and its histopathological basis. Gann Monogr. on Cancer Res. 14, 219-230 (1973).

Takahashi, M., Kawaguchi, A., Yasuma, T., Tanaka, M., Kawamata, K.: α-Fetoprotein by immunodiffusion and fluorescence antibody methods and histopathology of hepatoma (in Japanese). Med. Postgrad. 9, 249-260 (1971).

Takahasi, A., Yashi, A., Anzai, T., Wada, T.: Presence of a unique serum protein in sera obtained from patients with neoplastic diseases and in embryonic and neonatal sera. Clin. Chim. Acta 17, 5-12 (1967).

Tal, C., Dishon, T., Gross, J.: The agglutination of tumor cells in vitro by sera from patients and pregnant women. Brit. J. Cancer 18, 111-119 (1964).

Tal, C., Halperin, M.: Presence of serologically distinct protein in serum of cancer patients and pregnant women: An attempt to develop a diagnostic cancer test. Isr. J. Med. Sci. 6, 708-716 (1970).

Tappeiner, G., Denk, H., Eckerstorfer, R., Holzner, J.H.: Vergleichende Untersuchungen über Auftreten und Lokalisation des carcinoembryonalen Antigens (CEA) und eines normalen perchlorsäureextrahierbaren Dickdarmschleimhautantigens (NC) in Carcinomen und Polypen des Dickdarmes. Virchows Arch. path. Anat. 360, 129-140 (1973).

Tatarinov, Y.S.: Finding of an embryospecific α-globulin in blood serum in a patient with primary hepatic cancer (in Russian). Vop. med. Khim. 10, 90-91 (1964).

Terry, W.D., Henkart, P.A., Coligan, J.E., Todd, C.W.: Structural studies of the major glycoprotein in preparations with carcinoembryonic antigen activity. J. exp. Med. 136, 200-204 (1972).

Terry, W.D., Henkart, P.A., Coligan, J.E., Todd, C.W.: Carcinoembryonic antigen: Characterization and clinical applications. Transplant. Rev. 20, 100-129 (1974).

Thompson, W.G., Gillies, R.R., Silver, H.K.B., Shuster, J., Freedman, S.O., Gold, P.: Carcinoembryonic antigen and alpha$_1$-fetoprotein in ulcerative colitis and regional enteritis. Canad. Med. Ass. J. 110, 775-777 (1974).

Thomson, D.M.P., Krupey, J., Freedman, S.O., Gold, P.: The radioimmunoassay of circulating carcinoembryonic antigen of the human digestive system. Proc. nat. Acad. Sci. (Wash.) 64, 161-167 (1969).

Tillack, T.W., Rosai, J., Vervynck, D.J.: Immunologic studies of glycoprotein isolated from cell membranes of human lung carcinomas. J. nat. Cancer Inst. 52, 1059-1067 (1974).

Tom, B.H., Rutzky, L.P., Oyasu, R., Tomita, J.T., Goldenberg, D.M., Kahan, B.D.: Human colonic adenocarcinoma cells. II. Tumorigenic and organoid expression in vivo and in vitro. J. Nat. Cancer Inst. In press (1976).

Tompkins, W.A.F., Watrach, A.M., Schmale, J.D., Schultz, R.M., Harris, J.A.: Cultural and antigenic properties of newly established cell strains derived from adenocarcinomas of the human colon and rectum. J. nat. Cancer Inst. 52, 1101-1110 (1974).

Trouillas, P.: Carcinofetal antigen in glial tumours. Lancet 1971 II, 552.

Turberville, C., Darcy, D.A., Laurence, D.J.R., Johns, E.W., Neville, A.M.: Studies on carcinoembryonic antigen (CEA) and a related glycoprotein CCEA-2. Preparation and chemical characterisation. Immunochemistry 10, 841-843 (1973).

Turner, M.D., Olivares, T.A., Harwell, L., Kleinman, M.S.: Further purification of perchlorate-soluble antigens from human colonic carcinomata. J. Immunol. 108, 1328-1339 (1972).

Uriel, J.: Transitory liver antigens and primary hepatoma in man and rat. Path. Biol. 17, 877-884 (1969).

Uriel, J.: Fetal characteristics of cancer. In: Cancer 3. A comprehensive Treatise. Biology of Tumors: Cellular Biology and Growth (ed. *F.F. Becker*), pp. 21-55. New York: Plenum Press 1975.

Uriel, J., Aussel, C., Bouillon, D., de Néchaud, B., Loisillier, F.: Localisation of rat liver α-fetoprotein by cell affinity labelling with tritiated oestrogens. Nature New Biol. (Lond.) 244, 190-192 (1973).

Uriel, J., de Néchaud, B.: La recherche d'α-foetoprotéine en pathologie humaine. Etat actuel de la question. Ann. Inst. Pasteur 122, 829-839 (1972).

Uriel, J., de Néchaud, B.: An outline of the physiopathology of rat α-fetoprotein. Gann Monogr. on Cancer Res. 14, 35-47 (1973).

Uriel, J., de Néchaud, B., Dupiers, M.: Estrogen-binding properties of rat, mouse, and human fetospecific serum proteins. Demonstration by immuno-autoradiographic methods. Biochem. Biophys. Res. Commun. 46, 1175-1180 (1972).

Uriel, J., Loisillier, F., Szekely, A.M., Bismuth, H.: Autoradiographic localization of intracellular alpha-fetoprotein in primary liver cancer in man. Biomed. 21, 21-25 (1974).

Vogel, C.L., Primack, A., McIntire, K.R., Carbone, P.P., Anthony, P.P.: Serum alpha-fetoprotein in 184 Ugandan patients with hepatocellular carcinoma. Clinical, laboratory, and histopathologic correlations. Cancer 33, 959-964 (1974).

Wada, T., Anzai, T., Yachi, A.: Immunochemical studies of antigenic components common to carcinoma and fetus, and their diagnostic significance. With special reference to the connection with α-fetoprotein. Gann Monogr. on Cancer Res. 14, 157-166 (1973).

Waldmann, T.A., McIntire, K.R.: Serum alpha-fetoprotein levels in patients with ataxia telangiectasia. Lancet 1972 II, 1112-1115.

Weiler, E.: Antigenic differences between normal hamster kidney and stilboestrol induced kidney carcinoma: Complement fixation reactions with cytoplasmic particles. Brit. J. Cancer 10, 553-559 (1956).

Westwood, J.H., Bessell, E.M., Bukhari, M.A., Thomas, P., Walker, J.M.: Studies of the structure of the carcinoembryonic antigen – I. Some deductions on the basis of chemical degradations. Immunochemistry 11, 811-818 (1974).

Witebsky, E.: Zur serologischen Spezifität des Carcinomgewebes. Klin. Wochenschr. 2, 58-63 (1930).

Witebsky, E., Rose, N.L., Shulman, S.: Studies of normal and malignant tissue antigens. Cancer Res. 16, 831-841 (1956).

Yachi, A., Matsuura, Y., Carpenter, C.M., Hyde, L.: Immunochemical studies on human lung cancer antigens soluble in 50% saturated ammonium sulfate. J. nat. Cancer Inst. 40, 663-682 (1968).
Zamcheck, N.: The present status of CEA in diagnosis, prognosis, and evaluation of therapy. Cancer 36, 2460-2468 (1975).
Zawadzki, Z.A., Kraj, M.A.: Alpha-fetoprotein in hepatocellular disease and neoplastic disorders. Amer. J. Gastroent. 61, 45-52 (1974).
Zilber, L.A.: Study of tumor specificity of gastric cancer tissue. Ann. N.Y. Acad. Sci. 101, 264-270 (1962).
Zweibaum, A., Oriol, R., Dausset, J., Marcelli-Barge, A., Ropartz, C., Lanset, S.: Definition in man of a polymorphic system of the normal colonic secretions. Tissue Antigens 6, 121-128 (1975).

Subject Index

The numbers set in *italics* refer to those pages on which the respective catch-word is dicussed in detail

Index to Volumes 52–61 Current Topics in Pathology

MIX
Papier aus verantwortungsvollen Quellen
Paper from responsible sources
FSC® C105338

If you have any concerns about our products,
you can contact us on
ProductSafety@springernature.com

In case Publisher is established outside the EU,
the EU authorized representative is:
Springer Nature Customer Service Center GmbH
Europaplatz 3, 69115 Heidelberg, Germany

Printed by Libri Plureos GmbH
in Hamburg, Germany